Praise for *Sleep Easy*

sleep easy

BERNICE TUFFERY

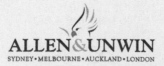

ALLEN&UNWIN
SYDNEY · MELBOURNE · AUCKLAND · LONDON

First published in 2021

Copyright © Bernice Tuffery, 2021

Disclaimer

Allen & Unwin
Level 2, 10 College Hill
Auckland 1011, New Zealand
Phone: (64 9) 377 3800

Email: info@allenandunwin.com
Web: www.allenandunwin.co.nz

83 Alexander Street
Crows Nest NSW 2065, Australia
Phone: (61 2) 8425 0100

A catalogue record for this book is available
from the National Library of New Zealand

ISBN 978 1 98854745 9

Design by Megan van Staden
Set in 15/15 pt Gazette
Printed and bound in Australia by McPhersons Printing Group

10 9 8 7 6 5 4 3 2

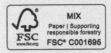

This book is for everyone suffering in silence through erratic sleepless nights. Take heart, you're not alone and there is a proven pathway through this. It's quite a journey, but, having done it myself, I assure you it's entirely worth it.

CONTENTS

FOREWORD

Insomnia sucks. Having treated thousands of insomnia sufferers in the past twenty years, I have witnessed how poor sleep can be debilitating. Many people with insomnia have become obsessed with sleep, worrying about sleep the moment they wake up in the morning. Some of my patients even develop a phobia or extreme fear of going to bed, with anxiety creeping in as soon as they think of sleeping or when the sun sets. 'Not another round of eight hours of torture,' some would say.

Many insomnia sufferers have tried innumerable potions, supplements, sleep hacks and sleep apps with not much improvement. Some will try yoga or meditation and find that it is not enough. Others will reluctantly resort to prescription tablets or purchase $10,000 beds touted to make sleep easy.

Good sleepers take for granted the complex process of sleeping. Many would ignorantly instruct insomnia sufferers just to shut their eyes then sleep. But sleep is not that simple once you have long-term insomnia. *Sleep Easy* takes into consideration the complexity of the sleep process without sounding too complicated.

Bernice's approach to this book is firstly from her personal experience of the horrors of insomnia. This can be very reassuring to the millions of insomnia sufferers. But what sets this book apart is her multi-faceted approach, which combines practical day-to-day management of insomnia, evidence-based CBT for insomnia, and techniques to manage overthinking and the tendency to beat oneself up. Many sleep clinicians focus solely on the techniques of CBTi but neglect the accompanying hyper-alertness and hypervigilance which afflict many people with insomnia. Mindfulness and self-compassion are effective approaches for these.

Even though her writing style is relaxed, casual and conversational, this book is full of recent scientific research and evidence-based recommendations. Whereas self-help books tend to pontificate, Bernice's *Sleep Easy* is more of a kind, helpful but very well-informed buddy.

This book provides hope without being too optimistic. It is realistic that certain approaches can be very difficult and require grit and perseverance. More than just an instructional manual of how to fix insomnia, this book guides the reader as to what attitude to adopt to increase the chances of the different interventions working.

Currently, this book is the most comprehensive self-help book on insomnia in the market. I would highly recommend it not just to patients, but also to primary care clinicians, nurses, and even other sleep specialists.

Dr Tony Fernando
Psychiatrist and sleep and insomnia specialist
Auckland, New Zealand

FOREWORD

Congratulations on picking up this gem of a book and congratulations to Bernice and her team at Allen & Unwin for a final product that is truly excellent—and likely to literally save lives and relationships.

Bernice approached me early into the first Covid-19 lockdowns in Australia and New Zealand, in April 2020, to let me know that she was writing a self-help book for people experiencing insomnia. Before then she had been unknown to me. Bernice asked me to help fact-check and look over some chapters from time to time, to which I said yes immediately, despite not having much spare time. My instincts often tell me to steer away from taking on too much, but I was immediately keen to support this project as I was instantly a true believer in *Sleep Easy* and its author.

This is a book of great courage and integrity—I am really pleased and honoured to have been able to provide some oversight of the research and current approaches to insomnia in Australasia. One of the main strengths of this book is that the community will have access to an accurate, heartfelt, sensible and sensitive self-help book written by someone who has a lived experience of the hell that insomnia can be. Not sleeping well for weeks, months or years on end can be extremely debilitating, and it's often an isolating and lonely experience for the sufferer. In the absence of obvious health markers of debilitation, such as crutches, bandages or a neck brace, people with insomnia often have no markers of their struggle—in fact, people can often look quite well. Bernice's accurate and poignant portrayal of this often silent personal suffering will resonate with readers who have shared that journey. It's enormously valuable that this book depicts not just a clinical or academic perspective on insomnia (although it does show due respect to the evidence and research) but also a personal tale of reckoning and triumph.

For a couple of decades I have worked with people in a clinical setting to help them improve their sleep, and I can confirm there is need for greater community education as well as more education and training among health professionals. This is long recognised and many organisations are putting out guidelines, education courses and fact sheets to help raise awareness and provide education about sleep. However, a multi-pronged approach is required and that is where good-quality, evidence-based and easily accessible books such as this one play a key role in reaching people who are often in desperate need of information and support. It can be very difficult to sort the treasure from the trash in the online multitude of products, all promising to provide a panacea for sleep. Bernice's narrative, on the other hand, is: 'I have something to offer you that I know, from the research and from personal experience, actually works. I am here to tell you it's not always easy but to stick with it!'

I wish all of the readers well in their journey toward improving their sleep. My sincere hope is that amongst these pages you will find some 'pearls' to help you to sleep well and to live well.

Dr Moira Junge
Health psychologist and clinic director
Yarraville Health Group
Melbourne, Australia

INTRODUCTION

Sometimes just getting up and
carrying on is brave and magnificent.

—CHARLIE MACKESY

Well done for finding your way here. If you've been experiencing persistent sleep difficulties (whether predictable or erratic) that are affecting your quality of life, and you simply don't know what to do about it, you're where you need to be.

Undersleeping is harsh. You've been living it, and you know the toll it takes on your energy, memory, concentration, productivity, performance and mood. It may be affecting you at work, at home or socially. Your quality of life may feel like it's being quietly eroded by an inability to sleep well. You may be noticing that sleep deficiency is impacting your looks, your weight, your fitness, your immunity, your health, even your overall sense of self. You know that sleep is essential, and you may be worried about the long-term effects of recurring sleep troubles on mental well-being and physical health.

Sleep may even be a nightly battleground. Something that you know you should be able to do, and yet, the more you try, the less success you seem to have. Your struggle to sleep might feel frustrating and unfair, given that sleep comes so naturally to some people; it may have even come naturally to you in the past. But now there's a problem.

Perhaps you're intensely focused on sleep and actively trying to sort it out: you've reached a point where you have lots of rules about what you can or can't do to avoid jeopardising your nights. But, despite all this, your sleep is still fickle and elusive.

Or things may have unravelled in a different way. Lack of sleep might have you feeling lost, disillusioned or disempowered. You may even be thinking that sleep is a lost cause—the problem has gone on for so long that it seems unsolvable, and you no longer have confidence in your ability to sleep. Perhaps you don't trust sleep any more.

Some of you will have been in touch with your doctor already. Some of you will be taking or will have tried taking sleeping pills. The medications may be helping, but for some they won't be the sustainable solution that you're comfortable with. You may have tried all sorts of alternative approaches to sleep and sleep support, been vigilant about your sleep habits, but nothing seems to work in a lasting, meaningful way.

When sleep remains hard to come by, or is short, fragmented, unsatisfying or inconsistent despite your best efforts and investments, it's easy to lose faith in the prospect of ever getting a good night's sleep. Cynicism and wariness towards products and services that promise miraculous sleep can set in.

Yet here you are with a self-help book in your hands. I applaud you. It takes courage and resilience to try one more thing. I know because I too have walked barefoot in the lonely midnight hours. Living with ongoing sleep deficiency sucks. I lived with it for far, far too long. But there's a way out: a proven protocol endorsed by the Australasian Sleep Association (ASA),[1] the Sleep Health Foundation,[2] the European Sleep Research Society (ESRS)[3] and the American Academy of Sleep Medicine (AASM)[4] called **cognitive behavioural therapy for insomnia (CBTi)**. It was my saving grace.

CBTi works. It's safe, and it provides sustained results with no side effects. As a treatment for ongoing sleep difficulties, CBTi has been extensively researched and validated, it's been around for decades, and it is prescribed throughout the world. However, most of us here in New Zealand and Australia have never heard of it. Even many of our healthcare professionals—through no fault of their own—are unfamiliar with CBTi. Sleep education within healthcare is much lighter and less consistent than we would like to believe.

The brilliant news is that CBTi can be self-taught. I'll be honest: it's quite a journey, but it's doable. When I taught myself CBTi, a few years ago now, I had to bushwhack my way through and find my own path. I didn't have access to a handy guidebook; there was a lot of trawling and researching as I navigated my way. While CBTi resources remain somewhat scarce, the information is out there. Internationally there are incredible sleep professionals committed to improving access to information about CBTi. Colin Espie, a professor of sleep medicine at the Nuffield Department of Clinical Neurosciences at the University of Oxford, has been advocating for a stepped-care approach to treating insomnia with CBTi for over ten years.[5] He recommends that those of us who can help ourselves get on and do it. To date, we don't have widespread public access to CBTi down under, despite the shocking prevalence of sleep problems in our countries. While our overworked, under-resourced sleep professionals are doing their best to help those most in need, those of us who are able can step up and help ourselves.

When relentless sleep difficulties were ruling (and ruining) my life, I wished for a CBTi guidebook on the shelves. That's why I wrote this book: an insider's guide to CBTi. I'm not a health professional; I'm a regular person who found their way from chronic sleep difficulties to confidently sleeping well. I have done my best to map out the information that will assist you on your journey towards sleeping well.

Two incredible, generous individuals from the sleep profession have championed and chaperoned this project: Dr Antonio Fernando, a psychiatrist and sleep and insomnia specialist in New Zealand, and Dr Moira Junge, a health psychologist in Australia and non-executive director on the board of the Sleep Health Foundation. Their belief in and help with this book assured me that there was a need for its existence. They gave me the confidence that there are many sleep-deprived people out there who are motivated and capable of helping themselves when provided with the information and techniques they need. And here you are.

I won't lie, CBTi can be challenging. It requires practical changes to your sleep habits, and it also requires a mind shift. But you're not alone: in this book I provide information, techniques and moral support to help you through the rough bits of the journey. It's important to remember that, compared to a lifetime of recurring sleep problems, a few bumpy weeks of CBTi is worth it. With this insider's guide to CBTi, you can be confident in the path ahead. The more you learn and apply these proven techniques and practices, the more you can let go of unhelpful habits, relax about sleep, and have confidence that your biology has your back. You have in your hands what you need to finally sleep easy.

**SLEEP EASY: to go to sleep without
(or be untroubled by) worries**

Turning the tide on 'sleep troubles'

The body's instinctive drive for sleep is so powerful that, when pushed to its limits, it can override logic and put life in jeopardy. This didn't seem plausible to me until I experienced it first-hand.

Floating in the bath at 2 a.m., I felt my soul surrender to the darkness, warmth and silence. At last I had found relief from the relentless wakeful nights that dictated the third trimester of my pregnancy. I closed my eyes. Sleep, seductively close, drew my swollen body deeper into the water. Warmth spread tenderly over my cheeks, my mouth, my eyes. I relaxed.

At last, the conditions for sleep. A whisper called from within: *Let go.* My heart feebly contested, *The baby.* The lulling voice reassured me, *You're together; you both need to sleep.* Released at last, I slipped beneath the surface of the water.

Despite usually being a rational, practical, upbeat person, in that split second my severe sleep deprivation put my life and that of my unborn baby at risk. I was lucky—I was in the bathtub and not behind the wheel. The moment I fell asleep, I inhaled a decent snort of water and became very conscious, very fast. After a few more sleep-deprived weeks, I became the mum I was meant to be to our glorious, life-affirming daughter, Lily.

But my battles with sleep had only just begun.

Sleep used to come naturally to me: a body rhythm needing no conscious thought, a simple occurrence at the close of each day. I fell asleep, I woke in the morning, no effort required.

Motherhood fundamentally changed that. With frequent waking in the night and long periods of settling, I fell into a pattern of very light and very broken sleep that went on for several years. By the time Lily started to sleep through the night, my ability to sleep had become severely compromised. A typical night involved passing out from exhaustion around 10.30 p.m., waking about 1 a.m. or 2 a.m., staying awake till 4 a.m. or 5 a.m., then sleeping intermittently until I was woken before six by our daughter. I averaged around 4 to 5 hours of sleep each night—a far cry from the 7.5 to 8 hours that my body and brain needed to function well. This continued for several years—far longer than what is a natural part of being a new mum.

It didn't occur to me that what I was experiencing was insomnia. My addled mind couldn't see the big picture. I just had trouble sleeping— nearly every night.

Ongoing sleep deprivation is a private hell. In our society, we receive kudos for being busy, always productive, always on. There's a pervasive 'sleep when you're dead' mentality: life's about having loads of energy, packing each day to the brim and being borderline invincible. Compare this with the phenomena experienced by the sleep deprived among us: dragging one's arse through the day, being 'tired', underperforming, making mistakes, forgetting things, being disorganised, withdrawing from social life and interests, having a short fuse, creating friction in close relationships, looking like hell, neglecting health, putting on weight, losing fitness, getting sick often, randomly crying with self-pity, and feeling hopeless, helpless and disempowered.

It's not the life story one wants to post on Instagram. Instead, we adopt a veneer: the mask of being okay. Humans are amazing; we adapt.

As an intelligent, responsible person, I wanted to get on with life—despite feeling like hell—and make the best of each day for myself and my family. To do this, I made good use of a multitude of readily available options that enabled me to get through the daylight hours while feigning my usual persona. I stripped back my life to the essentials: family, work, household chores. Caffeine (only in the morning) and carbohydrates (especially sweet ones in the afternoon and chocolate at night) became my two best friends. Despite being depleted, I powered on in a wired state of hyperarousal.

To solve my nights, I invested in a plethora of supplements and potions from pharmacies and health stores. My medicine cupboard was cluttered with products promising the miracle of sleep: half-empty bottles of tart cherry, valerian, passion flower, magnesium, and various combinations of vitamins and minerals with alluring names that evoked images of serenity, calm and tranquillity. Nothing worked. I sipped gallons of chamomile tea, which tasted like stinking daisies. I burned lavender oil. I tried yoga, meditation and mindfulness, but my efforts were sporadic and increasingly laced with cynicism.

At times I resorted to alcohol to at least numb me from the waking hell of another sleepless night. It was a roulette game that I only occasionally got away with; many times a squalling band of mind-monkeys would meet me after midnight and would not shut up till dawn.

I proactively visited my GP to address recurring colds and flu (which, I know now, were thanks to ongoing stress and a compromised immune system caused by lack of sleep), but I didn't raise the issue I was having with sleep. I knew I'd just be handed a script for sleeping pills in my fifteen-minute appointment. While sedatives are a great option for certain short-term scenarios (and I have embraced them post-surgery), I was after a natural, long-term solution. Oh, yes—I sat right up on my high horse about that.

Out in the world I continued to fake it, but my life was getting smaller. My tired-but-wired state was not sustainable. I had fewer interests, less contact with friends, less responsibility at work, less joy as a mother. I was becoming a ghost of my former self. Life had become about making it through the day.

I developed a love–hate relationship with my bed. While I craved it all day, I dreaded it at night, when I would face the reality of slipping between its untrustworthy sheets. Was it going to grant me the serenity that was promised when I bought it, or was it going to be a site of torturous wakefulness?

The night's aching hours had me tossing and turning, desperately trying to get back to sleep. I made conscious efforts to r-e-l-a-x. I irrationally resented my husband for *breathing* while he slept. The clock mocked me. Inevitably, my mind would start fretting, despite my best intentions. There'd be worrying, ruminating and, my personal favourite, catastrophising. Oh, the hell that I could conjure in those lonely pre-dawn hours.

Exacerbating the angst, I'd do 'night maths'. Arithmetic is not my strength by day, worse by night. Yet I was compelled to do elaborate, ever-changing calculations about how much sleep I'd had and not had, how many hours till morning, how much sleep I might squeeze in if I fell asleep instantaneously. I'd beg for mercy—just a half-hour of quality shut-eye before sun-up—then I'd ratchet things up with some algebra as to how wretched the coming day would be. It was exhausting.

Without meaning to, I'd become what I refer to as a 'lifestyle insomniac'. Sleep had become a battle, and I was losing.

But there was no medical or psychiatric basis for my sleep deficiency. I wasn't dealing with chronic pain or respiratory issues. I wasn't obese. I didn't have acid reflux, urinary problems, Parkinson's disease or any other medical conditions. I wasn't on any medications (prescribed or otherwise) that interfered with sleep. I didn't have anxiety or depression, post-traumatic stress disorder, psychosis, mania or dementia. I didn't have any of the symptoms of more dramatic sleep disorders: no sleep apnoea, no restless-leg syndrome, no sleepwalking, sleep talking, night terrors, exploding-head syndrome. I wasn't suffering from a neurological disorder, like narcolepsy.

I had run-of-the-mill, predictably unpredictable, shitty sleep that I'd been trying in vain to manage for a very long time. Officially, what I had falls under the clinical umbrella of *insomnia*—a sleep disorder where an ordinary person has difficulty falling or staying asleep. It might sound low-key on paper, but as a lived experience it's extraordinary and definitely unsustainable.

With none of my initiatives making any inroads, my sleep-salvation efforts became erratic, illogical and desperate. Putting my high horse out to pasture temporarily, I visited the chemist. I used my acting skills (aka 'lied', but I like to think of it as the late acting coach Sanford Meisner did: 'living truthfully under imaginary circumstances') to secure a pack of what I came to refer to as my true best friend: Blue Oblivion. That is not its pharmaceutical name or its intended purpose, but Blue Oblivion consistently sedated me when nothing else had worked. It was a last resort. A last resort that I began to use on an increasingly regular basis. Nightly.

Over time, and after many shameful chemist-hopping excursions, my conscience got the better of me. I conceded I was kidding myself— this was sedation, not sleep, and Lord knows what else it was doing to my system.

I went back to exploring permissible options. I just wanted a product, a potion, anything that would break the cycle and get me back to sleeping through.

One evening, I judiciously prepared a spoonful of equal parts sugar and salt to put in an eggcup beside my bed, ready for a highly probable 2 a.m. wake-up. According to an 'article' I had read, this combo was going to send me straight back to the land of Nod. Later that night, as I winced at the intense sweet-saltiness of my concoction, I reflected on how ridiculous insomnia had made me. I was now sucking pixie dust in the moonlight, rotting my teeth and raising my cholesterol with zero impact on my sleep. My sleep-deficient brain was clearly no longer capable of making decent decisions. I felt like I had become pathetic.

Unable to continue in this state, I decided to take action.

Paradoxically, I knew that I needed a reprieve from insomnia if I was to have any chance of applying my brain to dealing with it. For that, I needed professional help. I turned to an integrative GP who I'd worked with throughout my breast-cancer treatment and recovery the previous year. She understood my desire to find a long-term, natural and sustainable solution. She didn't have the answer, but she respected and encouraged my audacious goal to find a sustainable way to sleep naturally, as she knew so many other patients who needed this help. She understood my views on conventional sleeping pills, but, given the lack of alternatives available and the state of absolute depletion I was in, she introduced me to a short course of melatonin—a synthetic version of a natural sleep hormone. Grudgingly, I filled the script.

Melatonin, produced by the pineal gland, is known as the 'Dracula of hormones'—it only comes out at night. Its lovely job is to make sleep more inviting. And, thanks to melatonin tablets, inviting it became. Once we had the dosage and directions fine-tuned, a course of melatonin was life-changing. It reintroduced sleep into my life.

Previously, I had only fantasised about getting 6 hours of sleep a night for three nights in a row. Melatonin pills allowed me this luxury and more—for several weeks. I couldn't believe the difference that consistent sleep made to my life—once again I had energy, mental clarity and joy in my heart! I felt like Sleeping Beauty, finally awoken to her own life. Suddenly, filled with possibility, optimism and vitality, I was unstoppable. I would have happily taken melatonin forever—*Keep those scripts coming*, I thought.

Then the magical melatonin tablets stopped working. I had known it was only ever a temporary measure, but I was furious. I Googled to find out what was up with this product and was intrigued to discover that, while some research supported its efficacy in helping a patient fall asleep, other research suggested it was only as effective as a placebo.[6] *Hang on!* I thought. *Would I have been getting the same results if I'd stuck with my pixie dust, I just needed to* believe *in my pixie dust?* Then the possibility dawned on me—perhaps the ability to sleep is all in the mind.

The truth will set you free, but first it will piss you off.
—GLORIA STEINEM

I was outraged by this hypothesis, but my fury fuelled further action. Having tasted the sweet nectar of consistent sleep, I was on a mission to discover how to have it again, naturally and forever, and nothing would stop me. Sleep is one of the most fundamental human drives, the body needs it to survive, so I figured the body (or the mind) *had* to know how to do it naturally. I had to apply my brain to learn how to sleep again.

Highly motivated by my quest and a researcher by profession, I delved into the problem further. My first reading on the topic was Arianna Huffington's eye-opening book *The Sleep Revolution*. Those three hundred–odd pages were a call to action—so many nations around the world were in the midst of a 'sleep-deprivation crisis', we had to reclaim our sleep. I'd had no idea—I'd thought it was just me! As mentioned in the book, I typed the words 'Why am I' into Google, and was staggered to see that the super-helpful autocomplete function immediately prompts 'so tired' based on the most common searches in its universe. (That was back in 2016 and it still holds true at the time of this writing.)

It was strangely comforting to know that I wasn't the only soul on the planet feeling this wrecked and exhausted. Understanding how undersleeping had evolved in our society since the Industrial Revolution also helped me feel as though it wasn't all my fault. But I needed a practical action plan—what did I need to do to sleep well? I needed a manual, an insider's guide.

While searching for solutions, I kept finding two types of information in sources that people experiencing sleep problems were likely to happen upon:

1. Horror articles on the sleep-loss epidemic and the long-term effects of sleep deprivation on the body and brain, which created more anguish and offered no information on how to sleep or where to get help.

2. Tidy lists called things like 'Twelve ways to improve your sleep tonight' that were written by health journalists who all seemed to be good sleepers living sunny, upbeat lives. Having already tried most of these ideas without success, I had zero confidence in these stupid lists.

Faced with a lack of helpful information, I decided that there had to be experts in the field of sleep medicine who could show me, step by step, what to do. I tried another GP, this time spilling the beans on the extent of my sleep problems. She was shocked as she'd never had a sense of this previously (to my detriment, my mask of normality had been quite good), and she didn't have the answer either, but she suggested I visit a sleep specialist in Auckland.

A phone call later, I knew that demand was high. There was an eight-week waiting list, and I'd need a GP referral and a few hundred dollars to cover my *initial* appointment. It was likely I would need several sessions.

A check with my health-insurance company made it clear that, with my policy and its fine print, I was on my own.[7] Given the importance of sleep to my quality of life, now and down the track, I decided to invest.

Meanwhile, I had eight more weeks of insomnia to endure. As a practical, resourceful Kiwi, that didn't sit well with me. I was frustrated that there wasn't affordable, accessible help readily available, annoyed that the insurance company didn't have my back, and incensed that sleep deprivation was so pervasive in our society. I rolled up my sleeves and took those eight weeks as a personal challenge.

I decided to take a DIY approach while I waited, and I threw myself at the problem. My relationship with sleep had undergone an important shift: it was no longer about winning a fight. I'd become curious, open to new possibilities, and I was up for exploring. I read and researched, immersing myself in books, websites, articles, programmes, interviews and TED Talks. As a freelancer with occasional downtime between research projects, I was able to apply a serious amount of time to the cause.

The amount of information available on sleep can be overwhelming. There are brilliant doctors, specialists and academics around the world who have dedicated their lives to studying sleep, and new discoveries are being made all the time. While the knowledge is there, it's typically too daunting for the average sleep-deprived person to locate, process and, most importantly, implement. Even so, I decided to have a go— one practical step at a time.

Committed to changing my ways, I set myself up as a human experiment. I prioritised sleep and created realistic sleep goals for myself. Using applied wisdom and imperfect action, I started to think about and do things differently. I knew I had a lot to learn and that I was no sleep expert—my strengths were in the arts, not the sciences—but I needed to have a go.

Done is better than perfect.
—SHERYL SANDBERG

I started to keep a **sleep diary**, monitoring what *actually* went on with my sleep each night. In addition to hours of sleep, I began tracking my **sleep efficiency**. This percentage score captures total sleep time relative to time in bed (an important figure that for me started around 50 per cent and needed to be up around 85 per cent).

To kick things off, I used reverse psychology: I stopped caring about not sleeping. Rather than view insomnia as a problem, I looked at sleep as a source of fascination. I quit *trying* to sleep. It was clear that my efforts to force sleep were creating stress in my body, making slumber elusive. Proactively creating the conditions for sleep then letting nature do its thing became my focus.

Next, I took care of what specialists refer to as **sleep hygiene**. It sounds like washing sheets in boiling water with a splash of disinfectant, but sleep hygiene is about taking care of the basics most likely to mess with your sleep. I improved my **sleep environment** so that it better suited my needs—I made it darker, quieter, better ventilated, I adjusted the temperature, I simplified and decluttered. I removed the clock altogether, and phones and screens were forbidden. My bedroom was to be calm, a sanctuary for me to retreat to at the close of each day.

I decided to review coffee and alcohol. I didn't eliminate them—these were my friends who I liked and had relied on for a long time. I was the boss, and I simply used the black-and-white facts in my sleep diary to determine whether they were helping me or not. Surprise, surprise, it turned out they weren't that helpful. I modified things to establish how much and when was okay—it had to be workable while not jeopardising my nights. This was my journey, and I needed to have the freedom to choose. (Plus I had no intention of becoming a saint.)

Once I understood how important it was for my body to have a consistent routine, I set up a **sleep-wake schedule** that supported the possibility of good sleep but also worked in with my lifestyle. Creating this meant finally giving myself permission to wind down at the end of the day. Being sleep deprived had meant that I always felt like I was on the back foot and my evenings were often spent trying to catch up, before I panicked about how late it was and rushed off to bed. This time of relaxation became a non-negotiable. Previously, any wind-down time involved parking up in front of Netflix, but the research was clear: blue light is detrimental to sleep. It became easier to choose a good book.

I made friends with my bed. Like Pavlov's salivating dogs, I had developed all sorts of negative associations with my bed. It had been the site of much frustration and wakefulness, and, over years of insomnia, I had abandoned it many times to crash out on the couch or daybed. While those initiatives had solved the immediate crisis of the night, they had created an unhelpful pathway that told my brain that my bed wasn't a great place for sleep. My efforts to help myself had made things worse. I had to develop a new approach to my bed, so that it once again became a strong cue for sleep.

As I implemented these changes and continued to learn more, my sleep started to improve, and I felt empowered. My nights were heading in the right direction.

Next was **operation mind shift**. It was clear that I had been subconsciously holding myriad negative thoughts about sleep. As I exposed these to the light of day and reviewed them objectively, they lost their power over me. For instance, I'd thought that a day following sleep deprivation would be hideous and impossible. By reframing my thinking, I knew that, although they weren't the best days, I had proven time and again that they were in fact doable. Not ideal, but doable.

I'd also accumulated many misconceptions about sleep—there was now robust science to dispel sleep myths. I didn't necessarily need 8 hours of sleep a night; I learned to understand what *my* body needed.

For some it's a bit more, for others it's a bit less. If I'd had a bad night's sleep, I didn't need to go to bed super early the next night to 'catch up'—the body, given the right conditions, tends to sort itself out with better quality sleep, rather than quantity. Waking up for a period in the night is not impending doom—it can be part of a natural and necessary sleep process. This new knowledge about sleep allowed me to relax more and sleep came easier.

With my sleep improving markedly throughout these weeks of mental adjustments and behavioural choices, I had more energy, more clarity and, most importantly, more time. I liked where things were going with my sleep and I wanted that to continue as my appointment with the sleep specialist drew closer.

By then, during my research, I'd located an online sleep-improvement programme offered by specialists in the UK. Even though they sounded impressive, I didn't know a thing about Big Health or Sleepio and I wasn't keen to lay out the cash upfront. But I did offer to be part of a pilot study on another programme that they were developing, which in time gave me access to their sleep programme. It reinforced the information that I had discovered, validated the steps that I had already taken, and provided me with additional facts and action points to add to my sleep-recovery journey. Most importantly, it made me continue monitoring and evolving my behaviour, and I checked in with a weekly tutorial to continue my sleep education.

With more energy, I began to take a gentle interest in exercise again. Previously, I had been too exhausted to consider it. My eating habits started to improve, and my sweet cravings in the afternoon had become murmurs that could be ignored more often than not.

I found ways to incorporate relaxation into my life on my own terms. While I had aspirations of doing a mindfulness course and learning to meditate, for now walking in nature was working for me. Life got easier.

My sleep was in pretty good shape, with my sleep-efficiency scores consistently kicking up around 70 per cent, when my appointment with the sleep specialist finally came around. However, I still had two distinct parts to my night, and I wanted to reduce the time I was awake in the early hours of the morning. Under the direction of the online programme, I was about to embark on a protocol known as **sleep consolidation** (an important part of sleep improvement that sounds counterintuitive, but works on the principle that less can be more).

Given the price tag and the progress I'd already made, I considered cancelling my appointment. But I'd become passionate about sleep, the sleep-loss epidemic our nations are facing and the challenges of accessing help. I arrived at the clinic in my researcher, game-changer mode as much as my patient mode.

Looking at my sleep diary, health and happy disposition, the specialist questioned what I was doing in his office! He confirmed that the approach I was using was based on valid and respected principles known collectively as cognitive behavioural therapy for insomnia (even if my version was fairly loose and free-range). Then we discussed how I could safely use sleep consolidation to solve the final sleep challenge I was working through.

Within a couple of weeks of sleep consolidation, my broken sleep had knitted itself back together, and I was sleeping through the night. That's right: sleeping through the night. It felt like nothing shy of a miracle. Then it was just a matter of gradually increasing my sleep duration until I hit that glorious threshold of 7.5 hours a night on a very consistent basis. Hallelujah!

Over about twelve weeks of DIY research and experimentation with my sleep, I had turned the tide on nearly ten years of chronic insomnia (five years if you exclude those years of interrupted sleep caused by pregnancy and motherhood). After a few more weeks of implementing all that I had learned, I was confident that it was possible to reclaim sleep and that, to get there, CBTi can, for a lot of people, be self-taught. (For some people with pre-existing conditions, such as severe anxiety or depression, it's advisable to apply CBTi with the guidance of a qualified health professional, rather than try to do it solo.)

But it wasn't CBTi alone that saved me from the hell and high water of insomnia. I had unwittingly but instinctively applied principles and approaches of what I later learned were mindfulness and self-compassion in my sleep-improvement journey. **Mindfulness-based therapy for insomnia (MBTI)**, combining non-judgemental awareness and self-compassion with CBTi, is increasingly being proven as a highly effective treatment for insomnia.[8] Sure, my version of this incredibly valuable therapy was makeshift and improvised, but it enabled me to stick with a self-directed approach to CBTi.

What is CBTi?

Cognitive behavioural therapy for insomnia is a highly effective sleep-improvement programme that works without sleeping pills (but can be used alongside sleep medication). CBTi helps to identify thoughts and behaviours that have inadvertently been causing, worsening or perpetuating sleep troubles and replaces them with new knowledge and habits that provide the conditions for sound sleep.

The cognitive aspect focuses on reframing or eliminating unhelpful thoughts and sleep beliefs that keep us awake at night. The behavioural element concentrates on dropping any unhelpful lifestyle and sleep-schedule habits, while introducing or improving behaviours that are conducive to sleeping well naturally.

Unlike sleeping pills, CBTi addresses the underlying causes of persistent insomnia rather than just relieving the symptoms. In clinical studies, it has proven to be highly effective in the treatment of insomnia and the prevention of relapse. Unlike pharmaceuticals, CBTi is natural and sustainable, and has no side effects.

The five key components of CBTi are:

1. Sleep education
2. Sleep consolidation
3. Stimulus control
4. Cognitive therapy
5. Relaxation training

The core CBTi techniques are tough going even when supported by a qualified professional, and trying to implement them solo is ambitious and a recipe for non-compliance. If this book focused solely on CBTi, I would have had to give it a brutal title like *Sleep Bootcamp*. By including an introduction to mindfulness and self-compassion, the *Sleep Easy* approach to sleep improvement is more doable. 'Mindfulness' may sound a bit ethereal to you, but, for the sake of your sleep, it's worth putting reticence aside so that you can develop a mindset that supports adherence to CBTi. Doing this makes the sleep-improvement journey that much easier.

I continue to apply what I learned with CBTi (and makeshift mindfulness and self-compassion), and I have been sleeping well for several years now. My body and mind thrive on 7.5 hours a night, and I make sure I maintain the conditions that allow that to occur. Every morning I unconsciously reinforce my behaviour, quietly thinking, *What a great sleep!* or *I'm such a good sleeper*.

Of course life throws curveballs and, once in a while, I experience a wakeful night. In the past, one night of bad sleep could send me into a tailspin, and I'd be on the trajectory for many more bad and worsening nights. Now, I have road-tested knowledge and tools at my disposal, so the odd night of unsettled sleep is entirely manageable and does not herald the beginning of a bad patch.

The change that sleep has made to my life, brain, health, relationships and future is profound. Having overcome almost ten years of silent insomnia, I feel sincere gratitude for this transformation daily.

Chronic insomnia is a living nightmare. It's debilitating and disempowering, and it can be self-perpetuating. Thoughts and actions that you expect will help can actually trap you in the vicious cycle of poor sleep. Information on sleep can be challenging to access, overwhelming or conflicting, and specialist help for chronic insomnia is at this stage in limited supply, especially in New Zealand, and it can be prohibitively expensive. For most of us, we're on our own. With compromised cognitive function, memory and focus, along with depleted energy levels, it can be soul-destroyingly tricky for someone living with insomnia to wade through the options, apply themselves and navigate their way back to a decent sleep.

Learning how to sleep is liberating and empowering. Sleeping well is an essential life skill—a human right. Having achieved it for myself, I am wholeheartedly committed to encouraging others to turn the tide on their sleep troubles. When you're coming from a place of feeling ruined and depleted, the prospect of having to add 'learning to sleep' to the list can feel impossible. So congratulations, you are here exploring the possibility.

> *You're never ready for what you have to do. You just do it. That makes you ready.*
> —FLORA RHETA SCHREIBER

CBTi has been researched and used effectively for decades, and it is endorsed by sleep organisations throughout the world, including the ASA and the Sleep Health Foundation, both of which recommend CBTi as a first-line treatment for insomnia. In 2016, the American College of Physicians strongly recommended CBTi as a first-line treatment for adults with chronic insomnia, publishing their recommendation as an evidence-based clinical guideline in the *Annals of Internal Medicine*.[9] In 2017, the European insomnia guideline, developed by a task force of the European Sleep Research Society (ESRS), followed suit, stating:

Cognitive behavioural therapy for insomnia is recommended as the first-line treatment for chronic insomnia in adults of any age (strong recommendation, high-quality evidence).[10]

The challenge, highlighted by the ESRS, is that there is limited awareness of this highly effective treatment among those of us who most need it. A worldwide shortage of health professionals trained in CBTi means that it can be difficult or expensive to access.

While individual or group therapy may be the gold standard for CBTi, it can also be effectively conducted via phone, web-based options and self-help books. Having taught myself CBTi, I am a strong advocate for the DIY approach. You can step towards your salvation right away, without waiting for the healthcare profession or government funding to catch up with the sleep-loss epidemic that is occurring right here, right now.

What I love most about CBTi is that, at its very core, it feels like common sense. It gently encourages you to recognise, reconsider and disrupt thought and behaviour patterns that are unhelpful to sleep, and replace them with more useful alternatives. I'm a practical person (sleep-deprived pixie-dust and Blue Oblivion episodes aside), and the new thinking and alternative behaviours that CBTi required seemed so logical and sensible to me once they had been explained. What's more, they worked. I could see and track my progress, and I felt better. As I felt better, I was inspired to continue until I achieved my sleep goals.

> *What I like to offer is hope. If sleep difficulties are a learned behavior, that means you can unlearn them.*
> —DR CHARLES MORIN, PRESIDENT OF WORLD SLEEP SOCIETY (2018)[11]

I am not a sleep expert. I am an ordinary New Zealander who experienced ongoing sleep difficulties for far too long. I'm living proof that, when paired with mindfulness, CBTi can deliver sustainable sleep naturally with no side effects, even when applied imperfectly. However, making CBTi readily available and affordable for everyone who needs it will require significant investment in public health. Until that happens, those of us who can must call on our resourcefulness, ingenuity and pioneering spirit and take a DIY approach. Let's get on with helping to heal ourselves.

I have always loved that New Zealand is one of the first countries to see the sun and that New Zealanders start their days before everyone else on the planet. Now I think about how it also means, theoretically, we go to sleep before everyone else, too. With what I know now about the worldwide epidemic of sleep loss, and how ill-equipped New Zealand and Australian healthcare systems are to address it, I think those of us living down under could lead the way in a sleep renaissance. We have the potential to educate and upskill ourselves, so we can solve our sleep troubles first.

> *[CBTi] puts the patient in the driver seat of the entire process.*
>
> —DR CHARLES MORIN[12]

Is this book for you?

If you are sick and tired of sleeping poorly, *Sleep Easy* is for you. You may not want to take (or continue taking) sleeping pills. You are motivated to take responsibility for learning *how* to sleep well naturally, by following a practical, step-by-step approach inspired by CBTi.

The focus of this book is on the needs of people experiencing **chronic insomnia**, whose sleep problems are *not* the result of underlying psychiatric or medical issues.

What is chronic insomnia?

The definition of insomnia varies, but according to the International Classification of Sleep Disorders, third edition (ICSD-3),[13] chronic insomnia involves:

- dissatisfaction with the quantity or quality of sleep, e.g., difficulty falling asleep, difficulty staying asleep throughout the night, early-morning awakening,
- sleep difficulties occurring despite adequate opportunity and circumstances for sleep,
- suffering significant distress or daytime impairment,
- experiencing insomnia at least **three nights a week** for **more than three months**; and
- *not* having other sleep disorders that are causing what appears to be insomnia.

If you know or suspect that your sleep challenges run deeper than lifestyle choices or unhelpful thoughts and behaviours, please contact your GP, sleep specialist or sleep clinic. Go to your appointment armed with the sleep review that you'll complete in Chapter 1, and—if you have time—start keeping a sleep diary (Chapter 3).

If you're not sure what your situation is, Chapter 1 will help you figure out if CBTi is the right approach for you or if you need additional help.

For those of you enduring what seems to be 'just' chronic insomnia (with no underlying psychological or medical issues), you're in the right place. You have picked up this book because you're a smart, on-to-it person who's great to be around and aspires to a wonderful life on your own terms. But with all the tiredness, exhaustion and disempowerment, or the unsustainable 'wiredness', that accompanies sleep deprivation, you've been struggling to be your best self for quite a while.

This book will provide you with information, tools and encourage-ment to help you get your sleep—and yourself—back on track. Having successfully made my own journey to sleep recovery, I have used everything I learned along the way to map out a practical, step-by-step plan based on CBTi that incorporates some core principles of mindfulness and self-compassion. It's grounded in my personal experiences, extensive research into the field of sleep and insomnia, and interviews with a network of dedicated and generous sleep specialists and health psychologists in New Zealand and Australia.

How to use this book

Sleep Easy takes a divide and conquer approach. I'm all too familiar with how difficult insomnia makes it to find time, process information, remember things and follow through on commitments. The book is presented in three parts:

1. Sleep assessment and preparation.
2. The six-week programme.
3. Maintenance and follow-up.

Each part is broken into doable chapters that are designed to be read and worked through one by one, and each chapter builds on the one previous. Try not to feel daunted by how inadequate your sleep is currently, or how long your sleep troubles have been going on. Right now, your job is to make a start.

> *The best time to plant an oak tree is twenty years ago. The second-best time is now.*
> —UNKNOWN

You might be tempted to skimp on Part 1 so that you can get stuck into the action—the desire to 'do' something is understandable. But the very act of 'not doing' for a time matters. Part 1 dedicates time for you to sit back and learn what's really going on with your sleep and to open your mind to how sleep works. It will provide you with the foundation you need on your sleep-improvement journey. It will serve you well.

Along the way, consider this a workbook or a journal rather than a textbook. You're going to need to grab a pen, get stuck in to the pages and make them your own. Things are going to get personal—really personal. Make this book your sleep-recovery journal: highlight things, underline things, write notes, fill out the pages on your sleep habits and experiences, detail what's working and what's not. I struggle with writing in books, especially in pen—it feels like a small crime—but just do it. This book is replaceable; your sleep dictates your future. Let's go.

Make things a little easier for yourself

Head over to my website, Sleep Haven, and let me know that you've taken the brave and magnificent step of starting your sleep improvement journey. You'll get access to a handy sleep efficiency tool that'll make tracking your weekly progress easy.

www.sleephaven.co.nz

PART 1

Sleep Assessment and Preparation

CHAPTER 1

Review your sleep—screen for 'insomnia'

Faith is taking the first step even when you don't see the whole staircase.

—MARTIN LUTHER KING JR

The first step of your sleep-improvement journey is to understand what's happening with your sleep and assess how it's affecting your quality of life. This chapter includes a questionnaire that will enable you to take stock of your situation. The questions are based on the Auckland Sleep Questionnaire,[1] a sleep-disorder diagnosis tool developed and validated by Dr Tony Fernando and Bruce Arroll, Professor of General Practice and Primary Health Care at Auckland University and practising GP.

Let's leave the clinical diagnosis to the doctors, but this sleep review is useful to get you thinking about your sleep in new and helpful ways.

You won't score the answers or compare yourself with 'norms'. There are no grades to be achieved. Instead, your responses will enable you to look at your experiences in detail, so you can start to figure out the sleep issues you are facing.

This sleep review will also highlight if you need specialist support instead of (or in addition to) working through a self-help programme. Some medical and psychological sleep or health issues can present as insomnia, so this chapter and the next will encourage you to see a professional if the sleep symptoms you're experiencing raise any flags. Remember, CBTi is the recommended first-line approach for insomnia—if you have symptoms that suggest another type of sleep disorder, it is important to consult your GP, a sleep clinic or a sleep specialist. (And, with telehealth increasingly available, it's getting easier to access specialist sleep services wherever you live.)

Find a quiet place and start documenting what's been happening with your sleep. If you feel overwhelmed at any point, break down the chapter into doable chunks and complete them as you are able. If you feel hyped and ready to 'nail' this questionnaire, I ask you to ease up. Your 'wired' approach could well be courtesy of insomnia-related hyperarousal: a state of chronic activation, which makes the day intense and sleep at night elusive. If this sounds like you, just be aware of it, take a long, slow breath, and allow yourself to slow down. (Think tortoise, not hare—slow and steady wins the race.)

Your goal is to bring the essential facts together in one place—to support yourself in discovering a way forward, or to provide critical information to take to a healthcare professional if required.

The sleep-review questionnaire covers what is happening at night, and, as importantly, how you are going during the day. That includes:

- sleep patterns and behaviour
- sleep history
- daytime functioning
- emotional well-being
- life stage, lifestyle and physical health
- sleep initiatives explored.

This is your sleep, your story—as you go through the questions, just answer as best you can. It's common for sleep difficulties to be varied, with some nights better than others, or to have stretches when things are okay and times when they are really not. Opt for your 'best guess' based on your experiences. Trust that this will at least provide you with an overview of what's going on.

Be assured that there are no right or wrong answers. There's no magic diagnosis formula. This is merely an opportunity to gather some relevant sleep information in one place, to help you get a better perspective. Allow yourself time to contemplate the factors that can influence your sleep, so that you can look at your situation with fresh eyes and open your mind to new insights about your sleep.

SLEEP PATTERNS AND BEHAVIOUR

Think about your sleep over the last month and answer the questions as best you can.

1. How would you describe the quality of your sleep over the last month?
- ☐ Terrible
- ☐ Bad
- ☐ Average
- ☐ Good
- ☐ Excellent

2. How long does it usually take for you to fall asleep after lights out?
_____ minutes/hours

3. How many times do you typically wake up during the night?
- ☐ Never (*skip to Q5*)
- ☐ Once
- ☐ Two or three times
- ☐ Four or five times
- ☐ Six or more times

4. When you wake in the night, do you have trouble getting back to sleep?

☐ Yes

How long are you usually awake during the night in total?

_____ minutes/hours

☐ No

5. On an average night, how many hours do you actually sleep?

_____

6. How many hours do you stay in bed on a typical night?

_____

7. How many times a week do your sleep difficulties (falling asleep, staying asleep or sleep quality) affect how well you function the next day?

_____

8. What time do you usually go to bed and get up on weekdays?

Go to bed at _____ p.m./a.m.

Get up at _____ a.m./p.m.

9. What time do you usually go to bed and get up on the weekend?

Go to bed at _____ p.m./a.m.

Get up at _____ a.m./p.m.

10. How regular is your sleep schedule across an entire week (weekdays and weekends)?

☐ Very regular (*go to bed and get up at the same time throughout the week*)

☐ Fairly regular (*go to bed and get up at about the same time each day— within an hour*)

☐ Regularly irregular (*have a weekday sleep schedule and a weekend sleep schedule*)

☐ Erratic (*no schedule; bedtime and get-up times are highly variable*)

11. If you could set your sleep–wake schedule according to your body's needs, what time would you like to . . .

go to bed _____ p.m./a.m.

get up _____ a.m./p.m.

12. In terms of your body's natural rhythm, do you consider yourself a . . .

☐ morning person / a lark (*prefer to get up early and to be asleep before 11 p.m.*)

☐ evening person / an owl (*prefer to stay up late—midnight or later—and sleep late in the morning*)

☐ in between

☐ not sure

13. In the last month, have you been bothered by waking up earlier than you would like and being unable to get back to sleep before it's time to get up?

☐ Yes

How much earlier do you wake than you would like? _____

Does this happen more than three times a week? _____

☐ No

14. In the last month, have you been falling asleep much later than you'd like, even when you go to bed at a time that is suitable for your schedule?

☐ Yes

How long does it take you to fall asleep after lights out? _____

Does this happen more than three times a week? _____

☐ No

15. Which, if any, of these symptoms have you experienced *often* in the last month?

Your sheets or blankets are a crazy mess when you wake up in the morning.	Yes	No
You wake yourself up by kicking your legs at night.	Yes	No
You experience horrible sensations in your legs (aches, pains, creepy feelings).	Yes	No
You know, or have been told, that you are a heavy or loud snorer.*	Yes	No
You know, or have been told, that you seem to have trouble breathing while sleeping.	Yes	No
You know, or have been told, that you have frequent pauses in your breathing or wake gasping for air.	Yes	No
You grind or clench your teeth at night.	Yes	No
You wake with a sore jaw or teeth.	Yes	No
You walk in your sleep at night.	Yes	No
You need to pee often during the night (three or more times).	Yes	No
You sleep talk and interrupt your or your partner's sleep.	Yes	No
You have nightmares.	Yes	No
You wake in the night in panic, fright or terror.	Yes	No
You hear intense or loud noises that are not real as you fall asleep or wake up.	Yes	No
You have excessive night sweats.	Yes	No
You have a sense of being paralysed.	Yes	No
You experience hallucinations.	Yes	No

* If you don't know or aren't convinced whether you snore, you could use an app such as SnoreLab to get an overnight recording and summary of your snoring.

16. In the last month, how often have you been thinking or worrying about your sleep or ability to sleep?

☐ Not at all

☐ A little

☐ A moderate amount
☐ A lot
☐ All the time

17. How confident are you in your ability to fall asleep, stay asleep and experience good-quality sleep regularly?
☐ Very confident
☐ Moderately confident
☐ It varies—sometimes confident, sometimes not
☐ A little confident
☐ Not at all confident

SLEEP HISTORY

1. How long have you been experiencing sleep difficulties? _____

2. Did any particular event or factors trigger your sleep difficulties?
_____
_____

3. Did you have difficulties sleeping as a child or teenager?
☐ Yes
What problems did you experience?
_____
_____

☐ No

DAYTIME FUNCTIONING

Now that you've provided a thorough overview of your experiences during the night, and touched on what may have precipitated your sleep difficulties, let's think about the day.

1. Over the last two weeks, to what extent have you experienced the following?

	Not at all	A little	A moderate amount	A lot
Feelings of fatigue or exhaustion				
Feeling wired or hyperactive				
Feeling clumsy or accident-prone				
Morning headaches on waking				
Dry mouth on waking				
Difficulty with concentration and memory				
Accidentally falling asleep during the day				
Intentionally taking naps during the day				

2. Over the last two weeks, to what extent have sleep difficulties affected any of the following aspects of your life?

	Not at all	A little	A moderate amount	A lot
Ability to attend work or study				
Ability to function or perform at work or study				
Participation or enjoyment in social activities				
Participation or enjoyment in hobbies and interests				
Quality of relationships with partner, family or friends				

It can be a confronting process to work through these questions and realise the extent of your sleep problems and how they have been impacting your quality of life. Yet, when I did it, I also found it exciting to collate the information so at least I had a better handle on the scope and nature of what I was dealing with. It made me more aware of my own situation, and more aware that I needed to address it. Seeing everything in black-and-white on the page, rather than the shambolic day-to-day lived experience of it, I was able to look at my circumstances with less judgement and loads more compassion. It was apparent that what had been going on for me was not okay, and definitely not sustainable if I was to have the kind of life that I aspired to.

Let's take a breather here and work through what your answers might mean. First, we want to check whether what you have been experiencing is insomnia. Identifying sleep issues can be incredibly complex and involved, and, for some, it will require specialist investigation and in-home or clinical tests. However, the questions you've completed can provide an initial framework for understanding the fundamentals of the problem.

Does it seem like insomnia?

Last updated in 2014, the ICSD-3, created by the American Academy of Sleep Medicine, is a system that organises sleep disorders into seven broad categories:

1. insomnia
2. sleep-related breathing disorders
3. hypersomnolence (excessive daytime sleepiness)
4. circadian rhythm sleep–wake disorders (body clock)
5. parasomnias
6. sleep-related movement disorders
7. other sleep disorders.

The focus of this book is to empower people with chronic insomnia with insights, information and tools to help themselves, so let's check whether what you are experiencing has the signs of this very common sleep disorder. Keep in mind that many other sleep disorders can masquerade as insomnia, so it's essential that you also read Chapter 2, which provides an overview of the more complex sleep disorders and their associated symptoms. It also provides suggestions as to next steps if you suspect that your sleep troubles go beyond insomnia.

Insomnia describes a condition where a person has persistent difficulty falling asleep or staying asleep, and they are troubled by the duration or quality of their sleep (despite having given themselves sufficient opportunity to sleep well). The person also experiences some kind of daytime impairment as a result, and their sleep disturbances and associated daytime impairment occur at least three times a week.

Under the umbrella of 'insomnia', there are two main types of the condition to consider: short-term insomnia (symptoms last under three months) and chronic insomnia (symptoms are experienced for three months or more).

1. Short-term insomnia

Short-term insomnia is commonly associated with an identifiable cause or daytime stressors that have triggered sleep issues, such as a significant life event (e.g., a death in the family), a change of circumstances (e.g., caring for a baby, starting a new job, losing a job, going through a divorce), an illness or injury, changes in medication, or increased stress at work. Recently, the Covid-19 pandemic has been a trigger for sleep issues for many people.[2] With short-term insomnia, once the event or stress has passed, sleep generally settles back into its normal rhythm. Even though it's only temporary, short-term insomnia is no fun while you are in the midst of it.

What you can do: When you hit a patch like this, know that short-term insomnia in response to a life event or stress is not unexpected. Remind yourself that it will pass, and focus on looking after yourself as you try to deal with the cause or stressor that is compromising your sleep.

If this is you, it's brilliant that you are proactively exploring how to help yourself at this juncture. Dealing with insomnia in its early stages will help prevent the development of chronic insomnia. Here's a list of what you need to know and what you can do about short-term insomnia, summarised from the recent Australasian medical textbook *Sleep Medicine*.[3]

- Learn about sleep to better understand the cyclic nature of deep and light sleep. Brief awakening throughout the night is a natural part of the normal sleep pattern.
- Recognise that, during times of stress, it's common to increase caffeine or alcohol consumption. These substances aren't helpful for sleep or daytime well-being, so go easy on the coffee, energy drinks, cola, chocolate, wine, beer, etc.
- Know that it's normal for the time you're asleep to decrease during times of stress. If you take care of yourself and your approach to sleep throughout this period, your sleep will recover once the stress passes.
- Accept that daytime struggles, such as fatigue and irritability, arise from prolonged time awake in the night rather than sleep loss. (That is, from agitation, upset and stress about being awake in the night.)
- To improve the time it takes to fall asleep (and return to sleep during the night), match your time in bed to how much sleep you're actually getting.
- Develop practices such as mindfulness and relaxation that will help you manage your body's response to stress and support you through this challenging time.

While you won't need to do the six-week programme mapped out in this book, continue reading to gain a better understanding of your sleep and to understand how insomnia can develop. That way, you'll learn how to keep your current dilemma manageable and how to resolve it as quickly as possible. Do your best to maintain your sleep hygiene (these are the fundamentals of sleep outlined in Chapter 4), and pay particular attention to the chapters in Part 1.

It may also be worth supporting your system with natural remedies to encourage your sleep through this challenging period. It's important to note that empirical evidence to support the efficacy of herbal remedies is not strong at this stage.[4] Even so, I have heard very good things about certain naturopathic remedies, like SleepDrops and Nod. These products may give you a reprieve, enabling you to proactively address the stressors that are triggering your sleeplessness. Of course, everyone is different, so if you try something and it doesn't help, just move on.

If your insomnia symptoms are severe and unmanageable, it's worth seeking external support. Consider talking to your GP, and, if you are open to it, ask about a prescription for a *short* course of sleep medication. Remember: this is a temporary measure, just to get you through the rough patch. Read Chapter 8 on sleeping pills to understand the risks of tolerance and dependence with use beyond four weeks.

These actions are likely to see you through an episode of short-term insomnia. However, with life being what it is, extra pressures can become continuous and curveballs can keep coming, creating sustained or recurring bouts of short-term insomnia. In this situation, or if you have an ongoing health issue (or there's a global pandemic) messing with your natural equilibrium, sleep difficulties can become unrelenting. This persistence can wear a person down: the desire for sleep escalates, but confidence in the ability to sleep erodes. Thoughts and behaviours related to sleep can mutate, and the situation can gradually deteriorate into chronic insomnia.

2. Chronic insomnia

When the above sleep–wake difficulties hit the three-month threshold, they are classified as chronic insomnia (provided the symptoms aren't better explained by another sleep disorder or health condition). In the past, chronic insomnia was further classified based on suspected causes and triggers—medical issues, psychological issues, life stage or lifestyle factors, poor sleep habits, or inherited factors. The ICSD-3 classification has set these factors aside for now, as the recommended approaches for dealing with them are relatively consistent.

Once sleep issues have reached this three-month point, life can feel pretty grim. The cycle of bad nights can seem inescapable.

What you can do: CBTi is recommended by sleep experts internationally as the first-line treatment for insomnia. CBTi can be accessed through a trained CBTi professional (if this is something you can afford and have access to), or via an online programme;[5] or you can follow the approach outlined in this book. You could also explore MBTI, which formally combines the practice of mindfulness with CBTi. (If you are pregnant and have chronic insomnia, a mindfulness-based approach to CBTi is the preferable option for sleep improvement in my view.) If at any point you think you'd benefit from a more supported approach to sleep improvement, a list of resources is included in Appendix II.

When evaluating your insomnia, it is easy to jump to conclusions. But it's important to remember that a sleep disorder is classified as insomnia only *if the sleep–wake difficulties cannot be explained more clearly by another sleep disorder*. Be sure to read Chapter 2 to better understand other key sleep disorders before you commit to the approach outlined in this book.

Emotional well-being

The next section of the sleep review covers your emotional well-being. The following questions have been adapted from the Auckland Sleep Questionnaire, and focus on a really important question: are you okay?

As you work through the questions, be really honest with yourself. All too often we put on a brave face for the world, but this is a place where it's best to take a deep breath, drop the mask, and tune in to how you are actually feeling.

Once, I was blindsided by this razor-sharp question in a way that made me feel so vulnerable and, at the same time, genuinely seen. When I first met my friend's husband, Ian, he politely asked, 'How are you?' I responded with the usual mild, meaningless, but perfectly acceptable, 'Fine, great.' Before I could deflect attention to him by asking, 'And how are you?', he looked me straight in the eye and continued, 'And how are you, really?' The directness, kindness and respect with which he asked that question was truly disarming. Consider this next section your 'And how are you, really?' interlude.

Over the last two weeks, how often have you been bothered by the following problems?

	Not at all	Several days	More than half the days	Nearly every day
Feeling nervous, anxious, or on edge				
Not being able to stop or oontrol worrying				
Worrying too much about different things				
Having trouble relaxing				
Being so restless it's hard to sit still				
Becoming easily annoyed and irritable				
Feeling afraid as if something awful might happen				
Feeling down, depressed or hopeless				
Having little interest or pleasure in doing things				
Poor appetite, weight loss or overeating				
Feeling tired or having little energy				
Feeling bad about yourself, that you are a failure, or that you have let yourself or your family down				
Having trouble concentrating on things like work, reading or watching TV				
Moving or speaking so slowly that other people could have noticed				

	Not at all	Several days	More than half the days	Nearly every day
Being so fidgety or restless that you were moving around a lot more than usual				
Having thoughts of hurting yourself in some way or that you'd be better off dead*				

*If you feel this way, please seek help immediately and call one of the helplines listed in Appendix III: Other resources.

These are gritty lists, covering common signs of anxiety and depression, but it's vital to ask yourself these questions because there is a close link between sleep and mental well-being. What's more, the relationship goes both ways: if you are sleeping well, you are more likely to feel great in yourself. If you are feeling great in yourself, you're more likely to sleep well.

However, you are on this page because you're not sleeping well. Chances are, you will be experiencing some of the above symptoms. These 'not so well-being' symptoms may be occurring due to lack of sleep, but the lack of sleep may also be occurring because of existing anxiety or depression. You may know what started first; you may not.

Fear, worry and sadness are all part of life, and everybody experiences them sometimes. However, when these kinds of feelings intensify, happen all the time, cause you distress or interfere with your work, social or home life, it's essential to acknowledge that things are not okay, and to reach out and ask for support.

What you can do: Look back over your answers. If you are experiencing several symptoms or you have been experiencing certain symptoms frequently, you may be feeling that life's a struggle at the moment. You must take steps to seek help in addition to trying to improve your sleep. And there is help readily available—make an appointment with your GP, or check Appendix III, which has a list of agencies and helplines with trained professionals you can talk to, as well as a list of websites you can visit for practical information and advice.

It's worth continuing to learn how to improve your sleep at the same time, as better sleep can support your journey towards feeling okay again. Remember that good sleep and well-being go hand in hand.

If you are struggling, be assured that you are not alone—it's incredibly common to experience periods of anxiety and depression. About one in five New Zealanders have been diagnosed with anxiety or depression at some time in their lives.[6] According to Beyond Blue, it's estimated that almost half of people in Australia will experience a mental-health condition during their lifetime. Currently, around 3 million adults in Australia are experiencing anxiety, depression or both.[7]

LIFE STAGE, LIFESTYLE AND PHYSICAL HEALTH

Your sleeping needs and patterns will change throughout your life depending on your life stage, lifestyle and physical health. It's important to understand how and when this happens, and to adjust your expectations of sleep accordingly.

Life stage

1. Age: _____

2. Are any of the following factors affecting your sleep?
   ☐ New parent
   ☐ Sleeping with a bed-partner
   ☐ Pregnancy
   ☐ Perimenopause, menopause or postmenopause

The amount of sleep that a person needs is unique to the individual. Even so, there are healthy recommended ranges to aspire to, and these change with age. As we get older, we tend to require less sleep (but not radically so). According to the National Sleep Foundation, a US non-profit organisation that promotes public understanding of sleep and sleep disorders, the recommended sleep durations are as follows:

RECOMMENDED SLEEP DURATIONS

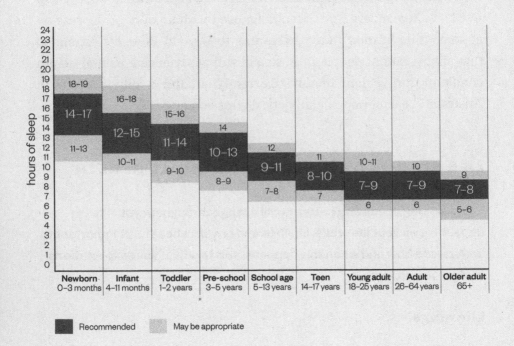

Recommended   **May be appropriate**

National Sleep Foundation's recommended sleep durations

The recommendation for working-age adults is at least 7 hours' sleep each night (although for some people 6 hours per night may be appropriate).

Before going into a tailspin about how little sleep you are getting in comparison to these recommendations, remember that your sleep is a work in progress. The guidelines are a little different for those of us experiencing insomnia. We at least give our bodies a chance to sleep, even if we don't achieve it to the extent that we hope. Dr David Cunnington, a renowned Australian specialist sleep physician, co-director of the Melbourne Sleep Disorders Centre and founder of SleepHub (an excellent online resource), says that among people with insomnia the risks associated with not getting sufficient sleep only occur if we're *averaging* less than 5 hours a night. So don't panic if you're not hitting the recommended norms just yet. You are being proactive; it is a healthy sleep-duration range that you will gradually build towards.

The other thing to keep in mind is that sleep patterns are likely to change with age. As you get older, it's normal for sleep to be lighter and for there to be more awareness and brief awakenings throughout the night. Don't be alarmed if you aren't sleeping like a log from bedtime till dawn like you did when you were young. That said, you shouldn't be feeling tired throughout the day.

Specific life stages also have the potential to interfere with your sleep. It may be the partner who snores loudly after having too many beers, or who starfishes in the bed. Maybe it's the relentless awakenings courtesy of the darling new baby in your life, or the late-pregnancy experience of trying to get comfortable in your body's temporary whale-like form. It may be the profoundly annoying 'tropical moments' of menopause. These life stages pose additional challenges for sleep and warrant further discussion. If any apply to you, please refer to Appendix I: Specific sleep challenges.

LIFESTYLE

The next questions relate to your current lifestyle and the choices that you are making. Think about your lifestyle habits over the last month.

1. Have you been taking naps during the day? _____

    If so, how long are your naps? _____

    What time of day do you tend to nap? _____

    How many days per week do you nap? _____

2. Which, if any, of the following caffeinated drinks have you regularly been drinking?

☐ Coffee

☐ Tea

☐ Soft drinks

☐ Energy drinks

3. How long before bed do you generally have your last caffeinated drink?

_____

4. Do you snack in the four hours before bed?

☐ Yes

Do these evening snacks include …

☐ rich or heavy food?

☐ sugary treats?

☐ chocolate?

☐ No

5. In the last week, how often have you exercised or been physically active?

☐ I haven't exercised (*skip to Q7*)

☐ Once

☐ Two or three times

☐ Four or five times

☐ Six or more times

6. Do you do moderate or strenuous exercise in the evening?

☐ Yes

What type of exercise do you do in the evening? _____

How long before bedtime do you complete your exercise? _____

☐ No

7. Do you smoke cigarettes?

☐ Yes

How many per day? _____

How long before bedtime do you stop smoking? _____

If you wake in the night, do you smoke a cigarette? _____

☐ No

8. Do you use recreational or non-prescription drugs?

☐ Yes

Do you think the use of these drugs is affecting your sleep (either while you take them or after you stop taking them)? If so, how?

☐ Yes _____

☐ No

☐ No

9. Which best describes your usual drinking behaviour?[8]

☐ Do not drink alcohol (*skip to Q12*)

☐ Low-risk drinking

Females: no more than two standard drinks per day; no more than ten drinks per week; and two or more alcohol-free days per week

Males: no more than three standard drinks per day; no more than fifteen drinks per week; and two or more alcohol-free days per week

☐ High-risk drinking

Drinking more than the above

10. How long before bed do you tend to finish drinking? _____

11. Do you use alcohol in the evening to help you sleep (as a nightcap)?

☐ Yes

☐ No

12. Are you a shift worker?

- ☐ Yes

    What type of shifts do you work?

    - ☐ Regular or fixed shifts
    - ☐ Rotating or alternating shifts
    - ☐ Long shifts (ten or more hours)

- ☐ No

13. In the hour or two before bed, do you typically engage in any of the following activities?

- ☐ Mentally stimulating activities
- ☐ Emotionally upsetting activities
- ☐ Wind-down or relaxing activities

14. How would you rate your bedroom on the following:

Temperature at night

Too hot • • • • • Too cold

Ventilation at night

Stuffy • • • • • Too breezy

Ambience of the room

Unappealing • • • • • Inviting

Comfort of your bed

Uncomfortable • • • • • Comfortable

Noise levels overnight

Noisy • • • • • Quiet

Darkness

Very light • • • • • Very dark

Peacefulness (effect of partner, kids, pets, etc.)

Interrupted • • • • • Peaceful

15. How long before bed do you switch off or stop use of all screens and devices? _____

16. Do you keep your phone in your bedroom overnight?
- ☐ Yes
  What do you use it for? _____
- ☐ No

17. Do you have a clock in your bedroom?
- ☐ Yes
  Do you 'clock watch' in the night? _____
- ☐ No

18. Apart from sleep, what else do you use your bedroom for?
- ☐ Reading
  - ☐ On a device or screen
  - ☐ A physical copy—book, magazine, etc.
- ☐ Watching TV / screens
- ☐ Listening to music or podcasts
- ☐ Thinking or planning
- ☐ Talking or conversations
- ☐ Worrying or fretting
- ☐ Eating
- ☐ Working
- ☐ Playing/gaming on screens, devices
- ☐ Exercise
- ☐ Sex

For now, these questions will encourage you to start thinking about how your current habits and behaviours can potentially impact your sleep, and make you more aware of your sleeping environment. Chapter 4 covers core aspects of sleep habits and environment, unpacking these topics in greater detail. Later in the programme, when the time is right, you'll work through any adjustments that need to be made in these areas.

If you are a shift worker, especially if you have rotating shifts or long shifts, it's worth reading Appendix I: Specific sleep challenges. The nature of your work can make sleep especially problematic, and you may need to take a different path towards improving your sleep.

OVERALL HEALTH AND MEDICATIONS

1. Do you have any physical health problems that may be impacting your ability to sleep well?

☐ Breathing difficulties, e.g., allergies, congested nose

☐ Coughing that troubles you at night

☐ Pain that keeps you awake, e.g., back pain, arthritis

☐ Indigestion, acid reflux

☐ Other _____

2. Are you taking any medication or non-prescription drugs (for non-sleep related physical or mental-health issues)?

☐ Yes

Names _____

☐ No

If you are experiencing health problems like those listed above, or you have other health issues that you suspect are interfering with your sleep, it's worth talking about these with your doctor and letting them know that your sleep is suffering.

Pain and disturbed sleep have a two-way relationship. Pain interferes with sleep—it can make it difficult to fall asleep, increase awakenings, and create problems or delay falling back to sleep. With less sleep, a person becomes more sensitive to pain. It's a vicious cycle: lack of restorative sleep adds to the experience of pain, and the pain makes sleep more elusive.

People living with pain can do things to deal with lost sleep that unintentionally perpetuate sleep difficulties, such as staying in bed longer, or napping to conserve their energy or recoup lost sleep. Behaviours that would usually help someone fall asleep, such as making the room quiet and devoid of distractions, can heighten focus on the pain. If you are dealing with pain as well as difficulty sleeping, you need to address both challenges. While exploring how to improve your relationship with sleep through the guidance in this book, it is essential to discuss pain relief with a health professional.

You can find practical tips and sound advice on pain management on the Sleep Health Foundation website, an excellent resource for questions and concerns about sleep. They have over 80 user-friendly fact sheets covering different sleep topics.

If you are taking prescription or over-the-counter medications, talk to your GP or pharmacist to establish if they contain ingredients, such as caffeine, that may be affecting your sleep. If they do, it's worth asking about alternatives to make your nights easier.

INITIATIVES EXPLORED

To round out your sleep review, reflect on what solutions you have sought for your sleep challenges.

1. Have you discussed your current sleep difficulties with your doctor?

☐ Yes

What did they suggest? _____

How well did that work for you? _____

☐ No

Is there a reason for this?

☐ I haven't seen a doctor since my sleep problems started.

☐ I didn't think it was important enough.

☐ I didn't think anything could be done.

☐ I didn't want to take sleeping pills.

☐ Other _____

2. Are you currently on any medication for sleep—prescribed or otherwise? (This may include sleeping pills, melatonin, antidepressants, antipsychotics, antihistamines, etc.)

☐ Yes

Name of medication being used for sleep: _____

Presoribed or over-the-counter? _____

How long have you been taking this medication? _____

weeks/months/years

How effective is this medication for your sleep now? _____

☐ No

☐ I haven't been prescribed any medication for sleep.

☐ I have tried medication for sleep and it didn't work.

☐ I have tried medication for sleep and I didn't like how I felt / I didn't like the side effects.

☐ I do not want to take medication for sleep.

3. What supplements or natural remedies have you tried for sleep? How helpful were they?

Supplement/remedy tried	Helpful	Unhelpful	No effect

4. Where else have you sought help for your sleep difficulties?

- ☐ Sleep clinic
- ☐ Sleep specialist
- ☐ Online sleep programme
- ☐ Psychologist
- ☐ Chemist
- ☐ Health store
- ☐ Naturopath
- ☐ Homeopath
- ☐ Acupuncturist
- ☐ Massage therapist
- ☐ Internet
- ☐ Podcasts
- ☐ Sleep apps
- ☐ Sleep trackers or devices
- ☐ Books
- ☐ Magazine articles
- ☐ Other _____
- ☐ I haven't sought help
  - ☐ I have been suffering in silence.
  - ☐ I've been too tired to figure out what I need and have just been getting through the day.
  - ☐ I don't really know where to get help for sleep.

5. Are there any other products or initiatives that you have tried to improve your sleep?

Product or initiative tried	Helpful	Unhelpful	No effect

It's common for people struggling with sleep difficulties to either head for the doctor to get sleeping pills, or to avoid the doctor because they don't want to take sleeping pills. While sleeping pills absolutely have their place (as will be discussed in Chapter 8), it's important to know there are other options that your GP can discuss with you once they understand what is happening with your sleep. A good GP can be a great place to start, especially if your sleep issues are more complex than insomnia and you need a referral to a specialist.

Digital sleep trackers can be fascinating and helpful for a general overview of sleep patterns. If you have persistent sleep issues, it can be tempting to use them to monitor what on earth is going on with your sleep—gaining insight into a specific problem and direction on what to do can provide a sense of control. However, the Sleep Health Foundation encourages people with sleep difficulties to be cautious about digital sleep trackers and realistic about their limitations.[9] Many devices and apps haven't undergone extensive scientific evaluation to determine their accuracy. People with sleep difficulties often have anxiety about the state of their sleep and a tendency to be vigilant about sleep matters. Becoming fixated on the detailed information generated by a sleep-monitoring device, especially if that information isn't robust, can exacerbate stress about sleep.

Many people with sleep difficulties have tried what feels like 'everything' to improve their nights. When initiatives don't work as well as hoped or within an expected time frame, they can create disappointment and frustration. This then adds to an already stressful situation, and it can feel like a solution will never be found. If you are in this camp, feeling disempowered and disillusioned like I was, that's understandable. Through no fault of your own, you haven't had the sound knowledge about sleep that you need to make effective choices. I'm glad that you found this book and set any cynicism aside, and that you're prepared to give this approach a go.

There's a difference between giving up and knowing when you have had enough.
—UNKNOWN

Chapter recap: what you can do

1. Complete the sleep review. Capture essential information about your sleep difficulties and how they're affecting your life, and identify factors that may be contributing to the problem.

2. Become curious and ready for action. Use the sleep review to learn what's going on with your sleep, highlight the need to take appropriate steps, and provide a summary for yourself or a healthcare professional if required.

3. Begin self-diagnosis. Do your sleep experiences seem like insomnia (short-term or chronic)? Remember other sleep disorders and health conditions can masquerade as insomnia.

4. Consider your emotional well-being. Could anxiety or depression be a factor in your sleep difficulties (as a symptom or a cause)? If so, seek help for these conditions while learning how to improve your sleep. Talk with your GP, check the resources in Appendix III for helplines or websites that offer support, or reach out for local advice.

5. Read on. The next chapter explores whether your experiences are better described by a different sleep disorder.

CHAPTER 2

Other sleep disorders to consider

People generally see what they look for, and hear what they listen for.

—HARPER LEE

Insomnia is only one of seven categories of sleep disorder identified in the ICSD-3, and some of the other sleep disorders can be tricky little buggers that present as insomnia, so it's important to learn about them to try to avoid being misguided in your self-diagnosis. If your sleep experiences could indicate a different or more complex disorder, it's time to seek specialist help and get a clinical diagnosis.

This chapter walks through characteristics of other key sleep disorders, primarily based on the ICSD-3 classification summary provided by the ESRS *Sleep Medicine Textbook*.[1] Using the information you have provided in the previous chapter, read through the different sleep disorders and evaluate whether any sound familiar to your experiences. Keep in mind that this information is to be used as an initial self-diagnosis tool only. Remember: you're just trying to figure out what might be going on, and you can use this information to seek specialist support if needed.

As you read this chapter, highlight any symptoms you are experiencing and anything that resonates with you, and take note of potential next steps and what you can do to help yourself.

Sleep-related breathing disorders

This is where it gets serious. Most sleep-related breathing disorders are different forms of **sleep apnoea**, a temporary suspension of breathing or a pause in breathing while sleeping. Breathing matters! An episode of sleep apnoea, where breathing is compromised or stalls, can last anywhere from ten seconds to two or three minutes. I haven't experienced an apnoea personally, but I have held my breath as I watched a video of a man during a sleep-apnoea episode. His pause was so long that I couldn't hold my breath for the duration and bailed out, lungs on fire, gasping for air. Some people's experiences of sleep apnoea are more subtle, with almost no snoring involved (especially women postmenopause). Still, noisy breathing and restlessness can indicate restricted breathing, which can have a serious effect on the quality and continuity of sleep.

So how do you know if you may have sleep apnoea? Key warning signs are snoring and excessive daytime sleepiness, but there can be many clues. According to Dr David Cunnington, the following are common symptoms of sleep apnoea.[2]

- Regularly snoring or breathing noisily during sleep.
- Changes in breathing during sleep, such as pauses or gasping.
- Waking up choking or gasping for breath.
- Feeling more tired during the day than expected.
- Having difficulties with memory and concentration.

- Feeling irritable or down when you usually wouldn't be.
- Needing to pee often during the night.
- Morning headaches on waking (that are not alcohol-related).

Sleep apnoea is more common than most people think: around 5 per cent of males and 3 per cent of females experience it.

The daytime effects of sleep apnoea don't just make life a struggle, they put safety at risk. Those with sleep apnoea are at much higher risk of accidents at work and on the roads. Based on New Zealand figures, the risk of having a motor-vehicle accident is four times higher for someone with sleep apnoea than someone without.[3]

If you snore, know that this doesn't automatically mean that you have sleep apnoea. However, most people with sleep apnoea do snore to a degree, and sometimes it can be what Rachel Lehen from Fit for Duty describes as 'heroic snoring'. If you think you might have sleep apnoea, this is not to be taken lightly—the long-term effects of restricted breathing during sleep are confronting, with at least double the risk of high blood pressure, heart attack or heart failure, and stroke.

What you can do: If you're experiencing or have been told that you're experiencing a number of the above symptoms, and you suspect that your sleep issues may be breathing related, you *must* make an appointment with your GP. It's vital to get these concerns checked out sooner rather than later.

If you're not sure, there are ways to double-check your symptoms. If you have a bed-partner, ask if they've noticed snoring or breathing-pause symptoms. If you're living independently, consider using the SnoreLab app. In terms of daytime sleepiness, check out the Epworth Sleepiness Scale online. This quick questionnaire provides an easy self-evaluation of the extent of your sleepiness.

If you find that your symptoms suggest sleep apnoea, see your doctor and take them through your sleep review, as well as the sleepiness and snoring information you gather. They may encourage you to see a sleep specialist, and you may need a sleep study either in a clinic or at home to establish what's happening with your breathing overnight.

Excessive daytime sleepiness (hypersomnolence)

The ICSD-3 defines hypersomnolence disorders as 'daily episodes of an irrepressible need to sleep or daytime lapses into sleep'.[4] Hypersomnolence goes well beyond feeling a bit tired and needing a nap after a bad night's sleep: the key words are 'daily', 'irrepressible' and 'lapses'. With hypersomnolence, the daytime need to sleep is persistent and non-negotiable—it can occur even after a good night's sleep.

You have most likely heard of one type of excessive daytime sleepiness: narcolepsy. Thanks to comedy TV shows and films, the word 'narcolepsy' tends to conjure images of people falling asleep at random in inopportune places. For people suffering from narcolepsy, the experience goes well beyond the odd gag. In addition to overwhelming daytime sleepiness, there may be other symptoms such as muscle weakness or loss of muscle control when awake, a feeling of being paralysed when waking up, and hallucinations.

This category of disorders also covers types of hypersomnia (excessive sleeping) that may be due to a medical disorder, medication or substance use, or may be associated with a psychiatric disorder.

What you can do: Obviously these disorders can be tough to live with. They leave a person feeling like they are missing out on their own life and, worse, feeling incredibly vulnerable and exposed. Falling asleep at unanticipated places and times can be dangerous—for instance, when driving a car.

If you are experiencing and are concerned about symptoms of excessive daytime sleepiness (especially if you have endured them for a few months) you must consult your GP or contact a sleep clinic. If you're unsure about the severity of your daytime sleepiness, check out the Epworth Sleepiness Scale online. Your health professional can provide a full diagnosis so that you can start working through the causes and explore ways to manage this problem.

Circadian-rhythm sleep–wake disorders

Essentially, these disorders involve a person's 24-hour body clock being out of whack with the local daytime–night-time cycle. With a circadian-rhythm disorder, you may find that you can sleep fine; you just can't sleep at the time you need to or are supposed to so that you can coordinate with the rest of society. You may find that you want to sleep long before anyone else and get up before the birds, or that you can't fall asleep until the wee hours of the morning and prefer to sleep till lunchtime. It may be that your body operates on a schedule that's longer than 24 hours, or that your rhythm is variable, which makes sleeping unpredictable and hard to coordinate with the standard light–dark cycle of the planet.

People with circadian-rhythm disorders tend to experience what they think is insomnia or excessive daytime sleepiness or both. They may feel that they are an extreme night owl or morning lark. Forcing themselves to fit in with standard sleep–wake times feels impossible because their bodies are so out of sync with local time. Because they still need to take the kids to school, get themselves to work or stay up for that function tonight, a circadian-rhythm disorder can feel incredibly stressful and debilitating.

Circadian rhythm sleep–wake disorders include:

- delayed sleep–wake phase disorder (falling asleep very late at night)
- advanced sleep–wake phase disorder (falling asleep very early)
- irregular sleep–wake rhythm disorder
- non-24-hour sleep–wake rhythm disorder
- shift work disorder.

What you can do: Circadian-rhythm issues that are enduring and distressing need a clinical diagnosis and specialist help to get the body clock realigned. Book an appointment with your GP or consult a sleep clinic.

In the meantime, there are helpful videos about circadian-rhythm disorders on the SleepHub website. Those with delayed sleep–wake phase disorder (often experienced by teenagers) can get help with melatonin and light therapy to realign their body clocks.

Circadian-rhythm problems that occur as a result of shift work warrant their own classification as a sleep disorder. For those of you who work shifts, especially if you are doing long shifts or rotating shifts, you will be very aware of the toll it takes on your sleep and your well-being. Be sure to check Appendix I for information on this sleep disorder, and consult a GP or sleep specialist to get help to manage your sleep.

Parasomnias

Parasomnias are quite common and don't tend to be confused with insomnia. While they may interrupt and disturb sleep, the symptoms are very distinctive. They cover abnormal or unusual behaviour that occurs during sleep, and include the below.

- **Confusion arousals:** a person seems to wake but is disoriented and unresponsive, and has slow speech or confused thinking.
- **Sleepwalking (somnambulism)** starts during deep sleep and includes sitting up in bed and walking around the room or house. It can also include leaving the house and even starting the car while still asleep.
- **Sleep talking (somniloquy)** can involve complicated dialogues or monologues, random words and phrases, complete nonsense or mumbling. There is no awareness or recollection of what was said.
- **Sleep terrors:** the sleeper experiences feelings of sudden intense fear, and may scream and thrash around in bed while remaining asleep.
- **Sleep-related eating disorders:** out-of-control eating and drinking in the night while still asleep. The sleeper isn't aware of what they are doing at the time but finds evidence of it in the morning.

- **Sleep paralysis:** a temporary episode of full-body muscle paralysis on falling asleep or awakening. The person is only able to move their eyes and breathe.
- **Nightmare disorder:** the sleeper experiences unpleasant dreams that can be remembered on waking.
- **Exploding-head syndrome:** a person imagines hearing intensely loud noises as they fall asleep or wake.
- **Sleep-related hallucinations:** vividly imagined events or experiences that seem very real to the person and are not recognised as a dream or nightmare.
- **Bedwetting (enuresis):** accidentally peeing in the bed while sleeping.

To the outsider these occurrences may seem extraordinary, yet parasomnias are common. Some people experiencing parasomnias find them quite manageable and even funny now and then. However, when parasomnias are severe or frequent, or feel unmanageable, they can be very disturbing. What's more, some parasomnias can pose a real danger to the individual and others.

What you can do: If you are experiencing night-time behaviour that seems to be a parasomnia you (or others) find distressing or unsafe, talk to your GP. You can also access valuable information about parasomnias and practical tips on how to manage and avoid triggering them on the Sleep Health Foundation or SleepHub websites.

Sleep-related movement disorders

It's normal to move in your sleep as you change position and get comfortable, or transition through different stages of sleep. You may also toss and turn if the temperature's not right or you're a bit worried. However, there are kinds of body movements that, in severe cases, can really interfere with your ability to fall asleep and stay asleep, and impact the quality of your sleep.

Among others, the sleep-related movement disorders category includes:

- restless-leg syndrome
- periodic limb-movement disorder
- sleep-related leg cramps
- sleep-related bruxism (teeth grinding).

If you feel like you just can't keep your legs still at night when you're heading to bed or trying to go to sleep, you may be dealing with restless-leg syndrome. This sounds quite innocuous, but it can be torturous. The irresistible urge to move the limbs can come out of a general feeling of restlessness or twitchiness, but, for many, it's to avoid horrible or painful sensations in the legs, like a crawling sensation.

If limb movements occur after you have fallen asleep, and are more rhythmic, and the pattern is repeated every 30 seconds or so, you may have periodic limb-movement disorder. While you possibly sleep through the experience, if they are significant movements they can be disruptive to a partner's sleep. Bed-partners might observe your feet rocking, toes pulling back or, in more pronounced cases, legs bending at the knees.

Sleep-related leg cramps are the sudden, involuntary and intense contraction of muscles in the leg—often in the lower leg or foot. They can be very painful, with the muscle becoming rock hard and spasming. (Ouch!)

Bruxism is grinding or clenching the teeth during sleep. While it's common, it's really hard on your teeth and can cause you to wake in the mornings feeling unrefreshed with a headache, an aching jaw or tooth pain.

To qualify as a sleep disorder, sleep-related movements must cause concern or distress for you (or your bed-partner!), and be severe or frequent enough to be detrimental to your sleep or negatively impact how you're feeling/performing during the day.

What you can do: If your experiences are severe or concerning, contact your doctor (or dentist in the case of bruxism). Discuss your symptoms and the impact they are having on you. This will enable your doctor to consider your symptoms in the context of your overall health, keeping in mind any medical, psychological or behavioural conditions that need to be taken into account. (In the case of restless-leg syndrome, it's also worth asking your doctor to check your magnesium and iron levels.)

You can also read up on a specific disorder using the excellent fact sheets on the Sleep Health Foundation website.

Now that you better understand the other main categories of sleep disorders, you will have a sense as to whether your sleep difficulties seem like insomnia or something else.

If your symptoms sound like one of the more serious or complex sleep disorders, visit your health professional for a clinical diagnosis and a referral if needed. Meanwhile, start on your sleep diary in the next chapter. Take your diary, your sleep review and any notes from this chapter to your appointment. This will give you a head start on explaining to your doctor the symptoms you've been experiencing and the impact of your sleep difficulties.

If you still can't figure out what's going on with your sleep, seek help from your doctor for a diagnosis. Remember, multiple things can go on at once—especially if you have other health conditions and medications in the mix, or are going through menopause. The ICSD-3 category 'other sleep disorders' is for those symptoms and experiences that fall outside the other criteria, so it's okay to be a bit unclear.

Chapter recap: what you can do

1. Form your initial self-diagnosis. Use the information in this chapter to clarify for yourself which sleep disorder your experiences align most closely with. Remember: some sleep disorders can present as insomnia, and different conditions sometimes coexist. While you might not be certain about what's going on, you will have a hypothesis and this gives you a great place to start.

2. Get started on next steps. The actions you need to consider taking from here depend on the sleep disorder you might have and the severity of your symptoms. If you suspect you might have any of the sleep disorders outlined in this chapter, visit your GP or a sleep specialist. If you think you might have a sleep-related breathing disorder, make your appointment as soon as possible. In the case of bruxism, visit your dentist. If you think you have chronic insomnia, continue on your CBTi sleep-improvement journey. You can do this with a trained CBTi professional, via an online programme or with the self-help DIY approach outlined in this book. Remember: MBTI is another option to consider, too.

3. Keep reading and learning about your sleep. The next chapter will introduce you to the art and science of keeping a sleep diary.

CHAPTER 3

Create a
sleep-diary
habit

Start by starting.

—MERYL STREEP

efore addressing your sleep troubles, you need to gather some data. While you may think you know what's going on, it's time to move from broad brush strokes into the reality of each night. To get there, you're going to keep a sleep diary to actively monitor your sleeping behaviour and experiences for the next one or two weeks, documenting the facts in black-and-white so that you can see objectively what's happening with your sleep. This will provide you with a starting point—your baseline sleep status.

You've got two options on how to proceed from this point. Option one: if life's challenging at the moment and you need time to psych yourself up, give yourself two weeks to prepare for the six-week programme—this will give you plenty of time to read Part 1 and complete a fortnight of sleep-diary information. Option two: if you can't tolerate sleep deficiency any longer and have the capacity to read Part 1 within a week, plan to keep a sleep diary for just one week to establish your baseline sleep status.

Whichever option you choose: brace yourself. People with insomnia tend to think about their sleeping issues as a whole—they recall the worst nights and overlook the better ones. It's easy to fall into the trap of overgeneralisation. Throughout my own insomnia, I'd wake in the morning acutely aware of the sleepless horrors of the night before—how much I hadn't slept, how dreadful I felt. As a result, my view of the problem became distorted—in my mind, all nights were a wash of dreadful sleep. Indeed, I had become an Eeyore about it: everything was gloomy and bleak.

After I had kept a sleep diary for two weeks, it was clear that things were bad, but they weren't desperately bad every single night. Some nights were a bit better, and some nights were a bit worse. The important thing was getting into the habit of jotting down what actually happened overnight, so that I could start seeing and working with my true sleep profile.

According to specialists who've studied people with chronic insomnia, 'patients tend to overestimate their sleep symptoms and underestimate their sleep duration'.[1] There's no need to get defensive or feel indignant about this—scientists know you're not intentionally making stuff up or exaggerating to garner their pity. It's just that human brains happen to have a 'negativity bias', meaning we're more likely to notice and be affected by the bad and overlook the neutral and the good.

A sleep diary is a tool to get your baseline sleep measurement—it's not rocket science. However, for it to have any value or meaning, it has to be completed in full, daily. It requires you to dedicate two minutes of *every* morning to writing down the key facts about your sleep the night before.

The process of keeping a sleep diary enables you to tune in to the reality of your sleep, become aware of and curious about your patterns and behaviours, and better understand causes and effects. You will learn how different things impact the duration, quality and consistency of your sleep. You will want to start doing more of the things that help you sleep well, and less of the things that sabotage your sleep. Knowledge is power. Remember, Dr Charles Morin, a world-renowned sleep researcher and pretty much a godfather of insomnia, encourages us to be in the driver's seat with our sleep-recovery efforts, so yes: you are the one who is going to be doing the work. Your sleep diary will be your key reference tool throughout the six-week programme.

Fear not, though. The questions that you'll ask yourself each morning are easy.

- What time did you go to bed?
- What time did you first try to go to sleep?
- What time did you fall asleep?
- How many times did you wake in the night?
- How long did these awakenings last in total?
- What time did you wake for the final time this morning?
- What time did you get out of bed for the day?
- How would you rate the quality of your sleep?
- In total, how many hours' sleep did you get?
- In total, how long were you in bed?
- Were there any factors that may have been unhelpful for your sleep?
- Were there any factors that may have helped your sleep?

When thinking about what may have helped or hindered your sleep, just base this on what you know or suspect so far. Your knowledge will grow as you learn more about sleep throughout the programme. When I started using a sleep diary, I diligently completed it each day. Still, I conscientiously avoided documenting my caffeine intake. I withheld that little fact from myself as long as I could, convinced that I was one of those fortunate people who had a really high caffeine tolerance. You too will own up to things in your own time.

Purposefully, there's only a small place to note your thoughts—

keep your comments brief. You don't want filling in your sleep diary to feel arduous (nor do you want to become obsessed with sleep or insomnia). Remember, it's often the initial, instinctive, unfiltered thoughts that are the most telling, so make sure you capture those!

When you're working with a sleep diary, please don't succumb to rigorous clock-watching—while this is typical of people with sleep difficulties, it's counterproductive. It creates stress, which reduces the likelihood of sleep. It might sound impossible, but the recommendation is to keep your bedroom free of any time-telling devices. That's right: no clock, no watch, no phone, nada. At first, this idea sounded a little unhinged to me, too. I felt anxious: how would I know what time it was? Or how much I had slept or not slept? Or how long I had left to sleep? And on it went. I realised these questions were the very reason I needed to go clock-free for a while.

Without a clock in your bedroom, you will learn to go by 'feel' instead. There is no need to be vigilant with the time—your best guess is all that's needed. Yes, there will be some discrepancies in your estimates, but that's all good. You're the one who is always going to be completing your sleep diary, so your differences will be pretty consistent.

Calculating your sleep efficiency

Sleep efficiency is a handy reference tool to establish your baseline sleep and monitor your progress as you work towards better sleep. It is an enlightening and helpful way to evaluate your sleep, especially while it's a work in progress. (Ordinary people tend to rely on measuring hours of sleep, but that's a fairly blunt instrument in comparison to sleep efficiency, so don't get fixated on sleep duration at this stage.) To work out your sleep efficiency, you will calculate a simple percentage that tells you the proportion of the time you spent in bed that you were actually asleep. Here's the maths:

sleep efficiency = total sleep time ÷ total time in bed × 100

Total time in bed is the difference between the time you first gave yourself the opportunity to sleep (in bed with the lights out, ready to sleep) and the time you got out of bed for the final time in the morning (any time out of bed throughout the night is counted as time in bed). For instance, if I was in bed at 10 p.m. with the lights out and got up in the morning at 6 a.m., my time in bed would be 8 hours. That's regardless of whether I slept like a log or was up and down like a yo-yo all night, and it's irrespective of how many hours I actually slept.

Measuring time in bed is important to make sure that you're actually allowing yourself sufficient time to have the chance to get enough sleep. Officially it's known as 'sleep opportunity'. If your body is crying out for 8 hours of sleep, you have to make sure that you are in bed for a minimum of 8 hours—and that's if you are one of those incredible people who fall asleep as soon as their head hits the pillow and bounce out of bed as soon as they wake! Most of us need a bit of wiggle room on the falling-asleep and getting-out-of-bed fronts. Now that I routinely sleep well, I always allow myself an additional 30 to 60 minutes in bed, beyond the 7.5 hours of sleep that I need. (I don't give myself more than 8.5 hours in bed as this decreases my sleep efficiency.)

Sleep opportunity determines whether you are technically *sleep deprived* or *sleep deficient*. This may seem pedantic, given most of us mortals think these two things are the same, but it's a distinction worth mentioning. If you are wrecked and ruined from too little sleep because you didn't have adequate opportunity to sleep, you are sleep deprived. If you are wrecked and ruined from too little sleep but did give your body plenty of opportunity to sleep, you are sleep deficient.

Inadequate sleep opportunity is not insomnia

If your low total sleep time is the result of inadequate time in bed, you haven't given yourself enough opportunity for sleep. This is sleep deprivation, not insomnia. Most people in this camp can fix their temporary sleep problem by creating a bigger sleep opportunity. Or, as our mothers would say, 'Just go to bed!'

Throughout this book, I use these two terms, sleep deprivation and deficiency, interchangeably as for most us they mean the same thing. But if you are in the sleep-deprived camp, make sure that you start rigorously using your sleep diary to track your time in bed. If you aren't giving yourself the opportunity to sleep, it makes it impossible for you to get the hours that you need, unless of course you are a horse, zebra or elephant and can sleep standing up! (Cows can too, but they mostly choose not to.)

Total sleep time refers to the total time you are asleep across the entire sleep period. It's the difference between the time you went to sleep and the time you woke up for the final time, minus the total time you spent awake in the night. So, if I eventually fell asleep at about 1.30 a.m. and woke up for the final time at about 6 a.m., but had been awake for about an hour in total throughout the night, my total sleep time would be 3.5 hours. Brutal.

If you are good at maths, these equations will be a breeze. If you are less maths-inclined, like I am, there's no shame in counting on your fingers to work these numbers out. Do it however is easiest and most natural for you—the important thing is to do it.

One way to make the maths straightforward is to write the times down in a format that makes sense to you, and to use 15 or 30-minute increments rather than getting down to the nitty-gritty of individual minutes.

At the end of each week, grab a calculator and set aside ten minutes to complete and review your diary, and work out your sleep-efficiency score for each night of the week. Don't worry, this isn't hard maths either but there are online sleep-efficiency calculators you can use to make life easy. Head over to my one at Sleep Haven (www.sleephaven.co.nz) or try www.mysleepwell.ca.

Let's take another run through the example above. I responsibly went to bed at 10 p.m. and got up at 6 a.m., so my time in bed was 8 hours, creating a pretty good sleep window. I finally got to sleep at 1.30 a.m. and dragged myself out of bed as soon as the alarm went off at 6 a.m., but I'd had about an hour of being awake throughout the night—so my total sleep time was 3.5 hours. Therefore, my sleep-efficiency sum would look like this:

$$\textbf{sleep efficiency} = 3.5 \div 8 \times 100 = 44\%$$

My sleep efficiency in this example comes out at 44 per cent (I was generous and rounded it up). If your figures are like this to begin with, don't get disheartened. It's essential to remain neutral and try to be accepting. They are what they are. Trust me, I had figures like this and plenty lower when I was starting out on my sleep-recovery regimen. It's not like school exams where 50 per cent is a pass. Your sleep efficiency is a measurement tool to help you track your progress towards the endgame.

In the long term, you want to be aiming for a handsome 85 per cent or higher. (Crazy, I know! When I started I thought I had no chance, but now I regularly hit those figures when I bother to do the maths.) While 85 per cent may feel like a very long way from where you are now, it's good to have lofty aspirations.

After calculating your sleep efficiency for all seven days on the chart, reflect on your sleep diary. Staying calm and non-judgemental, objectively review how your sleep was over the week. You may notice patterns—see if there are any clues as to what makes a particularly unsettled night for you, or what may have made a night work out a bit better.

Your diary may look like soup at this stage, and that's okay. When you are in the thick of insomnia, it's easy to look over a sleep diary and feel despair about how terrible your sleep is. When I looked at my first one I decided I was utterly useless; I couldn't even do the most basic thing that almost all lifeforms are naturally able to do. However, I have subsequently learned in my research that this kind of harsh judgement and personal contempt is utterly unhelpful in improving one's sleep.

Be compassionate with yourself and begin to develop curiosity about how sleep seems to work for your body (even if your sleep is suboptimal at this stage). Start thinking about how you might like things to be different in future, too. Do you fantasise about falling asleep more quickly at the start of the night? Waking less often throughout the night? Sleeping for longer? Changing the time you wake up in the morning? Perhaps your fantasy is about the quality or depth of your sleep. Maybe you'd like to sleep more consistently during the weeknights or sort out that Sunday-night insomnia. Plant the seeds in your mind now about what a good night or a good week of sleep would *actually* look like for you. Start thinking very gently about how you'd like your sleep to be down the track. Capture these notes and insights in your sleep diary for future reference.

Your sleep diary is a tool that, with daily use, will help you learn to sleep better. Think of it as your bedside companion. It's a friend that is there at your side to listen and observe without judgement, a place for you to kind-heartedly capture and document the truth about your sleep.

Once you start the six-week programme, your sleep diary will be the place to monitor your progress towards the kind of sleep you long to enjoy.

Creating the habit

For some, creating a sleep-diary habit will be a breeze, but, for others, building the new habit will feel a bit iffy. Sometimes, after we kick things off with gusto and commitment, our enthusiasm can wane, things can get sporadic and patchy, and soon our habit has disintegrated before it's properly formed. Lots of people have a tendency towards sketchy habit formation, and I bet it's even more prevalent among those of us with minds somewhat addled by sleep deficiency.

Fortunately, there is plenty of research on the formation of habits and the power of daily micro-actions to change our lives. Once a behaviour becomes a habit, it occurs instinctively and there is no conscious thought required.[2] From then on, you're on autopilot: there's no deciding to do it now or later or not at all—you just do it. There's no negotiating with yourself, no deals to be brokered, no internal excuses, no guilt, no angst. Having helpful unconscious habits can be game-changing.

The goal is to make updating your sleep diary as natural and automatic as having a shower or brushing your teeth each morning—you want it to be just what you do. Your sleep diary is going to be your progress-monitoring tool throughout the six-week programme, so you need to nail this little daily habit. To build the habit pronto and sustainably, let's embrace some handy shortcuts plucked from the brilliant work of habit-formation expert B.J. Fogg,[3] who runs the Behavior Design Lab at Stanford University, and behaviour-change writers James Clear, author of *Atomic Habits*,[4] and Gretchen Rubin, author of *Better Than Before*.[5]

Start by focusing on the habit that matters most. One of the first things Rubin recommends in *Better Than Before* is to concentrate your efforts on the habits that offer you the biggest payoff and sense of self-determination. These habits enable you to build a strong foundation for everything else that you aspire towards. Not surprisingly, forming habits that help to improve your sleep is number one on Rubin's suggestion list. Mastering sleep offers epic payoffs for your health and well-being in both the short and long term.

You're already under way building habits that will help you sleep. Your first habit is reading this book, and you've made it this far. Keep building that habit, as it's supplying you the information, tools and support you need to improve your sleep. The next habits to solidly embed: filling in your sleep diary *daily* and reviewing it *weekly*.

Scheduling is critical to robust habit formation—set a specific, regular time and place for the activity, to become the cue for the desired behaviour. With repetition, you create a mental association, which increases the likelihood of converting the action into a habit.[6] I recommend writing in your sleep diary when you wake each morning before you do anything else. Then, the information is freshest in your mind, so your data will be more accurate (remember it's just your best estimate). Then it's done and you don't have to try to remember to do it at an unspecified, slippery, 'probably won't get round to it' time later.

Accountability is another strategy you can use to form your sleep-diary habit. When we are held accountable, even if only to *ourselves*, we tend to exhibit greater self-command. If we think someone is watching us, we behave differently—usually for the better![7] To use this to your advantage, think about who cares the most about your sleep. Is it you, your future self, your partner, your children, your friends, your colleagues or your boss? Whoever it is, jot their name on the top of your sleep diary and draw a couple of eyes watching you. This may sound flaky, but Rubin writes that experiments have shown that watching eyes helps to trick us into feeling greater accountability.

Convenience matters if you are to start and stick with a new behaviour. The amount of time, effort and decision-making energy that goes into a new habit affects the likelihood you'll adopt and sustain it. Give yourself a head start in habit formation by making the new behaviour fast and easy to do.[8] The sleep diary is pared back to the essentials and can be filled out in just a couple of minutes, so you've got speed and ease on your side. To make it super convenient for yourself, and given that your sleep diary is best completed first thing in the morning, keep this book at your bedside with a pen. You'll have a visual reminder that will be noticed and is within easy reach—easy is good!

Treats are darling little pleasures enjoyed just because we feel like them. They are different from rewards because they don't need to be earned or justified by good behaviour—they are not carrots. Instead, treats are random acts of personal kindness. Forming new, constructive habits can be hard work initially, requiring conscious effort and self-discipline (until autopilot kicks in). This is draining for most people, but particularly taxing on those experiencing chronic insomnia. When we give ourselves treats, we feel happy and cared for. They put us in a better frame of mind, and we have greater self-command. In this state, we are more likely to continue our commitment to healthy habits. So, go ahead: treat yourself!

Treats don't need to be expensive or time-consuming, but once they are woven into your life, you start feeling more cooperative and able. When I was establishing my sleep-diary habit, I started allowing myself little treats. I had previously been too blinkered by insomnia to even know that my soul would enjoy them. I'd allow myself to sit outside while I had a cup of tea in the afternoon rather than at my desk. Those moments with the sunshine, the fresh air, the rustle of the wind in the leaves, were simple pleasures for me but so restorative. Sometimes I'd nip into a delightful little store in my neighbourhood that sells vintage French homeware. It wasn't about buying anything; it was about allowing myself a fragment of unstructured time to explore and be among fascinating items from a world away. If I was shy on time, my treat would be something as simple as washing my hands with beautifully scented hand soap.

Pairing can be used to piggyback a new habit on to an existing practice or activity that you already like doing, to increase the chance you'll adopt the new habit. You'll have rock-solid habits in your life that you do daily without giving them any thought—consider tagging your sleep diary on to one of these no-brainers. I linked my sleep diary to putting my feet on the floor: I'd swing my legs out of bed in the morning, and as soon as I sat up and felt my feet on the floor, I'd reach for my sleep diary and fill it in. I have a special relationship with putting my feet on the floor first thing in the morning. When I was a teenager, my mother would struggle to get me out of bed on cold, dark, winter mornings in Otago. She'd call out every five minutes for me to get my 'feet on the floor'. I'd ignore her calls until she was beside herself, then slither sideways in the bed and put my legs over the side, so my feet were technically on the floor. I could honestly answer 'They are on the floor!' to her hollers, even though I was still snuggled under the covers. Teenagers, eh.

Safeguards are essential to have in place when habit-building. Humans are gloriously imperfect, so we need to factor in a plan B for when our best intentions fail us or we rebel (both of which are normal). To protect the habit you are building, anticipate what could happen and know what you will do if that scenario occurs. That is, plan for failure.[9] This helps to prevent one lapse from turning into full abandonment of the new behaviour. For example, if you wake up later than expected and bolt out of bed so you're not late for work, school, or the train, what will you do? Or if you wake after a lousy night's sleep feeling like the world is against you? Even though your sleep diary asks only two minutes of you, when there's a train to catch or you're in a rotten frame of mind, the diary habit may get the flick. It happens. If that's the case, plan to fill it out in the evening when you get into bed. The data may have lost some of its immediacy and accuracy, but it's still there; just get it on the page. Having a backup plan for your habit means you won't have to expend any energy throughout the day thinking about it and wondering when or if you are going to do it.

Celebrate to reinforce a new behaviour and encourage the formation of a new habit. This might sound OTT, but there's solid neuroscience behind it! Fogg explains that habits aren't formed by mere repetition; it's the frequent association of positive emotion with a new behaviour that rewires your brain.[10] By celebrating in some tiny way the *remembering* to do, the *doing*, or the *completion* of a new behaviour, you'll feel happy and successful, so your brain (which is always on the lookout for patterns) is more inclined to remember and repeat the desired behaviour. The way you celebrate these little wins will be personal, but it's important to do something to acknowledge the new behaviour and to do it in the moment. Find a way that feels good for you—an enthusiastic 'Way to go!' or 'Go me!' self-talk, a quick fist pump, or a little victory dance. Even if it feels a bit bonkers to start with, go with it to help your brain embed the sleep-diary habit.

The helpful strategies outlined above will support you as you establish your sleep-diary habit. Adopt the tools that resonate with you, and they will strengthen your habit-building muscles—you're going to need these for the journey ahead.

The success of CBTi relies heavily on the breaking of unhelpful sleep habits and the creation of new, helpful ones. This includes habitual thoughts and habitual behaviours. We have so many quiet little habits nestled in our lives that may inadvertently be jeopardising our sleep. The six-week programme will encourage you to become aware of these habits in your thought patterns and everyday behaviours, and will provide you with information about habits that need review. Reading this book and filling out your sleep diary are the foundational new habits that will support you on your sleep-improvement journey.

Chapter recap: what you can do

1. Complete your sleep diary every morning to capture your sleep behaviour over the next one or two weeks. It will provide a baseline and set you up with a monitoring tool to use throughout the programme. Remember: it's not about exact times; it's your best estimate.

2. Review your sleep diary at the end of the week by working out your sleep-efficiency scores, reflecting on your sleep experiences with curiosity and self-compassion, and noting any patterns.

3. Consciously strengthen your habit-building skills. Use the following proven techniques to help yourself establish sustainable habits.

- **Focus**—prioritise the desired habit.
- **Schedule**—book in the desired habit at a regular time and place.
- **Accountability**—be clear about who you are doing this for, and don't let them down.
- **Convenience**—make it as quick and easy for yourself as possible.
- **Treats**—be nice to yourself with random acts of kindness.
- **Pairing**—link the desired habit with an established habit or behaviour you enjoy.
- **Safeguards**—anticipate slip-ups and have a plan B.
- **Celebration**—do or say something for yourself to associate the new habit with a positive emotion.

4. Continue your habit of reading this book to learn more about how sleep occurs.

SLEEP DIARY

Fill out your sleep diary every morning. Guess the approximate times, there's no need for clock-watching. On the next page, note any factors that helped with sleep or may have been unhelpful for your sleep. You're looking for clues and patterns . . .

Baseline Sleep— Week 1	Example	Night 1	Night 2	Night 3	Night 4	Night 5	Night 6	Night 7
Start Date _____ Day of Week								
What time did you go to bed?	9.45pm							
What time did you first try to go to sleep?	10pm							
What time did you fall asleep?	1.30am							
How many times did you wake in the night?	3							
How long did these awakenings last in total?	1hr							
What time did you wake for the final time this morning?	6am							
What time did you get out of bed for the day?	6am							
How would you rate the quality of your sleep? *(1 Terrible, 2 Bad, 3 OK, 4 Good, 5 Great)*	2							
Total Sleep Time In total, how many hours' sleep did you get?	3.5hrs							
Total Time in Bed In total, how long were you in bed?	8hrs							
Sleep Efficiency % (Total Sleep Time ÷ Total Time in Bed X 100 = %)	44 %	%	%	%	%	%	%	%

SLEEP DIARY

Baseline Sleep—Week 1	Night 1	Night 2	Night 3	Night 4	Night 5	Night 6	Night 7
Day of Week							
Start Date _____							
Any factors that may have been unhelpful for your sleep last night? (coffee, alcohol, stress, temperature, light, noise, disturbances, pain, medication, screen time, etc)							
Any factors that may have helped with sleep last night? (exercise, relaxation, supplements, sleep meds, etc)							

Observations & Insights:

SLEEP DIARY

Fill out your sleep diary every morning. Guess the approximate times, there's no need for clock-watching. On the next page, note any factors that helped with sleep or may have been unhelpful for your sleep. You're looking for clues and patterns …

Baseline Sleep— Week 2	Example	Night 1	Night 2	Night 3	Night 4	Night 5	Night 6	Night 7
Start Date _____ Day of Week								
What time did you go to bed?	9.45pm							
What time did you first try to go to sleep?	10pm							
What time did you fall asleep?	1.30am							
How many times did you wake in the night?	3							
How long did these awakenings last in total?	1hr							
What time did you wake for the final time this morning?	6am							
What time did you get out of bed for the day?	6am							
How would you rate the quality of your sleep? (1 Terrible, 2 Bad, 3 OK, 4 Good, 5 Great)	2							
Total Sleep Time In total, how many hours' sleep did you get?	3.5hrs							
Total Time in Bed In total, how long were you in bed?	8hrs							
Sleep Efficiency % (Total Sleep Time ÷ Total Time in Bed X 100 = %)	44 %	%	%	%	%	%	%	%

SLEEP DIARY

Baseline Sleep—Week 2	Night 1	Night 2	Night 3	Night 4	Night 5	Night 6	Night 7
Start Date _____ Day of Week							
Any factors that may have been unhelpful for your sleep last night?							
Any factors that may have helped with sleep last night?							

Observations & Insights:

CHAPTER 4

Learn the fundamentals of sleeping

Minds are like parachutes: they
only function when open.
—THOMAS DEWAR

With your sleep diary under way, it's time to prepare for the six-week programme by developing your curiosity about and understanding of sleep. This is not to kill time—sleep education is an essential component of CBTi. The better you understand sleep and what's needed for sustainable behaviour change, the better equipped you'll be to improve your sleep. In this chapter, you'll be getting familiar with what the experts refer to as 'sleep hygiene' and Gwyneth Paltrow's Goop calls 'clean sleeping'. I like to think of sleep hygiene as the fundamentals of sleeping: they lay the foundations for a decent sleep.

While there are several things to check and consider, don't feel pressured to make changes at this stage. If you're struggling with depletion or hyperarousal from lack of sleep, the last thing you need is more jobs on your list. We will explore sleep hygiene in more detail throughout the six-week programme and set up steps to take action then. However, if you're feeling up for it, you may choose to try some changes as you begin to prioritise and experiment with your sleep.

If you do start making modifications and adjustments based on the following information, it's essential to be realistic with your expectations. Making these changes will not miraculously cure chronic insomnia—you are simply starting to create the environment and conditions that will be *more conducive* to a good night's sleep. These changes set the scene for the CBTi-inspired work in the programme. This is preparation and education.

Dr Jade Wu, a US-based behavioural sleep medicine specialist, uses a dental-hygiene analogy to put sleep hygiene in perspective. She says, 'Treating insomnia with sleep hygiene is like treating a cavity with dental hygiene. Dental hygiene is great. Brushing and flossing will help prevent cavities. But once you have a cavity, no amount of brushing is going to get rid of it.'[1] She goes further, pointing out that sleep hygiene is often used as the placebo treatment in clinical trials for insomnia. So, while sleep hygiene is good and everyone needs to know about it, once you have chronic insomnia, you have to actually deal with the biological and psychological processes underlying the sleep problem.

To help people who want to improve their sleep, the World Sleep Society has created a set of 'commandments' for sleep hygiene.[2] We have all read those annoying lists in glossy magazines and on stylish health and lifestyle websites about transforming our sleep, but this is *the* list to take to heart.

The World Sleep Society is a collaborative international organisation comprising over 60 sleep societies and organisations across 40 countries, with a commitment to advancing sleep health worldwide. It's made up of scientists, physicians, psychologists, nurses, physician assistants, technologists, and other medical and research personnel all dedicated to the field of sleep—they know their stuff. They have done the research, conducted clinical trials with thousands and thousands of people with sleep difficulties, and completed systematic reviews and meta-analyses. These people know that these ten practices are non-negotiable if you want to start sorting your sleep.

1. Establish a regular bedtime and waking-time routine

This sounds infinitely boring, annoying and unnecessary, but it is the most important of the commandments. For those with chronic insomnia, getting a regular wake-time locked in is the priority. If you are only up for doing one thing at this stage, do this. (We'll learn that bedtime can be a little more fluid, but it's good to have a guide.)

Let's face it, most of us haven't been regular with our sleep schedule since our parents forced the issue when we were eight years old. Then, 7.30 p.m. bedtime was enforced regardless of what day of the week it was, so they could sit down and watch a bit of telly uninterrupted. Since then, you've probably chosen to be a bit loose with your bedtimes and wake-times—after all, you're the grown-up now.

Alternatively, and just as unhelpfully, you might be adamant that you have a regular sleep schedule, but your schedule includes a different set of rules for weekdays and weekends. So you are, in fact, regularly irregular!

According to the 2019 Philips Global Sleep Survey, an epic study of just over 11,000 people across twelve countries including Australia, it's pretty common for people all over the world to sleep longer on the weekends than they do during the week.[3] Over 60 per cent of adults sleep longer over the weekend to 'catch up' on sleep. In terms of sleep duration, people average an hour longer each night on the weekends than on weeknights.

While this seems like perfectly reasonable behaviour, even sensible, there's a deep flaw in this strategy. Having an irregular or changing sleep–wake schedule makes it difficult for your body's internal clock. Staying up late and sleeping in on the weekend may work in the short term, enabling you to snatch an extra bit of shut-eye, but it creates 'social jet lag' that contributes to insomnia. Yes, it contributes to insomnia.

Snoozing longer on Sunday morning messes with your wakefulness cycle. When you first get up and get going in the morning, your body temperature rises. Sleeping in delays the timing of exposure to sunlight and the rise in body temperature, which means that the natural drop in your body temperature (necessary for falling asleep) is also delayed that night. So falling asleep on Sunday night becomes trickier. What's more, if you're feeling a bit tired after late nights over the weekend, you might head to bed earlier on Sunday to try to catch up before the workweek. However, because your circadian rhythm is out of whack, it has other plans—according to it, you haven't been awake long enough for your body to fall asleep! So you lie there awake, even though you went to bed really early. This phenomenon is sometimes referred to as Sunday-night insomnia.

Sticking to a regular sleep schedule every day—even on weekends— is conducive to falling asleep, sleeping well and waking up with ease. It maintains the timing of your body's internal clock, and it means that your body has sufficient time awake during the day for 'sleep pressure' (your body's desire to fall asleep) to build to levels that make you feel sleepy at bedtime.

So how do you do this? People tend to be accustomed to setting the alarm for weekday mornings. You need to build on this habit and extend the use of the morning 'alarm' to weekend mornings. Plus, and this is worth being aware of, you need to retrain yourself to go to bed when your body wants you to. Many people become so mixed up in their sleep patterns, they lose touch with the fundamentals—like being aware of when your body is telling you it's ready for sleep. Some of us push on oblivious to our sleepy signals and some of us go to bed when we're 'tired' (feeling exhausted, depleted) but not 'sleepy'. Consider setting a nightly alert to remind yourself when it's a reasonable time to head for bed. While you may not physically need to go to bed at that time, it's a reminder to be on the lookout for your body's signals that you're sleepy—like yawning or rubbing your eyes.

Because you want to build sustainable habits that you enjoy, choose a kind ringtone. While it needs to get your attention, you don't actually want to be 'alarmed'—you simply want to be reminded. I listen to crickets these days, rather than sirens!

Remember, you aren't being made to go to bed earlier or later than you want to, and you aren't being forced to get up before you're ready. The World Sleep Society is merely asking you to be consistent. Make a call based on the reality of your life—choose a bedtime and a wake-time that you're confident you can stick with on both weeknights and the weekends while you endeavour to get your sleeping back on track. You are doing this for the sake of your body—so that it knows what to expect, when.

Having a regular routine provides structure and consistency for your sleep. However, be realistic and know that you're not able to sleep 'on demand'. Lying awake for ages in bed unable to fall asleep is unhelpful. There'll be the occasional night when you stay up a bit later until you're sleepy, or you get up in the night if you find yourself tired and wired in the wee hours. While routine matters, you also need to be flexible with it, especially as you're learning how to improve your sleep.

Implementing a consistent sleep–wake time doesn't make you boring; it's key to regulating your sleep and eventually your energy so that you can be more awesome. In the future, once you're confident that your sleep is operating the way it needs to, you'll once again be able to stay up late on a Friday night and go out dancing till sun-up. The difference is that it will be an active choice, and you will understand the sleep risks involved. It won't be a recurring unconscious phenomenon that corrodes your ability to sleep well.

2. Allow yourself a short nap, if you must

I have never mastered the art of napping during the day, except in the first trimester of pregnancy when my body would temporarily shut down in the afternoon if located somewhere semi-horizontal to curl up. Beyond this, I have simply not been able to nap—even when I need to!

While it's preferable to get all the sleep that your body needs at night, while you're learning how to do that you still have to get through the day on compromised sleep. Being exhausted is no fun. It impacts your ability to be productive, good company and to drive safely, so, if you can, it's worth considering taking a nap to help get through the really rough days. A nap can take the edge off lost sleep and offers a temporary coping mechanism for insomnia.

If you're lucky enough to be able to take a nap and you have the opportunity, you'll probably feel most inclined to do it in the afternoon, when a slump in mood and alertness can naturally occur. (It's no accident that the highly caffeinated energy drink V launched with the promise of being a 3 p.m. wake-up call!) If you do nap, keep it early in the afternoon (before 3 or 4 p.m.) and limit daytime sleep to under 30 minutes. This way you're likely to wake up more alert and energised, but you won't jeopardise your ability to fall asleep that night. Set an alert for 45 minutes, to give yourself time to fall asleep, and nap for a maximum of 30 minutes.

If the nap is nonessential, it's better to allow your body's sleep pressure to continue to build towards bedtime. A nap is like a release valve; it decreases some of the sleep pressure that builds throughout the day.

3. Curb the timing of your drinking (and smoking)

Alcohol is covered in detail in Week Five, but, for now, prioritise monitoring what happens to your sleep when you drink. Once you've been keeping your sleep diary for a few weeks, you'll be in a much better position to make an informed observation about how alcohol affects *your* sleep.

In the meantime remember that, even though alcohol is part of our social tapestry, at its core it's a sedative. Some of you will be enjoying or relying on a few drinks to help you sleep. A nightcap may help you feel relaxed and fall asleep more easily, but drinking—especially heavier drinking—tends to keep you in the lighter stages of sleep and it's more likely you'll wake in the night. For me, having a few drinks later in the evening is risky business for sleep. I typically end up with relentless bouts of daft and unproductive thinking throughout the night, and I feel incredibly ratty in the morning.

The World Sleep Society's view is that we should 'avoid excessive alcohol ingestion four hours before bedtime'. For the moment, be honest with yourself in your sleep diary about the amount of alcohol you're consuming (to establish what excessive means for your body), and focus on sticking to the recommended drinking cut-off time. If you're going to drink, you're much better to drink early in the evening than later.

If you binge-drink from time to time, be aware this messes with that vital sleep hormone, melatonin. According to the Sleep Health Foundation, a night of binge drinking affects melatonin levels for up to a week.[4] Factor this into your sleep observations on the nights after a big night out.

There are a million reasons not to smoke, but some of us still do. Having been a smoker in the distant past, I know it can be an arduous, erratic and at times humiliating journey to stopping. I have had to pour water on packs of cigarettes that I have thrown valiantly in the bin when I have 'quit once and for all', to prevent myself from reneging on my promise a few hours later and taking a drag on a binned cigarette. So there's no judgement from me.

If you're currently choosing to smoke, keep in mind that nicotine is a stimulant and is unhelpful for your sleep. It can often cause people to sleep only very lightly, and they may wake during the night or early in the morning because of nicotine withdrawal. The World Sleep Society recommends that you don't smoke during the four hours before bedtime. (And obviously, no smoking overnight.)

4. Establish a caffeine cut-off time

Caffeine is a stimulant, and well proven to interfere with the ability to fall asleep (and stay asleep). People have different levels of sensitivity to caffeine, and it's important to know your own body's ability to tolerate it. For many people, its effects take around six hours to wear off, but for some people it's a lot longer, taking twelve or more hours to leave their system. And caffeine is not just in our precious coffee—it's laced into colas, soft drinks, energy drinks, some teas, and chocolate.

Good coffee and dark chocolate are great friends of mine. I love them and have, at times, considered my relationship with each closer to an addiction than a daily pleasure. For me, they were and are non-negotiables. While I mostly relinquished drinking alcohol, I clung to coffee and chocolate and would not surrender them for the sake of my sleep. But, after experimenting and monitoring what went on with my nights, I had to concede that caffeine was definitely impacting my sleep. As a result, I made some modifications in my 'terms of use' for espresso and 80 per cent dark chocolate. I can live with that because good sleep is worth it.

While each person's caffeine tolerance is a little different, the recommendation of the World Sleep Society is to avoid caffeine six hours before bedtime. This is a good ground rule to work with. Once you've established your bedtime, you can work backwards to figure out your caffeine cut-off time. So, if bedtime is 10.30 p.m., caffeine curfew is 4.30 p.m. Use this as a guideline, but be aware that your body may be more affected by caffeine than most.

Later, you will use your sleep diary as a tool to monitor and fine-tune your caffeine threshold. I've learned that I can usually get away with a couple of bits of dark chocolate at night, but coffee is off limits from high noon (so much for my 'high tolerance of caffeine' theory). Learning where your boundaries are gives you a choice—there are days when I'm prepared to risk my sleep for a cup of coffee in the early afternoon, but other days I will protect my sleep at all costs and make the call to refrain, because I know the consequences just aren't worth it.

5. Lighten up on the bedtime snacking

It's challenging to sleep if you're hungry. If your stomach is growling and you're prowling the pantry, it makes sense to have a snack in the evening before going to bed. However, to be happy and fed without compromising your sleep, opt for light food choices. Think of it as something to tide you over till morning, rather than fill you up.

There are many good reasons to eat in the evenings—boredom, ritual, fun, comfort, socialising or a need to indulge. Enjoying good food is worth it, so long as it doesn't make sleep more elusive. To this end, if you want to have rich, heavy, spicy or sugary foods, be conscious of the time you choose to eat them. For the sake of your sleep, these foods are best consumed earlier in the evening rather than later. Keep them at least four hours away from bedtime.

6. Work out, but not right before bedtime

Being physically active during the day on a regular basis helps encourage better sleep at night. But when you're in sleep debt, exercise is one of those things on the to-do list that tend to fall away. If that's where you are now, so be it. Be kind with yourself—it's common and completely understandable. We'll talk about ways to integrate activity into your life further down the track.

If you're still managing to get exercise into your day, that's excellent so long as you aren't doing high-energy workouts right before bed. You want your body to be cool, calm and quiet as you wind down before slumber. Your body temperature naturally declines in the evenings, and, left alone, this biology makes you less alert and sleepier as the night progresses. You have an inbuilt thermostat that works with you to make it easier to fall asleep, so don't interfere with that if you don't need to. If night-time is your only window for exercise, explore gentler, slower options. Think yin yoga rather than body-attack-style training!

7. Make sure your bed is comfortable and inviting

Be aware of the need to truly feel good about the place you spend almost a third of your time. On a physical level, your bed needs to feel safe, warm, supportive and comfortable for your body. On an emotional level, your bed needs to be a place of calm and peace. It's crucial that your bed feels inviting for you personally. What this actually looks, feels and smells like will be as unique as you are.

Consider your bed and bedding and decide if it really is a

comfortable and inviting place to rest your weary head. Really look at the bed base, the mattress, the sheets, the pillows, the duvet or doona, the throws—do they feel right for you or are you making do? You want your body and soul to be able to relax fully, making it easier to surrender to the possibility of sleep.

When you have been struggling with sleep for some time, your bed and bedding can become associated with negative thoughts and feelings that are unhelpful in the quest for sleep. It may be worth changing things up in the future, and making your bed how you really want it to be.

I remember shopping for bed linen a few years ago and sharing a conversation with a woman in her sixties about our duvet-cover choices. We were both strong advocates for 100 per cent natural fibres. I'd opted for a soft shade of turquoise because the colour reminded me of the ocean and holidays in the sun. She, on the other hand, held a cover that was a symphony of spring flowers in every shade of yellow. She was clearly in love with it. She confided that, after forty-odd years of marriage, she had finally allowed herself to choose one that was genuinely what she wanted. Until then, she'd felt compelled to go with androgynous options even though her husband didn't care what it looked like, so long as it was the right weight.

At this stage, don't set yourself the expensive task of a bedroom makeover. You're in no state to Marie Kondo anything. Do what you can with what you've got, and only if you feel up to it. Start caring about your bed as a sleep environment, but give yourself permission to let it ride if needed—slowing down will be valuable in your journey towards better sleep.

8. Find a comfortable temperature and ventilate your bedroom

Body temperature changes throughout the day and night, but not radically—just a couple of degrees Celsius. All the same, core temperature is instrumental in the ability to sleep or not. As body temperature declines in the evening, you become less alert and drowsier.

Ensure that your bedroom honours your biology by supporting this natural temperature cycle that helps you to fall and stay asleep. The National Sleep Foundation recommends a room temperature of about 18 degrees Celsius (year-round). While there is some personal wiggle room, if your bedroom is too warm or too cold, it can prevent or disrupt your sleep.

I feel the cold—ridiculously so. I gravitate towards all things warm—the sun, heaters, cosy fires, woollen blankets and hot-water bottles have a special place in my heart. Yet, even for me, a too-warm bedroom is a no-no. If it's a few degrees above 18, there is no way I can fall asleep. Then, when my body temperature drops to its lowest a few hours before sunrise (as part of the body's natural cycle) I'm super sensitive to the cold, and it can wake me. I'm not keen on having a heater going overnight, so it's taken a fair bit of experimentation to get things right. Now I start the night with my room at the right temperature and have a warm blanket on standby just in case.

While I've been sensitive to the cold most of my life, things change, and we must adapt. Those of us in the throes of perimenopause or menopause are hyperaware of the impact of a dodgy personal thermostat. Random bouts of overheating in the night can wake you up—typically not in a great frame of mind. I'm facing these changes now, and it's seriously annoying given that I'd had things sussed. But, by understanding the vital role temperature plays in my body's ability to sleep, I don't even consider getting back to sleep while I'm overheated. My priority is to remain matter of fact and to cool my body down. Once I have managed that, I can return to sleep using the CBTi skills I've learned.

The World Sleep Society also advocates for good ventilation in the bedroom. If you can safely open your window a crack overnight without making the room too noisy, cold or hot, it's worth doing. This will provide you with fresh air, which makes for a better night's sleep. If you don't have that option, or don't feel comfortable with the window open at night, open the windows at some stage during the day to circulate air through your bedroom, to get stale carbon dioxide out and fresh oxygen in.

9. Create as much quiet and dark as possible

For most of us, it's easier to fall asleep when it's quiet and dark. However, our hyperconnected, busy, 24/7, screen-lit, always-on lives can make the silence, stillness and true darkness of night elusive.

Modern life has become somewhat disconnected from the natural cycle of day and night. Since the Industrial Revolution, the invention of electric light, the rapid evolution of technology and the internet, 'daytime' has been gradually extending, to create longer hours of light, productivity and connectedness. There's so much to do and get done. All of this comes at the expense of night-time—sleep gets sacrificed.

Mother Nature is no longer in charge of when night-time comes, so it's up to you. You're responsible for turning off your lights, your screens, your technology. It's not easy when there is so much to do and so much on offer—there's enough content out there to binge-watch forever. And there are endless distractions and diversions down the rabbit hole of your phone!

But, if you're serious about sleep, you have to start allowing the night to be the night. Become more aware of when the sun goes down and night is falling, the moon is rising, and the stars are out. These are nature's signals that you need to finish your day's work or play, and begin winding down and preparing for sleep. It can be helpful to dim the lights in the house once it's dark outside, to remind yourself that night is falling and before long it will be time for sleep.

The need for quiet and dark in the bedroom is imperative if you want to fall asleep quickly and allow your body to cycle uninterrupted through the stages of restorative sleep. You have to consciously turn off the lights and make sure that your curtains and blinds properly block any light that persists outside. If you can't achieve this to a workable level, consider using an eye mask and earplugs. (If you do, be nonchalant about giving these accessories a go—you want your relationship with them to be low key, rather than dependent or fretful.)

The most important thing for creating quiet darkness—and this is the bit you're most likely to struggle with—is to remove technology. Remove screens and devices from your bedroom to eliminate distraction and disturbances—from blue light, sound and *mental stimulation*. For many, this is a shocking prospect, which is why we eased into it with more doable things—like turning off the lights and pulling the curtains.

The reality is, screens and phones are the real troublemakers for sleep on the dark and quiet fronts. While the World Sleep Society doesn't expressly mention technology in their commandments for adult sleep hygiene, it's there in black-and-white in their commandments for children up to twelve years old. For those enduring chronic insomnia, it's best to take a hard-line approach to technology (like we would for kids with sleep challenges). You have to get rid of technology from the bedroom altogether while you are recalibrating your sleep patterns.

Dr Tony Fernando recently described mobile phones and technology in the bedroom as being *toxic* to sleep. I was relieved to hear that word; it's definitive. While writing this book, I started having difficulty sleeping—oh the irony. I was stressed about writing my first book— the responsibility of providing information that was up to date, safe and effective—and I was haunted by imposter syndrome. *Who am I to write this*? I thought. *I'm not a sleep specialist or an academic.* I started waking in the night, worrying about all of the above, so I began taking my phone to bed to access sleep meditations I knew worked well for me. Even so, my nights were deteriorating. I was worried I might not be able to get my sleep back on course.

When I next met with Tony, to ask if he'd provide expert guidance throughout the writing of this book, I felt tired and like a total fraud. Then, the technology-in-the-bedroom conversation came up, and Tony revealed that he, too, had been having trouble sleeping lately because of his damned phone! Even people who've dedicated their lives to sleep health are susceptible to the lure and distraction of phones in the bedroom. I imagine Tony was doing something more intellectual on his phone than going to Headspace via Gmail, Facebook and Cats of Instagram, but the end result for both of us was the same— compromised sleep!

Mobile phones in the bedroom
are toxic to sleep.
—DR TONY FERNANDO

So the challenge is to get your devices out of the bedroom. The intensity of your resistance, justifications and defensiveness is probably correlated with how important it is that you break the overnight tech habit. Cold turkey tends to be the best approach: get the devices physically out of the room.

'Oh, but what if . . .' I hear you say. Absolutely. Some urgent calls or messages may need to be taken in the night, especially if you are responsible for teenagers or elderly parents. Consider putting your phone outside the door of your bedroom. It's still within earshot in case of an emergency, but it's physically out of arm's reach.

Argue for your limitations and
sure enough, they're yours.
—RICHARD BACH

If you need your phone to know the time overnight or to hear your alarm in the morning, remember that, if you have trouble falling asleep or find yourself awake in the night, relentlessly monitoring the clock can be your nemesis. You need to retrain yourself to trust that if it's dark, it's night, and it's an opportunity for rest and sleep.

Beyond the physical and mental distraction posed by technology, blue light from electronic devices and screens suppresses the body's production of melatonin. Avoid screens to give yourself the best chance of producing melatonin naturally, so you don't have to go to the doctor to get a prescription for a synthetic version that may or may not work!

Using screens in the evening delays sleep onset. Since you've been experiencing sleep difficulties, be conscious of your screen use. If you are watching or using screens at night, set blue-light-filter options where you can and consider wearing blue-light-filtering glasses. Do what you can to prevent your brain getting wake-up signals when you are on the trajectory towards bedtime.

External sounds are comparatively easy to silence to create the quiet recommended by the World Sleep Society, even if you have to use earplugs. Those of us who know insomnia intimately will appreciate that there is also a need to create quiet internally. When you lie awake at night, internal talk—thoughts, worries, stresses, fears—often creates noise inside your brain and prohibits you from finding the inner calm you need to relax and allow sleep to occur. Quietening this inner noise is essential for sleep, and considerable attention is paid to this throughout the six-week programme. More than anything else, learning to sleep is an inside job.

10. Reserve your bed for sleep and sex

For many people, bedrooms have become multipurpose living spaces. With televisions, mobile phones, laptops and e-readers, a bedroom soon begins to function as an office, a TV room, a recreation room, a second lounge and a library.

Using bedrooms for these wakeful activities creates unhelpful messages and associations in your brain. Rather than being a place where your body instinctively knows it can withdraw from the world, relax and sleep, your bedroom becomes linked with alertness, engagement, mental stimulation, even stress. If you want to make sleeping easier, you need to think of your bedroom as a sleeping room. It should be defined by its primary purpose, and be treated like that.

Aside from sleep, the World Sleep Society concedes that we can use our bedrooms for sex. Phew.[5]

The World Sleep Society's ten commandments for sleep hygiene for adults

1. **Establish a regular bedtime and waking-time routine.** Set a bedtime and wake-time that you stick to on weekdays *and* the weekend.

2. **Allow yourself a short nap, if you must.** Any daytime sleep should be completed before 4 p.m. and keep your nap brief (under 30 minutes).

3. **Curb the timing of your drinking (and smoking).** If you're drinking, go easy in the four hours before bedtime. If you're smoking, keep the four hours before bed smoke-free.

4. **Establish a caffeine cut-off time.** Avoid caffeine for at least six hours before bedtime.

5. **Lighten up on the bedtime snacking.** Light snacks are okay. Keep any rich, heavy, spicy or sugary foods well away from bedtime (by at least four hours).

6. **Work out, but not right before bedtime.** Keep evening workouts low key or away from bedtime.

7. **Make sure your bedding is comfortable and inviting.** Make your bed a little more lovely for you.

8. **Find a comfortable temperature and ventilate your bedroom.** Keep the temperature around 18 degrees Celsius, and get some fresh air into the room.

9. **Create as much quiet and dark as possible.** Keep all electronics—TV, laptops, cell phones—out of the bedroom, and limit screen time before bed.[6]

10. **Reserve your bed for sleep and sex.**

Chapter recap: what you can do

1. Continue filling out your sleep diary each morning on waking. Work on this behaviour until it becomes an automatic habit that requires no thought. You want it to be just 'what you do' first thing in the morning.

2. Review the World Sleep Society's sleep-hygiene commandments. These aren't a bunch of 'shoulds'—they're merely sleep information to consider. Approach them with curiosity—you're in control of what you do or don't do. You're free to experiment with the practices and find out how they work for *you* and *your* sleep.

3. Include notes on sleep hygiene in your sleep diary to capture further clues about what may be helping or hindering your sleep.

4. If you feel like it, make some adjustments to your sleep hygiene. If you do want to make some changes at this stage, prioritise setting a consistent bedtime and wake-time, and getting your phone out of your bedroom overnight. Remember not to expect too much—you're laying the foundations for sleep, these adjustments won't miraculously give you a good night's sleep.

5. Keep reading, keep learning and stay curious about your sleep.

CHAPTER 5

You are not alone

Insomnia is lonely, but you are definitely not alone.

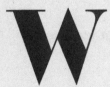hen I used to roam the house at 2 a.m. or sit staring out at the darkness, it was easy to feel lonesome. Like the mournful 'sessions of sweet silent thought' in Shakespeare's Sonnet 30, these dark and lonely hours were times I felt forlorn, isolated and forgotten. Why couldn't I be asleep like everyone else? It was night, for heaven's sake. I knew my husband and our daughter were in deepest slumber. Even our dear wee ginger cat was curled up asleep in her favoured cat-ball position. Across the neighbourhood, the street was deserted, the homes shrouded in darkness. With no lights glimmering, I was sure I was the only one still wide awake in the tiny hours. Everyone else was out to it, softly snoring or dreaming. Not another soul was up and about; it was just me and the moths. On nights like this, self-pity and self-blame would settle in. *What is wrong with me?* I'd think. *Why can everybody sleep except me?*

While the individual experience of insomnia is indeed solitary, the prevalence of poor sleep is astounding. Those suffering sleep problems are anything but alone. Each night people in every town, city and country all over the world share these symptoms. Sleeping poorly is staggeringly common, and insomnia is the most prevalent of all sleep disorders.[1] It's important to get perspective on this—it helps to recognise the scope of the problem worldwide and to know that sleep issues are shared across humanity.

Even Shakespeare's characters couldn't sleep

Shakespeare was an insightful observer of the human condition. Throughout his works he depicts numerous clinical disorders, including common sleep disorders.[2] His characters suffer from insomnia, sleep apnoea, sleepwalking and nightmares, making them achingly human. Lady Macbeth was a sleepwalker, and King Henry IV's nights were riddled with insomnia. 'How many thousand of my poorest subjects are at this hour asleep! O sleep, O gentle sleep,' he cries in *Henry IV, Part 2*. Sleep was a blessing denied to many of Shakespeare's characters.

According to Dr Ashley Bloomfield in the *Director-General of Health's Annual Report on the State of Public Health* (2017), nearly a third of adults in New Zealand are not getting the recommended amount of daily sleep.[3] Findings from key health insurers in New Zealand, which monitor health habits and lifestyle trends, reinforce this. In 2015, Sovereign Insurance (now AIA) conducted research that found a third of Kiwis report that they're not getting enough sleep or that the quality of their sleep is compromised.[4] Southern Cross Healthcare Group report over a quarter of adults feel tired or fatigued *every day*.[5] A study in 2019 using data from a survey tracking the health of 15,000 Kiwis revealed even higher figures, with 37 per cent of people reporting an average of less than 7 hours' sleep per night over the previous month (remember: 7 hours is the nightly *minimum* recommended for adults).[6]

If New Zealand's poor sleepers gathered together in one place, they would represent the entire population of the country's largest city, Auckland. Even so, each person with persistent sleep difficulties experiences it alone.

I feel annoyed and jealous. I know everyone else
has slept well, but I haven't. I have sleep envy.
—RACHEL (67, RETAIL MANAGER)

Across the Tasman, Australians are doing it hard too. A 2019 report for the Sleep Health Foundation provided robust insights on the prevalence of chronic insomnia among adults.[7] It found two of every five people had difficulty falling or staying asleep and exhibited daytime functioning issues, such as fatigue, exhaustion, compromised memory or concentration, irritability and reduced productivity. These combined symptoms are the main criteria for insomnia. More than half of these people had lifestyles that didn't allow enough opportunity to sleep most of the time, which means they were suffering from sleep deprivation. The remainder were struggling with sleep despite giving themselves an appropriate sleep window, so they were genuinely sleep deficient—meaning one in seven Australian adults in the study met the threshold for a clinical diagnosis of chronic insomnia.

And the figures don't stop there. The National Sleep Foundation in the US states that around one in three Americans has at least mild insomnia.[8] Director of the Stanford Sleep Epidemiology Research Center Dr Maurice Ohayon confirms, 'One third of the population is concerned over their sleepiness as it affects their lives and ability to perform their jobs.'

Dr Charles Morin puts the prevalence of sleep disorders in his home country of Canada at around 40 per cent, with nearly one in seven adults displaying the symptoms to diagnose chronic insomnia.[9]

People in the UK are also struggling. GP Online, an NHS England programme to support and inform general practice, estimates 30 to 50 per cent of the UK population are experiencing symptoms of insomnia, and around 8 to 12 per cent are expected to fit the criteria for chronic insomnia.[10]

The list goes on. The Philips 2019 Global Sleep Survey, representing Germany, France, the Netherlands, Canada, the US, Brazil, India, Japan, South Korea, China, Singapore and Australia, reports that 37 per cent of adults sampled across the world stated that insomnia was impacting their lives.[11]

The data has been gathered and the patterns are there—regardless of the country you live in, sleep difficulties are incredibly common. The World Sleep Society refers to the prevalence of sleep problems as a global epidemic.[12] The current estimated number of individuals living with insomnia around the world is 2 billion. (Oh, and I'd been thinking I was special!)

The World Sleep Society refers to sleeplessness as a global epidemic.

Sleep issues have been increasing over time, with numerous longitudinal studies tracking a steady upward trend in insomnia.[13, 14] Recently, the Covid-19 pandemic has been playing havoc with sleep on a global scale. Stress levels and fear are rising as the world experiences unprecedented levels of contagion, sickness and death. Ongoing anxiety about the pandemic and its disruption of daily schedules has been sabotaging sleep in many countries, making things worse for those with existing sleep difficulties and generating a new wave of people with troubled sleep. The pandemic has triggered a significant increase in the prevalence of acute and chronic sleep problems, making them even more common.[15]

While problems with sleeplessness are rife, most people would like to improve the quality of their sleep. The Philips Global Sleep Survey puts this figure at a handsome 80 per cent.[16] The challenge, of course, is *knowing* what to do to get results, then actually *doing* it. However, 60 per cent of these survey respondents who were keen to improve their sleep tend not to seek help from a medical professional.

In 2019 the Sleep Health Foundation report *Chronic Insomnia*

Disorder in Australia had similar findings, including the observation that 'relatively few Australians speak to healthcare professionals about sleep, despite almost half of the population reporting inadequate sleep'.[17] This was even the case for people experiencing symptoms consistent with chronic insomnia. We can be tight-lipped about our sleep problems, even when the situation is physically rough, emotionally raw and ongoing. The same report stated that more than half of those with insomnia that do visit a medical professional don't initiate discussions about sleep in their appointment, even though they may be feeling physically or emotionally unwell, aware of being sleepy or unfocused, or worried about their ability to do daily tasks like working or driving. A New Zealand study conducted in GP waiting rooms found that 41 per cent of patients visiting the doctor experienced difficulty sleeping (whether this was raised in their appointment or not).[18]

Reticence to visit or talk to a doctor about sleep may be linked with an underlying perception that the only option a doctor will offer is sleeping pills, which could be based on experience or suspicion—it may be true, it may be profoundly false. A recent trans-Tasman review of healthcare professionals, including GPs, nurses, psychologists and pharmacists, found that 'all healthcare disciplines currently receive limited training in addressing deficient sleep'.[19] Furthermore, it revealed that GPs and primary-care physicians in New Zealand and Australia 'have variable training, experience and skills in sleep disorder diagnosis and management'. So perhaps it's little wonder that a lot of people aren't taking a punt at the medical centre. The Philips Global Sleep Survey identified that two-thirds of people turn to Dr Google for information and help with their sleep rather than a physician or sleep specialist.

Among those people who *do* discuss sleeping difficulties with their doctor, many accept (even expect) the option of sleeping pills for an immediate reprieve from insomnia or other sleep disorders. In 2013 in the US, around 16 per cent of adults with a diagnosed sleep disorder used prescribed sleeping pills.[20] More recent figures in Australia put the occasional or regular use of prescribed sleeping medication at 19 per cent among adults exhibiting the symptoms of chronic insomnia.[21]

In my view, a lot of people with sleeping difficulties don't consider going to the doctor initially because they don't understand how vital sleep is, and they don't think anything can be done to help them (beyond sleeping pills). With this kind of thinking, it becomes difficult to justify the consultation fee. There isn't widespread public appreciation of the importance of sleep to physical and mental health, and awareness of different types of sleep disorders and treatment options is lacking. Only when sleep debt becomes dire or manifests as some other physical or mental health problem do people relent and make an appointment at their local medical centre.

Indeed, there is a tendency for those with sleep difficulties to suffer in silence. The National Sleep Foundation found that inaction on sleep issues is common, with two-thirds of Americans going for the 'shake it off' approach to sleepiness.[22] (Down under, our cultural equivalent is a bit less flamboyant and more stoic—we harden up and tough it out.) I fully support this high-spirited Taylor Swift 'shake it off' philosophy for some crap in life. However, it doesn't address persistent symptoms of sleep deficiency or resolve chronic insomnia.

Though sleep issues are pervasive, we don't open up and speak with one another about them. In modern culture, where incessant productivity prevails, mentioning your sleep issues—and the accompanying tiredness, lack of energy and poor concentration— feels like exposing yourself as substandard, weak or flawed. At work, it seems safer to keep it to yourself and get on with the job as best you can. Mentioning chronic sleep issues socially can feel like owning up to being drab, boring and no fun. (How many haggard-looking selfies do you see on your Facebook feed?) If you do risk bringing up chronic sleep difficulties, it can trigger well-meaning but unhelpful responses: pseudo-empathy ('Oh, I'm a bit tired too!'); questionable advice on quick fixes, sleep remedies and supplements ('You must try this great sleepy tea'); or, worse, pity. There are many good reasons to keep quiet about ongoing sleep challenges.

Another complicating factor is that many people aren't even

aware that they're short on sleep. They convince themselves that they 'only need' or 'can get by on' five or six hours a night. Sleep can erode gradually, and sleep deprivation sneaks up on people. Over time, they adjust to living on less, until short or poor-quality sleep becomes the baseline. They become accustomed to experiencing life with low levels of exhaustion, unaware of how their daytime functioning is impaired—mentally, physically or emotionally. Millions of people all over the world are unsuspectingly carrying out their lives in a suboptimal state, oblivious to the actual sleep needs of their bodies.[23]

While there are a few souls who genuinely flourish on little sleep (under 6 hours each night), they represent an infinitesimal proportion of society (a fraction of 1 per cent) and owe their short-sleeping super power to a rare gene.[24] For everyone else living on less than seven hours and feeling fine, scientific research makes it clear that they're kidding themselves. Down the track, the sleep debt will catch up with them and there will be a physiological and psychological day of reckoning. Yet it's common to have no clue that sleeping under 7 hours a night is not viable.

> *You do not know how sleep-deprived*
> *you are when you are sleep-deprived.*
> —*WHY WE SLEEP*, MATTHEW WALKER

Given all these factors—the lack of awareness about sleep deficiency and the prevalence of sleep problems; the tendency not to seek professional help; the real barriers to talking about sleeplessness among colleagues and friends—it's not surprising that so many of us feel isolated and despondent when sleep problems endure.

Like so many others, I made do with diminishing sleep, thinking I was okay. When my sleep duration, quality and continuity deteriorated to the point that it was clear there was a problem, I unconsciously adopted the silent harden-up approach, even though this made my difficulties worse. In the early days, I didn't think my sleep was 'bad enough' to warrant a trip to the doctor, and I had little faith in their ability to help as I wasn't keen on sleeping pills. I thought I knew what to do to sort myself out: I could take supplements, cut back the coffee, restrict alcohol, go to bed earlier, have a nap, listen to music, drink herb tea, do yoga, not watch TV too late, listen to a meditation app. I had plenty of things to try, and try I did. The problem was they didn't produce results, which led to greater frustration and entrenched my fear that there was no way out. I thought it was just me—my problem alone. I felt lost, helpless and on my own.

It turns out there's a crowd of around two billion of us! It's common to have sleep problems, it's common to suffer in silence, it's common to avoid seeing the doctor about it, and it's common to do nothing about it or try an array of mildly useless initiatives without success. Know that you are not alone. There is a well-researched path ahead and you are on your way.

Chapter recap: what you can do

1. Take comfort in the fact that you're not alone. Nearly one in three adults around you has problems sleeping.

2. Break the silence. Ask around trusted friends, family and colleagues to find who else in your circle is experiencing *ongoing* sleep difficulties (longer than three months). Share what you're discovering, and let them know they're not alone and there's a way forward. (Filter out any pseudo-helpful advice from those who haven't experienced *chronic* sleep problems—shake it off.)

3. Identify yourself as someone taking action. Having made it this far in the book, you are actively committed to sleep improvement. If you take ownership, your new habits (your sleep diary and continued learning) are more likely to stick. We're more successful when we believe new practices are part of who we are: 'I'm a person committed to improving my sleep.' Own it, and keep living it.

4. Continue completing your sleep diary each morning and review it at the end of the week. Give attention to *any* areas where your sleep has been a *little* better. Notice incremental improvements, where your sleep is heading in the right direction. You're looking for *progress*, not perfection.

5. Be curious and keep reading to discover that, while sleep issues are common, they are not 'normal'—they defy our biology, compromising our bodies, minds and spirits.

Supporting your sleep-improvement journey

LETTING GO OF 'TRYING' TO SLEEP

You may be feeling like you need to get stuck in and do something about your sleep. As frustrating as it is, you need to let go of the notion that your sleep is somehow broken and that you need to fix it. If you must *do* something, your job is to let go of trying to sleep.

The act of trying, in whatever form it takes—thought, behaviour, expectation—is a disaster. Trying means that you're exerting effort of some kind, even if your efforts are to lie still with your eyes closed. *Effort* creates tension and stress, which gets in the way of your body being able to fall asleep. A fixed goal—such as falling asleep—means that you have a set expectation and you're attached to that specific outcome. When you try to fall asleep, you unwittingly set up falling asleep as a performance; something that you must *try* to achieve. If you fail at your performance, you will be awake. You may be stressed by the prospect of being awake in the night or worried about the impact it will have tomorrow. Even though your goal is to look after yourself, this unintentionally creates *performance anxiety* about falling asleep. This causes internal stress that physiologically works against the possibility of sleep.

Exerting effort to sleep inhibits the natural sleep process. Sleep is not a matter of will—it occurs involuntarily. People who sleep well don't *try* to sleep. For them, sleep is not a performance or goal to be achieved each night. They don't have strategies to make sleep happen; sleep just occurs. If you ask a good sleeper how they get to sleep, they stare at you blankly, flummoxed that you asked such a question. Follow their lead. You mustn't try so hard—in fact, you need to allow yourself to let go.

ACTION WITHOUT EFFORT

The idea that you need to quit trying to sleep might sound absurd and counterintuitive, even alarming. Before you throw this book at the wall, consider giving the paradoxical-intention protocol a go. This is the idea that, rather than chase sleep, you must let it come to you. (Yup, you've got to play a little hard to get.)

This psychological technique has been around since the 1970s and is still recommended to people desperately trying to sleep. Dr Charles Morin and Professor Colin Espie include it in their clinical guide to treating insomnia.[26] If the term 'paradoxical intention' sounds confusing, think of it as a kind of reverse psychology—you're trying to outfox your own mind.

Morin and Espie suggest that you surrender all efforts to fall asleep and replace this with a gentle intention to remain passively awake for as long as you can.

Tonight, lying comfortably in bed with the lights out, keep your eyes open for as long as you can. When your eyes start to drift, or your eyelids begin to close, remind yourself to keep them open *just a little while longer*. Even if it feels like you're awake for ages, that's okay—that's what we're hoping for in this exercise, so you're doing well. Don't prevent sleep from overtaking you by actively rousing yourself—just play a little hard to get, and allow sleep to come to you. Give it a go, and see if it helps you let go of trying to fall asleep.

CHAPTER 6

Understanding sleep and insomnia

Knowledge is learning something every day.
Wisdom is letting go of something every day.
—UNKNOWN

You'll be all too familiar with what your own particular version of unsatisfying sleep looks and feels like. You know it intimately because it's horrible and you continue to make its acquaintance at night. But do you have a clear sense of what constitutes healthy sleep? Do you have realistic expectations of your sleep? The '8 hours of sleep a night' mantra has been drummed into us all, but you now know that this is only an average. In truth, there is a perfectly acceptable range of sleep durations. Striving for 8 hours is unnecessary and even futile for some, and efforts to achieve 8 hours of slumber when it's more than your body requires could create stress that makes nodding off more elusive.

What else have you been misinformed about or accidentally misconstrued? Where are the gaps in your knowledge about sleep? This chapter will help you get your bearings on how sleep works (or doesn't work), so you can start thinking about your sleep needs from a better-informed vantage.

With a deeper understanding of how sleep works, it becomes easier to grasp how insomnia can evolve. Struggling with chronic insomnia can feel like an endless cycle of deteriorating nights, efforts to improve the situation that get you nowhere, and outcomes that continually degrade your confidence in helping yourself. You must understand this cycle to reverse it—by being aware, or mindful, of your thinking and behaviour you can change it for the better.

The components of sleep

Duration is the most common yardstick used to monitor and judge sleep, but healthy sleep is officially comprised of three key elements—duration, continuity and depth. When working well and harmoniously, these elements combine to create healthy sleep that supports your body and mind in functioning optimally. For people with insomnia, reliability is also an incredibly important factor.

ELEMENTS OF SLEEP QUALITY

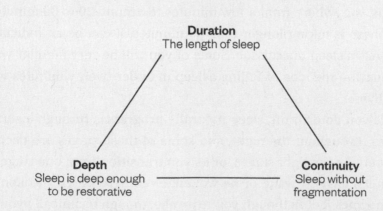

Duration
The length of sleep

Depth
Sleep is deep enough
to be restorative

Continuity
Sleep without
fragmentation

Duration

As outlined in Chapter 1, the National Sleep Foundation in the US recommends 7 to 9 hours of sleep overnight for adults aged from 18 to 64 years. For some adults, a total of 6 hours may be appropriate, but anything under this is not advisable on an ongoing basis. The recommendation for adults 65 years and over is 7 to 8 hours. (For some older folk, 5 to 6 hours may be appropriate.) You are most likely reading this book because your sleep duration routinely falls shy of these recommendations—you feel like you are absolutely not getting 'enough' sleep. However, it's essential to be realistic about the amount of sleep that you aspire to, and to also consider the quality of your sleep, not just the quantity. That's where continuity and depth come into play.

Continuity

It's common to imagine sleep continuity to be an idyllic experience of nodding off easily and sleeping right through the night without interruption. No forcing oneself to sleep, no random wake-ups, no hours of staring at the ceiling, no prowling the house. Just solid, non-stop slumber. While this is a sublime ideal, it's worthwhile understanding the process a little better.

Sleep continuity includes the process of falling asleep—the time it takes from lights out and settling down for the night to actually entering the first stage of sleep. This is sleep onset, and in healthy sleep this phase occurs quite quickly depending on how *sleepy* a person is—anywhere from a few minutes to around 20 to 30 minutes. If this phase is taking longer than 30 minutes, it can be an indicator that there's a sleep-onset issue. Some of you will be very familiar with this scenario—the idea of falling asleep in under twenty minutes will sound divine.

Once you do drift off, sleep naturally progresses through a series of stages throughout the night, and some of these stages are deeper than others. In the light stages, or as you transition from one stage to another, it's easy to wake or be woken. Even if you aren't woken, it can sometimes *feel* as though you're awake, though technically you're asleep. It's helpful to keep in mind that surfacing throughout the night is a natural part of the sleep experience. In healthy sleep, these periods of nocturnal wakefulness are brief, and may or may not be recalled.

When sleep is healthy, waking in the night is a low-key affair. You surface as you transition between sleep stages or awaken for practical reasons—a visit to the bathroom, a sip of water. There may be some adjusting of the body and bedding, followed by a simple settling before you drift back to sleep. There's no drama, just a gentle acceptance about surfacing as part of the sleep cycle and trusting patience as the next phase of sleep unfolds. There can be multiple brief awakenings throughout the night, even in healthy sleep. Some you will recall, others not. All up, night-time awakenings are likely to be under 30 minutes.

If you're experiencing insomnia, sleep can often be fragmented with periods of sleep interspersed by unwanted episodes of wakefulness. Some people have trouble with frequent brief awakenings, others struggle with one or two prolonged periods of being awake during the night. Some will struggle with early-morning awakenings—being awake at 4 a.m. or 5 a.m. and having difficulty falling back to sleep before the alarm.

For those with sleep-continuity issues, CBTi offers initiatives focused on knitting unravelled sleep back together to help with sleep onset and sleep maintenance. Later, as you work towards improved sleep continuity, remember that even healthy sleep can involve taking some time to fall asleep and can include brief interludes of waking in the night. Knowing that periods of lighter sleep and brief awakenings are a natural part of the sleep cycle can be reassuring, helping you to have a more realistic perspective on a good night's sleep and be less critical of your current sleep patterns.

Depth

Sleep occurs in a series of stages, cycling through lighter and deeper sleep repeatedly throughout the night. Each stage has different characteristics and is responsible for various functions necessary for restoring and caring for the mind, body and soul in preparation for the next day and in service of the long haul of a healthy life ahead.

The body needs the opportunity to cycle through each of these stages to wake feeling refreshed and restored. Throughout the night, particularly during deeper sleep, the body and brain attend to myriad functions, including physical renewal, hormonal regulation, growth, immunity, memory processing and emotion synthesis. REM sleep is the state where dreams are made and higher-level thought occurs.

In healthy sleep, a person naturally spends sufficient time in each of the sleep stages, to ensure they get the depth of sleep required. When sleep is abbreviated or interrupted, or you don't go entirely offline, it's more challenging for your body to take care of itself and perform to its potential. While you will get some core sleep, your body may not have as much time, continuity or depth to do all that can be done. Instead, it must improvise and make do in some of the caretaking, maintenance and optimisation work. Your body is smart and will do the best it can with the sleep it gets. While you'll be feeling far from fabulous on your current sleep, rest assured that your body is covering the basics.

Reliability

Reliability is the sense that you can depend on your sleep and have confidence in your ability to sleep. People who regularly experience healthy, quality sleep have an innate trust in their own sleep and their ability to sleep. For them, decent sleep is a given. It comes naturally most of the time, and if they have an unsettled or disrupted night they tend to be able to explain it objectively or brush it off as an anomaly. These are the annoying bright-eyed, bushy-tailed people we hear boasting, 'I'm a great sleeper, I always sleep well' and we feel a small part of ourselves shrivel and wither as we reflect on our troubles and deficiencies in this realm.

For those with persistent difficulties sleeping, sleep can seem unreliable, unpredictable and even untrustworthy. It can come with a sense of helplessness or disempowerment—the feeling that you can no longer relax and trust a fundamental bodily function because it seems erratic or fickle. By learning how sleep occurs, and repeatedly proving to yourself that progress is possible, your reliability will improve.

It may not be perfect, but you will be sufficiently knowledgeable to understand what is going on and confident that you can do things to support yourself.

> *So much of sleep lies in a person's confidence in their ability to sleep.*
>
> DR ALEX BARTLE, SLEEP WELL CLINIC

As you move through the programme, you can expect improvements in all areas of your sleep—duration, continuity, depth and reliability. There will be some aspects of sleep that are more important to you than others. For me, continuity, duration and reliability were priorities. I believed that, when I was asleep, I got some deep sleep. Falling asleep was fine at the start of the night, but maintaining sleep throughout the night was iffy, with long stretches of being awake during the wee hours and early-morning wake-ups. Plus, the reliability of my sleep was shot to ribbons. It was predictably unpredictable, which made it very difficult to be relaxed, especially on nights when I knew I needed to be on my game the following day. Understanding the components of sleep meant that I had some reassurance there were parts of my sleep that worked just fine (sleep onset and depth), and this gave me hope and a bit of a foothold. It also gave me clarity about the areas of my sleep that I wanted to improve, and I gained a more realistic perspective on what progress would look like.

The stages of sleep

When sleep is healthy, you go through the initial stage (N1) when your thoughts wander and your body surrenders in a transition towards sleep. You drift into a drowsy, relaxed state where you're not quite awake, yet don't feel as though you're asleep. Your breathing and heart rate slows, your eye movements decrease, and your muscle tension reduces. There's a drifting feeling of letting go. You may experience thought fragments, but you don't pay them much mind, and you might enjoy a sensation similar to daydreaming. It feels as though sleep is close, but you're not quite there. You may experience the odd body twitch (hypnic jerk), which jolts you briefly back to consciousness before you settle down again.

You're easily awakened from this state, and, if that happens, you'll maintain that you weren't actually asleep. In healthy sleep, the N1 stage lasts between 5 and 20 minutes, depending on your sleepiness. The sleepier you are, the faster you'll crash out when sleep is healthy.

After this initial stage of sleep, you'll transition through more stages of NREM (N2 and N3) and REM sleep. Don't be intimidated by the labels—they just refer to what your eyeballs are doing: while you're in NREM sleep, your eyes remain peaceful and still (non-rapid eye movement); and, you guessed it, in REM sleep your eyes dart about even though the lids are closed (rapid eye movement). When sleeping healthily, about three-quarters of the night is spent in NREM sleep, and the remainder is made up of REM sleep.

The characteristics of each sleep stage are briefly outlined below.

Sleep stage	Characteristics
N1 NREM: light sleep	The transition from being awake to the first stage of sleep A profound calm settles over the body Brain waves start slowing down Increasing detachment from thoughts and environment The brain makes a few attempts to hang on to awareness before tuning out Consciousness dissolves Loss of muscle activity Still reasonably easy to wake in this stage
N2 NREM: deep sleep	Brain activity changes to slow brainwave patterns Shut off from surroundings Breathing slows, heart rate and blood pressure decrease Body temperature drops More difficult to wake Most of the night is spent in this sleep stage
N3 NREM: deepest sleep	Brainwaves transition into a very slow pattern Shut off from the outside world Breathing, heart rate and blood pressure continue to decrease Entirely offline and very hard to wake

REM: dream sleep	Brainwaves escalate The mind becomes very active, similar to a waking brain Dreaming takes place Eyes move rapidly behind closed lids (following the dream action) Heart rate, blood pressure and breathing increase and can be irregular There may be slight finger and face twitches Large body muscles are virtually paralysed (so dreams can't be acted out, phew!) May wake after REM sleep and recall the dream

Throughout the night, a sleeper cycles through these four stages every 90 or so minutes. Ideally, about five of these cycles occur overnight, and the lengths of the stages vary. The first half of the night favours NREM sleep, and the second half leans towards REM sleep. But, whatever part of the night you sleep, in whatever fragments, your body will endeavour to cycle through and secure some of each sleep stage to do its best to look after you.

Matthew Walker, a British scientist and professor of neuroscience and psychology at University of California, Berkeley, who has dedicated most of his career to understanding the impact of sleep on human health, provides a helpful overview of what your brain is up to overnight during the NREM and REM phases, summarised below.[1]

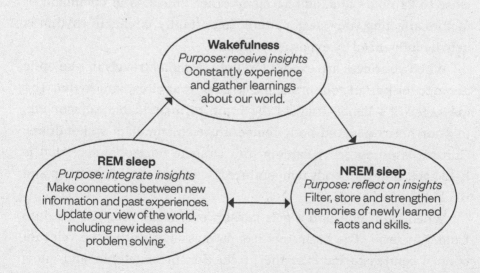

Wakefulness
Purpose: receive insights
Constantly experience and gather learnings about our world.

REM sleep
Purpose: integrate insights
Make connections between new information and past experiences. Update our view of the world, including new ideas and problem solving.

NREM sleep
Purpose: reflect on insights
Filter, store and strengthen memories of newly learned facts and skills.

Sleep is profoundly important to the ability to assimilate experiences in life so that you can effectively learn, grow and have a crack at life the next day. When I look at this cycle, it makes me think, *This is why so much of my life with insomnia felt like some weird melange of the movies* Groundhog Day *and* Memento. (In *Groundhog Day* Phil, played by Bill Murray, keeps reliving the same tedious day over and over, and in *Memento* Leonard, played by Guy Pearce, has a type of amnesia that means he can't form new memories.)

While your body and brain are doing what they can with the sleep they get, chances are you're feeling suboptimal these days. By improving your sleep, you'll be giving your body the opportunity to cycle naturally through the different stages of sleep, and spend plenty of uninterrupted time in each stage across the course of the night. The benefits of this will be evident in how you feel when you wake each day, as well as in your health and well-being longer term.

The two biological systems that regulate sleep

1. Circadian rhythm: the glorious body clock

Your circadian rhythm is a biological system driven by a part of your brain that plays a vital role in governing when your body wants to be awake and when it wants to sleep. This internal clock runs on a cycle close to 24 hours and, among many other things, is in command of factors affecting your sleep pattern. Importantly, circadian rhythm is heavily influenced by exposure to light.

When your eyes are exposed to light, a signal travels up the optic nerve to the part of your brain in charge of your circadian rhythm. The message—'it's light'—triggers the brain to make some adjustments to your hormones and body temperature to stimulate wakefulness. Cortisol is produced, melatonin (the Dracula hormone) secretion is held back, and your body temperature rises, so you feel pepped up and ready to go.

When night falls and it gets darker, your brain receives that info from your eyes. The brain then sends messages out to the relevant control centres to increase the production of melatonin and allow your body temperature to fall. The presence of the sleepy hormone combined with a cooler body temperature slows you down, and the sensation of sleepiness naturally unfurls.

To help healthy sleep occur, you need to work in harmony with your natural circadian rhythm. That means that you need to be mindful of your exposure to light (daylight or otherwise) so that it's working in sync with your body clock, rather than accidentally throwing your body out of time. In short: sunlight first thing in the morning and throughout the day is helpful, artificial light and blue light from screens before sleep is unhelpful.

People have inherent differences in their body clocks that affect when their bodies are naturally inclined to fall asleep and wake up each day. Overall sleep needs (duration, continuity and depth) are the same, but the timing of when sleep is best varies depending on whether you're a night owl or a morning lark. This natural pattern, or chronotype, is believed to be partly determined by genetics. One chronotype is no better than another: work and education schedules are geared in favour of morning people, but city nightlife is suited to evening people. I'm a morning person through and through—give me a 6 a.m. spin class any day over partying till 1 a.m. (I want to crawl into a hole and be asleep by midnight—even New Year's Eve is a challenge!)

2. Sleep–wake homeostasis: precious sleep pressure

The other key driver in sleep regulation, sleep–wake homeostasis, is a system that keeps track of your biological need to sleep.

As soon as you wake in the morning, your body helps you out by stimulating hormones (including cortisol) that kick you into gear for the day. At the same time, your body releases a chemical called adenosine that builds up in your brain during wakefulness. Adenosine quietly slows down brain activity, causing the feeling of drowsiness. First thing in the morning, when adenosine levels are low, you feel more alert. But, as the day goes on, adenosine levels rise, increasing your sleep pressure. The longer you're awake, the higher adenosine levels rise, and the drowsier you feel. When you've been awake for a long time, sleep pressure accumulates, and you feel an increasing desire to sleep. When you sleep, the adenosine breaks down and the cycle starts over the next day.

Sleep pressure also regulates the intensity of sleep required to stabilise the body. The longer you have been awake, the stronger the compulsion to sleep, which can cause a person with healthy sleep to sleep longer to bring their body back to its natural sleep–wake equilibrium. Furthermore—and this is the exciting bit—there's a self-correcting aspect of the system. In the case of sleep deprivation or sleep debt, the system encourages the body to *sleep deeper* to restore the balance. So, when you are underslept, stabilisation comes from the depth of the sleep your body instinctively induces, not merely from how long you sleep. When we think about catching up on lost sleep, we tend to think only of hours and minutes, but our bodies are smarter than that—they can generate deeper sleep to help compensate for sleep loss on our behalf!

The sleep–wake homeostasis system naturally strives towards ensuring that you maintain enough sleep overnight to get you through the hours of being awake. When it's working well, this restorative system means you feel most alert at the start of the day, then, as the day progresses, your wakefulness levels gradually wane as sleep pressure begins to build. Understanding that your body's inbuilt sleep–wake homeostasis system has an innate drive to balance your sleep and wakefulness is encouraging. Sleep is best thought of as a 24-hour cycle: your wakefulness during daylight hours matters just as much as your nights, and your daytime choices will affect how sleepy you are come nightfall.

These two remarkable biological systems have the capability to naturally regulate your sleep—biology has your back. Granted, they may not be operating how you would like at this point, but it's fortifying to know that Mother Nature is actually on your side. You just need to find a way to tune in to your biology and these systems will serve you as intended.

The cycle of insomnia

How it begins

Chronic insomnia generally kicks off as a seemingly harmless bout of short-term insomnia, often triggered by an identifiable cause. But, with sustained pressure, recurring stressors, or ongoing health or pain issues, insomnia can become unrelenting or make a comeback. The desire for sleep escalates and the inability to sleep restoratively creates stress, making sleep more elusive. You cast about trying different measures to improve your sleep but make little sustainable headway or unintentionally make things worse. Negative thoughts about the situation and your ability to sleep set in, your confidence in being able to sleep erodes, you start identifying yourself as a person with sleep difficulties or as an insomniac, and on and on it goes as you get increasingly desperate for sleep. The cycle that underlies your sleep difficulties is vicious and unforgiving, and it has been instrumental in allowing insomnia to take hold.

Unhelpful thoughts:
Focus on the negative and extrapolate—for example, I didn't sleep a wink ... today will be a disaster ... I won't cope ... I'm such a bad sleeper ... I've tried so many things but nothing works.

Unhelpful behaviour:
Take actions to get through the day or to sort out sleep that *unintentionally* perpetuate sleep difficulties or make them worse.

THE VICIOUS CYCLE OF POOR SLEEP

Unhelpful emotions:
Feel terrible—for example, worried, frustrated, stressed, disempowered, angry, desperate, afraid.

Seeking solutions and getting nowhere

In your attempts to cope with or combat ongoing insomnia, you might feel like you've tried countless options. Recall the items you mentioned back in Chapter 1, when you reviewed the ways you've been attempting to help yourself. Many compensatory strategies make sense at the time and seem like entirely reasonable initiatives. In fact, lots of them will have been suggested by well-meaning friends and family, or found online or in magazine articles. They may have been recommended at the chemist or health store, or perhaps they were the go-to solutions that 'everyone knows' for sleep difficulties.

For chronic sleep difficulties, many of these initiatives are ineffective or don't provide sustained improvement, and they contribute to stress about sleep. This is a fundamental pattern that keeps people stuck with insomnia. It's like an invisible force that traps you, even though you are conscientiously attempting to help yourself. It sucks.

Dr Moira Junge often tells her patients, 'This is the cruel irony of insomnia. In all other aspects of your life and health, it usually stands true that the more effort you put in, the better the results. But no, not with sleep.'

Many of the efforts we make to help ourselves perpetuate our insomnia.

Dr Michael Perlis, director of the Behavioral Sleep Medicine Program at the University of Pennsylvania, and his colleagues provide a helpful summary of common compensatory strategies that can perpetuate insomnia.[2] As you read through the list, tick those endeavours that you've tried. As you progress through the six-week programme we'll come back to many of these and unravel why they are hindering, not improving, your sleep, and you'll learn alternative strategies that will lead you towards better, more consistent sleep.

PERPETUATING FACTORS OF INSOMNIA

Extending sleep opportunity
- ☐ Going to bed early
- ☐ Sleeping in (waking up later)
- ☐ Napping

Counter-fatigue measures
- ☐ Increased use of stimulants—coffee, tea, chocolate, energy drinks, or cigarettes
- ☐ Using stimulants later in the day to get through
- ☐ Decreasing or avoiding physical activity to conserve energy

Sleep rituals and sleep strategies
- ☐ Increase in non-sleep behaviours in the bedroom to 'kill time', e.g., TV, phone, work
- ☐ Sleeping somewhere other than your own bed or bedroom—couch, spare room
- ☐ Use of 'special rituals' hoped to induce sleep, e.g., special herbs, teas [or, in my case, pixie dust]
- ☐ Avoidance of behaviours thought to hinder sleep, e.g., sex, exercise

Self-medication or sedation
- ☐ Increased alcohol intake or alcohol each night before bed (including a nightcap)
- ☐ Cannabis use
- ☐ Overuse of over-the-counter sedatives [hmm, that's my Blue Oblivion right there!]

When insomnia begets insomnia: common symptoms

People enduring persistent sleep difficulties often operate in **a state of hyperarousal.** This is a stress response that means the body and brain are running 'on alert' at all times.[3] You may experience it by day as rushing or pushing, being always 'on' or perpetually on edge—you might feel irritable and intolerant, or have difficulty concentrating and remembering things. By night it may manifest as an inability to switch off—even though you're knackered from months of shonky sleep, you're on high alert and can't seem to calm yourself down. It's that extraordinary feeling of being simultaneously 'tired and wired'—ready to fight or flee in a nanosecond. For some, it means powering through a to-do list despite insufficient sleep. For others it means being relentlessly busy while making little headway. Regardless of how hyperarousal plays out, it makes sleep (even a daytime nap) elusive and is simply not sustainable long term.

Another classic symptom of chronic insomnia is **a preoccupation with sleep**.[4] As my sleep deteriorated, I became obsessed. I started to think that I would never be able to sleep well. Fixating on sleep comes from a genuine desire to 'fix' the problem. You want to avoid anything that will make it worse and do all that you can to make it better. You may develop set routines and rituals that you refuse to deviate from in case it jeopardises your sleep. Indeed, it's possible to become a control freak about sleep—and I say that with love as I was in this group when my sleep truly bottomed out.

A touch of perfectionism can sometimes be adding to the insomnia cocktail. People with a high propensity to experience 'concern over their mistakes' or have 'doubts about their actions' can be predisposed to insomnia. Plus, these tendencies can feed into the persistence of sleep difficulties.[5]

People experiencing ongoing insomnia may have **a tendency towards overthinking**. This includes worrying or ruminating about sleep and fretting about the 'ghastly' daytime ramifications of sleep difficulties. This hawk-eye focus on sleep is problematic because such thinking is predominantly negative and unhelpful. It feeds into the cycle that you are trying to escape from.

All of these tendencies can be common when you're living with insomnia. If you're experiencing any version or hint of them, know that you're not alone. While hyperarousal, preoccupation with sleep, perfectionism and overthinking make sleep more challenging, it helps to be aware that they are in the mix. Accept that they are fairly standard for people with insomnia. Step back, create some breathing space for yourself, and work with what you've got. Understanding and accepting that these are just part of the journey gives you choices moving forward.

Reversing the cycle

In the late 1800s, the people of Chicago realised that the rivers flowing through the city and into Lake Michigan posed an ongoing threat to the water supply. The residents' drinking water came from the lake, yet the large waterways that ran through the city were at risk of being polluted by industry and sewage in an extreme weather event. Left unchecked, the natural flow of the rivers could become poisonous.

The good people of the city wanted to be able to confidently and safely drink water from the lake during good weather and storms. In an epic feat of civil engineering, the direction of the Chicago River system was reversed. Rather than running into the lake, the waterways now flow in the opposite direction, into the Mississippi River and journeying on to the Gulf of Mexico. A hundred years later, in 1999, this radical achievement was described as the 'Civil Engineering Monument of the Millennium' by the American Society of Civil Engineers.

Notice they did not stop the rivers—those rivers were always going to flow. The city used the natural power and flow of the rivers to their advantage. That's what you need to do. Your thoughts are like the rivers: they are incredibly powerful, but the direction they are currently flowing is unhelpful.

Look at things strategically. If you harness your propensity to focus on sleep and to overthink, you can use it as a strength. Use it to pause the cycle by seeing it for what it is, and actively apply your thinking to learning about insomnia, sleep and how to do things differently. Beneath your tiredness and exhaustion, you are intelligent, motivated and capable of reversing this cycle.

Central to this switch is *mindful awareness* of your thoughts, emotions and sensations. Be non-judgementally conscious of your current headspace and the state you are in. This will allow you the opportunity to make different choices moving forward.

Overthinking is generally not recommended, but, for now, use your tendency to overthink to your advantage. You might not be able to stop overthinking initially, but you can alter the course to use it constructively so that it no longer feeds a cycle that's unhelpful to your health and well-being. (In time, you will explore ways to reduce overthinking and quiet your busy mind, but for the moment embrace it and use it wisely.)

Helpful thoughts:
Learn about sleep, understanding how it works and what you can do to improve it. Focus on progress and realistic aspirations.

Helpful behaviour:
Take constructive actions to make the most of the day and create conditions conducive to sleep at night.

USING THE CYCLE TO IMPROVE SLEEP

Helpful emotions:
Feel encouraged, hopeful, inspired, empowered.

As you reorient your thinking about sleep, you must be kind to yourself. Sleep is fundamental to health and well-being, but most of us have never learned about it—what healthy sleep looks like, how sleep works and how it can unravel even when you are trying your best to help yourself. Even frontline healthcare professionals—GPs, psychologists, pharmacists and nurses—receive minimal education on sleep.[6] In the US and Canada, medical students receive an average 3.1 hours of training in sleep education, and indications are that training down under is similarly lacking.

Understanding what constitutes healthy sleep provides you with a more realistic perspective. Don't use it to harshly critique everything that is 'wrong' with your sleep or to reflect on how 'bad' things are—this will only add to feelings of frustration and failure. Instead, use your knowledge to notice *any* aspects of sleep that are working pretty well and any areas you'd like to make progress. Now you know how sleep works, cut yourself some slack. For instance, knowing that surfacing throughout the night is a natural part of the sleep cycle, or that having periods of sleep that seem light (almost as though you are awake) is natural, can make you feel much better about your sleep.

You have an opportunity to turn your thinking around. Instead of construing your tendency to overthink as a flaw, use it to your advantage to break the unhelpful cycle of insomnia. Instead of looking at your sleep as something that's derailed, start noticing things that are okay. Reassure yourself that you have excellent biological processes in place that are looking after you as best they can and *want* to help get you back on track. And, finally, have confidence that there is a proven process for working with your thoughts and actions that will provide you with momentum towards sleep improvement.

Chapter recap: what you can do

1. Celebrate. You have stepped back from the vicious cycle of insomnia, you've looked at it for what it is, and you know that you have what it takes to reverse it.

2. Focus on the positive. Note *any* aspects of your sleep that are actually okay, even if they are shaky. Focus on the areas of sleep where you'd like to see progress, while being realistic about what healthy sleep actually looks like.

3. Be kind to yourself. Cut yourself some slack—loads of medical students and frontline healthcare professionals have minimal sleep education. Know that it's common to adopt strategies that perpetuate insomnia.

4. Keep building your sleep-diary habit. By now you may have collected enough information to review the first week of your sleep diary—look out for any patterns, things that are helpful to your sleep, things that are unhelpful.

5. Keep reading, keep discovering and stay curious.

Supporting your sleep-improvement journey

BE PATIENT WITH THE PROCESS

You may be starting to get impatient at this point, itching to get on and start *doing* something about your sleep. While reading and monitoring baseline sleep may feel like nothing, trust me, it has incredible value. For now, you are quietly working on your thoughts and your headspace. This preparation phase may feel like a delay, yet it's quietly growing your impetus to begin.

Building curiosity about sleep and the possibility of sleep improvement creates an impulsion—an essential willingness to make valuable changes, a readiness to experiment with different thoughts, different ways. If you currently feel unsettled, it will serve you well. Breathe and be patient with yourself and the process. You *are* on your way. For now, the priority is to continue to calmly track your sleep and keep reading, learning, and opening your mind to new approaches.

DOING LESS CAN BE MORE

In *Insomnia: A clinical guide to assessment and treatment*, Dr Charles Morin and Professor Colin Espie refer to a process called 'thought-blocking'.[7] Right now the prospect of thinking of nothing, or completely clearing your mind, may seem impossible if not ridiculous. You will be very familiar with the relentless parade of intrusive thoughts that can arrive as you wait to fall asleep or when you lie awake staring at the ceiling in the night.

However, there's evidence that, if you give your mind something meaningless or mindless to do, a simple, stress-free task blocks the path of other thoughts. A process known as articulatory suppression means that while something is being said, memory can't work properly at the same time. It's almost as though, in this scenario, your brain can only hold one thought at a time.

Experiment with giving your mind an easy, repetitive task to do, or a word to say silently, so it's tricky for your memory to conjure up taxing things to think about. I've had success with slowly counting backwards from 50 or repeating the word 'rest' every couple of seconds for five minutes or so. (This may be why counting sheep is a thing for sleep!) It doesn't matter if your mind drifts off track: just gently escort it back to the no-stress job at hand.

CHAPTER 7

Finding your true north— prioritising sleep improvement

*You can't go back and make a new
start, but you can start right now
and make a brand-new ending.*

—JAMES R. SHERMAN

arly detection saves lives. It doesn't always save breasts. When I was diagnosed with breast cancer at 47, I was given the grim choice of having a mastectomy or taking a punt and waiting it out. The cancer was at an early stage, but there was a lot of it. If I delayed, there was a greater chance that it would get the upper hand and slip into my lymph system. When pressed, my specialist gave me the sobering odds of those pervasive precancer cells later cutting loose in my tissue and causing havoc: an estimated 80/20 in cancer's favour. I like to think I'm an optimist, but in this scenario I really didn't like my chances. If I postponed, I was staring down the barrel of not only a mastectomy but also chemotherapy, radiation and possibly the loss of my life.

I hate hospitals. I faint at the sight of blood, and I have a deep, deep fear of knives slicing through my flesh. I loved my well-worn but wonderful body as it was. There was no part of me that wanted to give the go-ahead to colossal surgery and deeply personal disfiguration. After extensive research and soul-searching, I knew what had to be done. I called it Operation Everest. It was my world's highest mountain, and it was an expedition that I absolutely did not want to be on. I knew I'd be climbing that final peak solo, and the air at the top would be thin.

To survive the ordeal, I had to have a reason, a driving purpose that was going to provide me with lasting motivation throughout the entire journey—not just to the summit, but safely home again. It needed to act as my true north, providing direction even when I felt disoriented and lost.

At that time, my daughter, Lily, was five and loving her first year of school. One day, when the dreaded first surgery date was looming, I sat nestled beside her on the daybed on our sunny deck, a library book poised in her small hands as she read out loud, every ounce of her committed to figuring out and forming those fledgling words. When she finished, she looked up, eyes sparkling, face beaming. I was so proud of her and so inspired by her. I looked at that beautiful soul with so much heart and so much life ahead of her, and my purpose became clear—I would do everything I could to make sure this girl would grow up with a mother.

It was this thought that I returned to time and again throughout the harrowing months of biopsies, surgeries, tests, mind-bending reconstruction and painfully slow rehab. The words 'Lily is not growing up without a mother' were like a talisman. They kept me going, kept me on track every day as I gradually recovered physically and emotionally. I got the all-important five-year all-clear a few years ago, and it feels so good to have that experience behind me. It taught me many things, and one of the most profound was that having a purpose that resonates throughout every fibre of your being makes even the impossible doable.

Knowing this, when it came time to deal with chronic insomnia, I instinctively applied the same approach. Trust me, learning how to sleep better is far easier than surviving a mastectomy and surgical reconstruction. Even so, when in the thick of sleep issues and feeling helpless and disempowered, the road ahead can look daunting—near impossible. It's all very well to be told that you must prioritise sleep; the big question is *how* do you prioritise sleep?

Being crystal clear about *why* you are embarking on your sleep-improvement journey makes it fundamentally easier and improves your chances of success.[1] It makes learning to sleep a priority and gives you lasting motivation. Not only does it help get you started, but it also strengthens your resolve, keeping you committed even if progress slows or you experience setbacks. Sleep recovery is non-linear—you need to be realistic and anticipate that there will be some frustrating and disheartening nights along the way. You want to go in well-equipped to keep at it, doing what needs to be done, till you reach the desired destination with your sleep patterns.

In this chapter, your job is to discover the true north for your sleep-improvement journey. There is a wide array of short- and long-term effects of sleep and insomnia that might matter to you. While reading, take note of any sleep benefits that resonate strongly ('Hell, yes!') or any insomnia risks that reverberate and rattle you *in a constructive way* ('Hell, no!').

According to Sigmund Freud, the founder of psychoanalysis, all human behaviour is motivated by the pain and pleasure principle. Whatever you do, you're either running away from pain or running towards pleasure. It doesn't matter whether you feel more motivated by avoiding the risks of sleep deficiency or by wanting to ace the rewards of better sleep. What matters is that you find something that will keep you on course. You will know it when you read it.

As a side gig throughout my life, I have studied and performed as an actor. Acting is doing; it is not pretending. You can't act truthfully from your head, working with what you think should move you. Instead, you must work from your heart, with what truly does move you. If you work from the heart, your acting becomes effortless and organic—you instinctively do what needs to be done. To empower yourself as an actor, you have to take a scenario and make it real for yourself. To do this, you find a way to make it very *personal* and very *specific*, and you put it *in your own words*.

My 'surmounting cancer' mantra was not a generic 'if I don't do this, I will die'. That was entirely meaningless to me, even though I thought it should compel me. It felt conceptual rather than real. But once I made it personal and specific, by thinking through the implications for Lily, the risk of my mortality started to have weight and depth. I played around with the wording of this notion until I struck a raw nerve—'growing up without a mother'. That hit home. I would do everything I could to prevent that from happening.

You will know when you are in the zone of something that has the potential to really motivate you. Then, make it personal and make it specific so that it really gets into you. Sometimes it's a matter of finding the right way to articulate *why*. Play around with the words— they are powerful.

You want to have a compelling purpose that will propel you all the way through your sleep-recovery journey, so let's take a look at the risks of insufficient sleep and the benefits of better sleep to help you find your mojo. This summary draws on Matthew Walker's fascinating book, *Why We Sleep*.[2]

As you read on, make sure you take the information in the way that it's intended—to help you find your *why*. These risks and benefits are scientifically proven, but some of them will matter to you and others will seem less personally compelling. Still other insights may help explain your experiences.

A big note of caution: do not look at this list in its entirety and get freaked out. That would be entirely counterproductive—it will add to your stress and make sleep more elusive. Stay positive—you are here reading this book, educating yourself about sleep and preparing to actively improve your sleep. Go, you! Use this list as a tool only, to find the *why* that will make you prioritise sleep improvement.

Some of you may be wondering if my years of compromised sleep caused breast cancer. From everything I have read on the topic, there is no *causal* link between sleep deficiency and cancer, or any of the other long-term health impacts outlined below. There are correlations between being underslept and an increased probability of these health conditions—but they are links, not causes. This is an important distinction. Poor sleep does not *cause* terrible health outcomes. Instead, improving your sleep reduces some key health risks, giving yourself better odds of shoring up your longevity and your future self's quality of life.

Before getting to the significant long-term gains of sorting your sleep, let's check in with the here and now. What's in it for you in the short term? The quick wins, if you like.

Short-term insomnia risks and sleep benefits

Physical

Food consumption and weight stability

On those days after your sleep has been especially sketchy, you might have noticed your appetite, cravings and eating behaviour go haywire and, at the time, you don't really care! Several biological factors are going on behind the scenes to make this happen. When you reach for a second piece of ginger crunch in the afternoon and it seems a brilliant idea, you're not being greedy or weak-willed. Lack of sleep has hijacked your body's natural food desires *and* your mind's ability to override and regulate things. It affects your feelings of hunger, your ability to feel full, your cravings and even the types of food that you gravitate towards.

> *The less you sleep, the more*
> *likely you are to eat.*
> —MATTHEW WALKER

Inadequate sleep can interfere with the balance of two appetite-controlling hormones—ghrelin and leptin.[3] Ghrelin triggers a strong feeling of hunger and a desire to eat. Leptin signals satiety and lets your body know when it's had enough. Even a couple of days of short sleep can interfere with the balance of these helpful hormones, whether it's more ghrelin making your body cry hunger, less leptin obscuring your sense of feeling replete, or some crazy combo of the two. When you are shy on sleep, you're likely to want to eat more—and even when you do you may not feel satisfied. Bring on the buffet!

Short sleep can also increase levels of endocannabinoids circulating in your bloodstream.[4] This groovy chemical triggers your appetite and your desire to snack, snack, snack. When this happens, you may feel like you have the munchies and catch yourself patrolling the pantry, endlessly grazing the fridge, or with your hand deep in a box of high-sugar cereal.

There's likely an unhealthy shift in the type of food you eat when sleep deficient, too. Rather than tucking into a big salad and some grilled fish, a person short of sleep is more likely to be pulled towards high-sugar, high-carb or salty snacks. In Walker's research, this altered food preference was explained by unhelpful changes to parts of the brain. The region controlling judgements and decision-making is muted by a lack of sleep, and, without your prefrontal cortex diligently supervising your behaviour, cake, biscuits, chocolate, bread, pasta and chips can seem like excellent options. (Or you may know they're not great choices but go for them anyway!)

Many factors affect what happens on the scales, but sleep is definitely a contributing factor. The impact of short sleep on food consumption increases your probability of gaining weight. What's more, trying to effectively lose weight while wrestling with insomnia is more difficult. Research shows that, on a strict low-calorie diet, people can lose weight when they are underslept, but the body tends to shed most of the weight from the lean body mass, not from fat stores.

While suboptimal sleep can sabotage our good intentions when it comes to food and nutrition, sleeping well helps bring the appetite back to equilibrium. It restores the balance of your hunger or satiety hormones, keeps the 'munchies' chemical at bay, and restores the impulse-control part of your brain. Good sleep provides a stronger biological and neurological foundation for food consumption—it will support you in making better choices about what to eat, how much to eat and when to step away from the kitchen.

Does this matter to you? If yes, be specific about why.

☐ _____

_____

Exercise: the likelihood of getting out there

The less you sleep, the less likely you are to feel like putting on your Lycra. When you're tired and fatigued, the prospect of a run or an exercise class seems too hard and horrible; you want to conserve the little energy you have for the essentials. Research shows that people with insomnia symptoms are less active and tend to have lower cardiovascular fitness.[5] Short sleepers also tend to be more sedentary. With less activity, there's less energy used, meaning fewer calories get burned up. Improving your sleep will improve your chances of feeling inclined to get your body moving.

Does this matter to you? If yes, be specific about why.

☐ _____

_____

Exercise: physical performance

Nothing beats sleeping well before exercise to enhance your performance. Sleep has been shown to significantly improve motor skills across a wide variety of sports. It helps with coordination, reaction times, stamina and strength. Post-performance, a decent night's sleep supports physical recovery—including muscle repair and inflammation recovery.

Conversely, athletes getting less than 8 hours of sleep a night prior to performance, and especially those getting less than 6 hours, don't do so well. They tend to get physically exhausted faster, and have lower aerobic output and decreased muscle strength. They can't jump as high or throw as far. So forgive yourself if you're not operating at peak levels—improving your sleep will help you realise your performance potential.

Does this matter to you? If yes, be specific about why.

☐ _____

_____

Accidents and injury

Whether on or off the sports field, the likelihood of having an accident or being physically injured is higher if you haven't slept well. You're probably already familiar with bumps and bruises due to dumb-clumsiness from being mildly uncoordinated after a night or two of substandard sleep. If you're playing sports, operating machinery or driving a vehicle, the risks are higher—reaction times are slower and the outcome can be dire.

Concentration is seriously compromised by sleep deprivation. Even being a bit shy on sleep makes it easy for the mind to wander, but being chronically sleep restricted puts you at risk of having microsleeps. These are momentary lapses in concentration, where for just a few seconds your eyelids partially or fully close, and you nod off. For the briefest moment you become oblivious to the world around you, and all of your senses—sight, sound, smell, taste, touch—go entirely offline. Yep, total blackout. In those brief seconds that you're out to it, you don't have a clue what's going on, and, more critically, you have no 'decisive control of motor actions'.[6]

This doesn't matter so much if you're in the comfort and safety of your lounge, but if your microsleep occurs when you're behind the wheel of a car, those two seconds can be fatal. Roadside billboards encouraging you to stay awake and not drive tired are there for a damn good reason. As is the case elsewhere, vehicle crashes rank highly among leading causes of death in New Zealand.[7] A New Zealand Ministry of Transport investigation into motor-vehicle crashes found that one in ten fatal crashes is caused by fatigue alone—no alcohol, no speed, just fatigue.[8] Furthermore, in one out of every two fatigue-related crashes where the driver dies, a passenger or another road user dies too.

To put driving under the influence of too little sleep into perspective, consider this: the National Sleep Foundation in the US describes drowsy driving as similar to drink-driving. Being awake for eighteen hours straight makes you drive like you have a blood-alcohol level of 0.05 grams per 100 millilitres. This is the legal blood-alcohol limit for driving in both New Zealand and Australia. For those with persistent sleep difficulties, it's pretty easy to clock up several days in a row when you've been awake for over eighteen hours.

Improving your sleep is vital to keeping you physically safe. Better sleep reduces the risk of accident and injury. When it comes to driving, being well slept is a responsibility. It gives you a much better chance of keeping yourself and your loved ones alive on the road and helps to prevent accidents that may haunt you.

Does this matter to you? If yes, be specific about why.

☐ _____

_____

Immunity

Experiencing recurring coughs and colds, or coming down with the flu more often than is usual, is a common complaint among those getting by on insufficient sleep. Throughout my foggy years of addled sleep, there were winters when I felt like I was always coming down with something or just couldn't get rid of my cold.

Sleep and immunity go hand in hand. People who are underslept are more likely to have compromised immunity. Lack of sleep can make your body more susceptible to picking up viruses and infections, and less resilient in shaking them off. Research shows that after exposure to the common cold virus, infection rates are considerably higher among people who have been sleeping about 5 hours a night in the week prior (almost 50 per cent), compared to those who've enjoyed 7 or more hours a night (only 18 per cent).[9]

Improving your sleep gives you greater protection from common infections. And, if you do succumb to a bug, better sleep supports your immune system in fighting against the illness and getting you well again more quickly. It's no coincidence that, when you do get sick, your body demands that you crawl into bed and sleep.

Does this matter to you? If yes, be specific about why.

☐ _____

_____

Libido

You'll be all too aware that insufficient sleep leaves you feeling tired, exhausted and generally not that fabulous, and this interferes with your ability to feel in the mood for anything beyond a good night's sleep. Your priority is sleep, not sex. If your partner happens to be a good sleeper who crashes out instantly after making love, it's easy to run with the 'Not tonight, darling, I have resentment' strategy. If you're a bloke, being underslept reduces levels of testosterone, dulling your libido and the likelihood of a great sex life.[10] But all is not lost—improving your sleep can help awaken your libido.

Does this matter to you? If yes, be specific about why.

☐ _____

_____

Mental and emotional

Focus and concentration

It doesn't take much of a reduction in sleep for your focus and concentration to crumble. You will know from experience that you simply aren't as sharp and on to it following a night of shabby sleep, and that your attention span deteriorates markedly with each subsequent night of iffy sleep. Drifting away with the fairies and trying to haul yourself back on task may be an all-too-familiar feeling.

Restricted sleep not only creates confusion, it also slows reaction times and, more concerningly, it causes brief interludes where you stop responding altogether. Sleep deficiency doesn't have to be extreme for these lapses of concentration to kick in, as demonstrated in an experiment measuring reaction times and response lapses in participants enduring different levels of sleep deprivation, recounted in Walker's book. Those lucky folk in the research group enjoying 8 hours of sleep each night performed consistently well throughout the two weeks of testing. As could be expected, the performance of those who had to stay awake all night was a disaster. Their concentration lapses increased by 400 per cent after one night, and the incidence of microsleeps got progressively worse with each night without sleep. Surprisingly, the concentration of people getting 6 hours of sleep a night became so severely impaired after ten nights that they performed as poorly as the group of people who had pulled that first all-nighter. (Six hours of sleep a night for ten nights can seem highly aspirational to people with sleep difficulties.)

Retraining yourself in the art of sleeping well will help to improve your ability to focus and concentrate on the tasks at hand. The ability to stay mentally with it and on track is central to productivity. With decent, regular sleep, you'll be in a much stronger position to power through your to-do list efficiently.

Does this matter to you? If yes, be specific about why.

☐ _____

_____

Memory

Overnight, if you give your body sufficient time and depth of uninterrupted slumber, your brain can efficiently perform some truly incredible tasks. During sleep, your mind:

- **sifts** through your short-term memory bank (your hippocampus) and reviews the information that you have acquired that day
- **filters** out the facts that are no longer needed and disposes of them
- **identifies** the facts and information tagged as keepers, and
- **transfers** these valuable short-term memories to the more permanent long-term storage site in the brain (the cortex), carefully preserving them so you don't forget.

By doing this each night, your brain wakes refreshed. Sleep enables you to clear space in the short-term memory bank, so there is storage capacity for new learning tomorrow. Plus, it allows you to convert important information to long-term memories, so that you have a rich archive of life learnings that you can use for future reference.

Keep in perspective that this is a *nightly* process of clearing, creating space for new learning and consolidating information so that it's not forgotten. This has implications for studying, learning and growing as a person. The neuroscience makes clear that you are better able to absorb new information on a day after you have slept well, and you will better retain what you learn in a day if you have a decent sleep that night.

Some days following nights of dreadful sleep, I felt like my brain had turned to mush. I was befuddled, forgetful and couldn't think straight—it felt like my IQ dropped radically with a succession of broken nights. At these times, my workdays were challenging—I'd have to work longer hours and try so much harder just to do the expected amount of work. I set high standards for myself, and I worried the quality of my work was underwhelming. It was reassuring to learn that this was not some personal flaw or a sign of dementia—it was just one of the many neurological consequences of undersleeping.

Improving your sleep allows you to improve your memory, expanding your capacity to learn and grow and, equally importantly, strengthening your ability to remember.

Does this matter to you? If yes, be specific about why.

☐ _____

_____

Creativity

During sleep, your brain does an incredible, borderline magical, thing on your behalf. In the REM sleep stage, when dreaming occurs, your brain throws together a fantastical concoction of fragments of information from your memory warehouse. It wantonly puts together disparate ideas and far-flung facts to see what flies. This process defies the logic of the waking brain and daytime inhibitions, exploring possibilities and helping to solve problems beyond your daylight capabilities.

This process can often seem like nonsense, but sometimes on waking there is a real Eureka moment to celebrate. You may have experienced this, when you struggle with a problem, give up working on it in frustration and decide to sleep on it. In the morning, you discover a viable solution thanks to the nocturnal efforts of the subconscious mind.

Does this matter to you? If yes, be specific about why.

☐ _____

_____

Mood and emotions

Those who have lived with sleep deficiency know the impact it can have on mood. Lack of sleep can take you down into the pit, hoist you up to a delirious high, have you operating on an extremely short fuse or make you vacillate wildly across the spectrum. Undersleeping plays havoc with moods and emotional reactivity—to the point where you may not feel like yourself. It's disorienting and awful for those who are living it, and no one feels good about the impact it has on those nearby. Partners, children, friends and colleagues can all be affected by the fallout.

How lack of sleep messes with emotions

Moods, mood swings and reactivity are based on biology rather than feeling. Know that it's not something wrong with you and it's not that you need to get a grip.

Sleep deprivation can affect the brain in the following ways.

- **Angry or afraid?** The amygdala, a primitive part of the brain that triggers strong emotions, is highly reactive to negative stimulus. It is linked to the fight-or-flight response and revs you into gear when it perceives danger or threats, and it can fire you into anger, rage, aggression and hostility.

- **Excited or exuberant?** The striatum, an emotional centre associated with impulsivity and reward that's bathed in the 'feel good' chemical dopamine, can go into overdrive, making you hypersensitive to pleasurable experiences.

- **No filter?** The part of the brain responsible for rational, logical thinking and decision-making (the prefrontal cortex) loses its usual connection with the amygdala and striatum. This takes away the brain's ability to reality-check and restrain any over-the-top or out-of-line emotional responses.

The moods and reactivity you experience with insufficient sleep depend on how your brain is being affected. It's very complicated, and the effects can be extreme. While volatility does come with the territory with insomnia, if you or those close to you feel that your moods and emotional reactivity are extreme or concerning, please seek professional help (relevant resources are provided in Appendix III).

Resolving your sleep challenges may help calm the emotional centres in your brain, returning them to a more manageable and predictable emotional equilibrium.

Does this matter to you? If yes, be specific about why.

☐ _____

_____

Anxiety and depression

Unsurprisingly, given the effect of sleep on mood, ongoing insomnia is associated with increased symptoms of anxiety and depression. Initially this may manifest as being worried or stressed out, or feeling down about things, but over time inadequate sleep can really take a toll on mental well-being.

Insomnia and depression often coincide. While poor sleep can be a symptom of depression, insomnia can increase your risk of depression. When negative moods become extreme or pervasive, the situation can deteriorate into debilitating feelings of worthlessness, helplessness and hopelessness. None of us want to go there if we can help it.

Improving sleep can help prevent the development of depression, and, if depression has already taken hold, improved sleep can alleviate the symptoms." The same holds true for anxiety.

Does this matter to you? If yes, be specific about why.

☐ _____

_____

Take a moment to review the short-term risks and benefits that have resonated with you. Do they affect your quality of life? Your ability to be the person you want to be, as a partner, parent, employee or friend? How do they affect your ability to achieve what you want for yourself in this life? Consider how these sleep impacts may be holding you back or, conversely, how they could transform your life. Remember: the more personal and specific you can be, the more powerful your *why* will be.

Much of this process is about waking yourself up. When you are sleep deficient, you can become very adept at getting by on limited sleep. You can become oblivious to how it's affecting you and those around you. You may not notice that your world has shrunk or that your aspirations are muted.

You may have already identified some key insomnia risks or sleep benefits that really resonate with you. These may be sufficient for you to prioritise sleep and give you the momentum you need to commit fully to improving your sleep. If you haven't yet found something that will drive you forward on this journey, read on—your true north may lie in the longer-term impacts of sleep on your life.

Case study: Donna

A couple of years ago, I worked through this process with Donna, who had been struggling with her sleep for a year or so. She just wanted to fix her sleep and she was keen to get on with the programme.

As we explored what was behind her need to improve her sleep, she discovered that, deep down, she worried she wasn't being the mum she wanted to be to her two young children. While she fed, clothed and took good care of her kids, she realised she wasn't wholeheartedly there for them—she lacked energy, her moods were a bit off, she got impatient at times, and she preferred resting to playing with them. As a mum, she felt that she had 'lost her happy'.

This revelation was a game changer for Donna. She wanted her kids to have more of her than that. With a clear true north, she committed 100 per cent to the sleep-improvement programme and transformed her nights and her days in under six weeks.

Long-term insomnia risks and sleep benefits

Physical

Virility and fertility

If you and your partner are in the baby-making mode, slipping between the sheets is obviously a priority—not just for great sex, but for great sleep too. Getting sufficient shut-eye helps with a healthy libido, as you know, but Walker also cites studies in his book that highlight how vital sleep is for reproductive health. For guys, sleeping too little or having poor-quality sleep can contribute to a considerably lower sperm count. For women, routinely sleeping less than 6 hours a night is associated with a notable drop in follicular-releasing hormone (this hormone peaks before ovulation and is necessary for conception).

If both partners lack sleep, achieving conception can be even more challenging, and delays and difficulty with conception are heartbreaking. The epidemic of sleep deprivation is linked to subfertility or infertility, which makes improving your sleep a high priority if you're planning a family.

Does this matter to you? If yes, be specific about why.

☐ _____

_____

Obesity

Given the impact of sleep loss on food-consumption behaviour, the propensity to exercise, and weight gain, increased risk of obesity is not a surprising outcome for ongoing sleep deficiency. While many factors contribute to obesity, there is longitudinal evidence that sleep loss is a factor. Over time, people who sleep less have a higher likelihood of being overweight or obese.

Mastering sleep gives you a better chance of being able to manage your food consumption and physical activity levels, and avoid accidental weight gain.

Does this matter to you? If yes, be specific about why.

☐ _____

_____

Diabetes

Short sleep can impair the body's ability to regulate blood-sugar levels. Blood sugar, or glucose, circulating in the body is essential, provided it's kept in balance. When you eat, your blood-sugar levels naturally increase, and in a healthy, well-slept body the hormone insulin will trigger cells to absorb excess blood sugar, making sure that glucose is kept within safe and helpful levels. When you are underslept, your cells can become less receptive to insulin—almost like they start ignoring the message to drain surplus glucose from the bloodstream. Excessive blood sugar puts the body into a prediabetic state of hyperglycaemia. If this condition persists, the body can develop type 2 diabetes over time. Over weeks or years, excess blood sugar is harmful to body tissue and can eventually damage organs.

Chronic sleep deprivation is now recognised as a significant contributor to type 2 diabetes. Currently, 5 per cent of the New Zealand population is diagnosed with diabetes, 90 per cent of these people have type 2, and it's estimated that one in four people are living with undiagnosed prediabetes.[12] Based on self-reported data collected in 2017–18, it's estimated that 4.9 per cent of Australians have diabetes.[13]

While there are other variables at play in diabetes (many of which are predetermined), improving your sleep removes a contributing factor. Sleep is one area where you can help yourself towards prevention.

Does this matter to you? If yes, be specific about why.

☐ _____

_____

Heart attack and stroke

Sleep loss adds an unhealthy load to the cardiovascular system. Being underslept can increase your heart rate and raise your blood pressure.

Staggeringly, it doesn't take much sleep loss for these effects to occur. Even being short of a few hours of sleep each night puts more pressure on your cardiovascular system, thanks to the effect of sleep loss on the sympathetic nervous system.

The sympathetic nervous system is responsible for the fight-or-flight response. When you instinctively believe you are under threat or your life is at risk, the sympathetic nervous system kicks into top gear to help save you from the perceived danger (physical or psychological). The system can trigger action from numerous parts of the body, such as breathing, stress chemicals (like cortisol), blood pressure, heart rate—whatever it takes to get you mobilised into saving yourself. Back in the day, when humans had to be on the lookout for sabretooth tigers loitering around the cave, this was incredibly helpful. These days, when threats are not so life-or-death, you'd hope the sympathetic nervous system might chill out a bit, but no. Our superintelligent bodies see lack of sleep as a life-or-death issue and go into overdrive.

The problem is, this system is only supposed to be activated for a relatively short time to solve the crisis at hand (slay the tiger or sprint into the cave and hide). When sleep loss is not being remedied, the sympathetic nervous system vigilantly remains 'on'. When a person is underslept, their sympathetic nervous system will be overactive, and it stays that way until sleep deficiency is resolved.

Being in a state where the sympathetic nervous system is supercharged and stuck on puts additional strain on the body. Over time it takes its toll, and it can wreak hell with the cardiovascular system— blood pressure, heart rate, calcification of arteries, constriction of blood vessels. When left unchecked, this can increase the likelihood of a heart attack or stroke down the track.

We love our hearts, we love our brains—we need them for the long haul and we can choose to look after them. Calming your nervous system and improving your sleep is crucial to support your body in healing the cardiovascular system, doing what you can to keep clear of life-threatening cardiovascular diseases.

Does this matter to you? If yes, be specific about why.

☐ _____

_____

Cancer

Nobody likes the C-word. As one of the leading causes of disease and death in developed nations, cancer strikes fear in the heart. It's horrifying for anyone facing a cancer diagnosis—the arduous treatment, the uncertainty and the prognosis. I know, I lived it, and I was on the low-key, 'lucky' end of the spectrum.

There is still more to discover about cancer—how to prevent it, how to slow its growth and spread, how to help the body fight it. But we do know some things already about the role sleep plays with this disease, and it makes a strong case for improving sleep.

Regularly sleeping well strengthens your immune system, and, in the case of cancer, strong immunity is vital. Within your immune system, you have natural killer (NK) cells (yes, this is their official medical name—I double-checked!), which are like the elite force when it comes to white blood cells. Among other things, NK cells can target cancer cells, pierce their surface and inject a protein that destroys malignancy. With healthy sleep, we have strong reserves of these incredible immunity cells. But, if sleep is compromised, it can markedly reduce the numbers of these heroic bad boys.[14]

We know insufficient sleep fires up the sympathetic nervous system, and this can create a sustained inflammation response from the immune system. While inflammation has a temporary role to play in looking after you when needed (e.g., in anticipation of the tiger fight), if it remains on and you stay in a chronic state of non-specific inflammation, you are susceptible to numerous health problems. And cancer cells have been found to cunningly use inflammation to their advantage—to help with tumour growth and spread.

Improving your sleep is an important step to take in the battle against cancer. Sleeping well can reduce the risk of developing cancer, and, if cancer does occur, it puts your immune system in a stronger position to stymie the survival and growth of these dangerous cells.

Does this matter to you? If yes, be specific about why.

☐ _____

_____

Mental

Alzheimer's disease

Alzheimer's, the most common form of dementia, is suffered by one in ten adults over 65, and the World Health Organization projects that the prevalence of this disease will continue to rise.[15] Sleep disruption has long been recognised as an early indicator and symptom of the disease, but insufficient sleep is now also being investigated as a risk factor.

Alzheimer's disease is associated with build-up of a toxic protein within the brain. These amyloid proteins form into sticky clumps, or plaques, which are poisonous to the surrounding brain cells—they kill them.

Each night during sleep, an amazing cleansing process occurs in the brain. There is an extensive network called the glymphatic system within the brain, made up of glial cells, which collects and drains waste and contaminants that are by-products of brain activity. While the system does some daytime cleaning, it does its heavy-duty sanitation overnight. One of the toxic wastes that the system flushes out during deep sleep is that troublesome, sticky amyloid protein.

Without sufficient sleep, these toxic proteins build up in the brain. In a cruel twist, the proteins tend to build up in the area of the brain that is responsible for generating the deep sleep needed to activate the cleaning system (deep NREM).

While there is more neurological research being conducted in this area, already there are strong signals that prioritising sleep throughout our lives is one essential variable in reducing the risk of Alzheimer's disease.

Does this matter to you? If yes, be specific about why.

☐ _____

_____

If, having read through this chapter, you're still searching for your *why*, consider the impact insomnia is having on your sense of self—your identity and feeling of agency in your life. In my experience, the overarching risks that insomnia poses to a person's sense of self (or the opportunities that improved sleep offers) can be critical in helping an individual to truly prioritise their sleep.

Identity

Over time, compromised sleep can leave you feeling like you're not yourself. It might be hard to articulate to an outsider, but it can feel like you are less than you were, as though you are there in person but not in spirit. I felt like I was almost a ghost or hologram of myself while sleep deprived. I was going through the motions of life, rather than living it heart and soul. I'd drifted into a state of getting through life, rather than truly embracing it.

Years later, when I read some of Brené Brown's insightful work, the term 'wholehearted' really stood out to me.[16] When you are once again consistently sleeping well, it feels like you have come home to yourself and you are living your life wholeheartedly, whereas on insufficient sleep it can feel like you're living half-heartedly.

Sleep allows you to feel like you're your whole self once again—fully present, fully engaged, unstoppable.

Does this matter to you? If yes, be specific about why.

☐ _____

_____

Agency

After years of living on insufficient sleep, I felt like I had lost momentum in my own life. It was like being on a treadmill: I couldn't gather the internal resources to break free and move forward in a meaningful direction. I felt powerless to make change. If I did get my act together to get clarity on what I wanted, I couldn't find the inner strength and resolve to make things happen. I began to feel like a passenger in my own life rather than the driver.

Once I had a clear purpose and had made learning to sleep a priority, things started to change. Committing fully to learning to sleep gave me focus and direction that truly mattered. Then, as my sleep improved, I gained confidence in my ability to go after what I wanted and actually make things happen in my life. I developed a strong sense of agency, which has proved invaluable. I don't know if it was sleep itself or learning how to sleep that created this, but now that I've found that self-determination I'm never going back.

Does this matter to you? If yes, be specific about why.

☐ _____

_____

Prioritising sleep and being clear on your motivation gets your mojo working. It will help you do what needs to be done to improve your sleep. (Even when what needs to be done is sometimes doing less and not trying so hard!)

Remember that the path to improved sleep is quite a pilgrimage. For some people, having a clear motivation may not be enough to implement and sustain all the behavioural changes and mental shifts needed to resolve persistent sleep difficulties. If that turns out to be your scenario, it's all good. Hold on to your true north and call in reinforcements. CBTi with professional support is another option that you can explore to make the journey easier.

Chapter recap: what you can do

1. Reflect on the insomnia risks and sleep opportunities that resonate. Revisit them and identify the ones that matter most to you. Narrow down your list.

2. Explore your list from different angles. Notice if things have more power when you look at them as risks or opportunities. Let your imagination play with this. Explore your fears or fantasies to make the purpose more meaningful—make the scenario *personal* and *specific*.

3. Select the *why* that hits home, and hone it. Explore different ways of articulating it, until it feels 100 per cent you and you feel viscerally moved by it.

4. Having found your true north, write it below.

My purpose for prioritising sleep and committing fully to improving it is:

_____

_____

_____

_____

5. Keep up your sleep-diary habit.
Complete it each morning and review it at the end of the week. Use the sleep-efficiency calculator to make it easy.

6. Keep reading, keep learning and stay curious about sleep. Educating yourself about sleep is central to your sleep transformation.

Supporting your sleep-improvement journey

APPROACH THE JOURNEY WITH AN OPEN MIND

As you continue to make your way towards better sleep, develop an attitude of openness and curiosity—as though you're learning things anew. You will already have plenty of thoughts and beliefs about sleep, but throughout this process you'll let go of some of those perceptions and become acquainted with new and different ways of approaching your days and nights.

Letting go of preconceptions and expectations can make you feel unsettled at first, even vulnerable. Yet there is wisdom in uncertainty. It provides you with a blank page upon which a different and more helpful sleep story can unfold.

So far, your sleep has been unreliable, erratic and not how you want it to be. You may be fed up and want concrete solutions and guaranteed outcomes to give you clarity, certainty and control over your nights. Yet that's not how sleep improvement comes about—it needs almost the opposite approach. CBTi provides education and sleep-improvement techniques, but it's your receptivity to the process, your willingness to explore these ideas with an open mind and change your relationship with your difficulties, that will influence how your sleep will be.

ACCEPT THAT THINGS ARE DIFFICULT AT THE MOMENT

As much as you want your sleep to be different (and different fast), you are getting a little ahead of yourself. In your journey towards sleep improvement, you need to acknowledge and accept where you are and what you are experiencing. Your sleep, as different as it is from what you want, is what it is. Be okay with this for now. No amount of forcing it to change or railing against it will improve the situation. Resistance tends to make it worse. This is not a battle; there is no winning or losing. With acceptance, you acknowledge your experience simply as it is—even if it feels unpleasant, uncomfortable or difficult at the moment.

It's important to distinguish acceptance from giving up or quitting. Acceptance is being aware of what's truly going on, acknowledging it in all its imperfection, and being honest with how that is for you. From this place, you can pause, take a breath and consider making different choices for yourself.

CHAPTER 8

Sleep medication —to take or not to take

Reality simply consists of different points of view.
—MARGARET ATWOOD

The safest and most sustainable long-term treatments for persistent insomnia are non-drug strategies (such as CBTi), but for some people there *may* be a role for medication. Some of you will already be taking sleep medication as you embark on this sleep-improvement endeavour and will be wondering whether to continue or stop the meds during the programme. Others of you will be keen to start the CBTi programme but may be feeling so overwhelmed by sleep debt that you want a reprieve from your insomnia to be able to gather the strength to begin.

You will know in yourself whether sleeping pills feel like the right course of action for you. It's very personal. You might be taking them and value the difference they are making in your life at this time. Or you might be taking them but they feel at odds with what you want for yourself. Some of you will be considering trying them, and others still will be avoiding sleeping medication at all costs. Different people need different things at different times in their lives. Regardless of where you are on the continuum, what matters is to be informed and, in consultation with your healthcare professional, to do what's right for you based on the facts of sleep medication and your specific situation. (This is critical when other mental or physical conditions are involved, such as anxiety, depression or medical issues, and when other medications are being taken.)

Sleeping pills

Let's be clear: sleeping pills do not induce natural sleep.[1] They provide you with a form of sedation—a proxy to sleep, but not actual sleep. (Having worked in market insights for most of my career, it's clear to me that calling out the consumer benefit of 'sleep' is a lot more enticing and less concerning than referring to them as 'sedating pills'. It's a much easier sell—marketing 101.)

'Sleeping' pills go to work on pathways in the brain that regulate whether you are awake or asleep. Different types of sleeping pills work in different ways.[2] Most of them work by encouraging the 'sleep pathways' to be more active (e.g., temazepam, zopiclone and zolpidem), whereas others work on dulling the 'wake pathways' (e.g., suvorexant). Regardless of which route they take, the user expects that they will deliver much better sleep. But are these expectations realistic?

When people reach the point of taking sleeping pills, things tend to be feeling unmanageable, even desperate. They don't believe they can do their nights alone any more—they need salvation from the hell of ongoing sleep deficit. It can be a cry for help or a proactive move to regain control. According to Dr David Cunnington, when a patient wants sleeping pills, their expectations tend to be high. They are after a magic pill that will get them to sleep quickly, deliver a much-needed stretch of continuous, high-grade sleep, and allow them to wake fully refreshed and ready to embrace the day. And, of course, they don't want any unpleasant side effects—and absolutely no risk of dependency or withdrawal, thank you very much!

We also want these miraculous sleeping pills to maintain their effectiveness over time so we can stick with the original dose and get the same effect whenever we choose to use them—we don't want to build a tolerance to them. We want the pills to be predictable tools that we have control over, so that we can get brilliant sleep results on demand.

But we are dreamers: pharmaceutical companies have not been able to create a medication that delivers anything close to this so far. Each drug has a different profile, delivering in some areas but falling short or posing issues in others. So we need to align our expectations with the reality of sleeping medications, and have our eyes wide open about what they can and can't do for us.

A recent textbook for Australasian healthcare professionals, *Sleep Medicine*, highlights that research on the most commonly prescribed sleep medications shows they can provide some of the following benefits to sleep.[3]

- Reduce the time it takes to fall asleep by 15–30 minutes.
- Provide an additional 15–30 minutes' sleep per night.
- Reduce the number of awakenings throughout the night.

Importantly, this refers to improvements in participants' *actual* sleep, rather than their *perceived* sleep. I don't know about you, but I find these improvements underwhelming.

An extensive research study referred to in Matthew Walker's *Why We Sleep* provides even more reason to doubt the efficacy of these medications. In 2013, a review of all published studies on the effectiveness of the newer forms of sleeping pills that are commonly prescribed for adult insomnia was completed. It found that, while people believed sleeping pills gave them better sleep than a placebo, the actual recordings of their sleep showed their improvements (in the time it took them to fall asleep) were not significantly different from when they used a placebo. Walker concludes that common prescription sleep medications for adult insomnia are only *minimally helpful*.[4]

There are times when a bit of help is better than nothing. A prescription for sleeping pills can feel like a helper, a safety net, even a lifesaver to a desperately sleep-deprived person—even if most of the benefit is psychological rather than physical. For those people experiencing difficulties falling asleep, a sleeping pill that is fast-acting and doesn't last long in the system can be an option. For those who experience waking in the second half of the night, a slow-release or longer-lasting alternative may be preferable. There are also sleep meds available that offer support in both sleep onset and continuity.

While sleeping pills may provide incremental improvements, it's important to be honest with yourself and know that none of them are going to perform miracles. The benefits may primarily be in your mind. At best, you will get a temporary reprieve from wakefulness—they do not address the cause of your poor sleep.

Sleeping pills come with risks

All sleeping pills come with a dark side worth considering when making your 'to take or not to take' decision. Being aware of the risks enables you to make an informed choice about starting, staying on or coming off sleeping pills.

Side effects

The morning after using sleeping pills, unwanted side effects can include grogginess, forgetfulness and slowed reaction times, especially when the medication is intended to provide support in sleep continuity in the second half of the night, or if a person is taking a dose that is above the minimum level they require. (This can happen if a person plays around with their prescribed dosage or frequency in an attempt to *better* self-medicate.) Oddly, the after-effects of sleeping medication can feel similar to the aftermath of not sleeping well, or even akin to a hangover.

Some people counter these unwanted effects by doing things to make the post-sleeping-pill day a bit easier, like staying in bed a while longer, grabbing a double-shot espresso, avoiding the gym, tucking into comfort food or taking a nap. Then, at night, they might go to bed earlier to have another go at getting more sleep, or have a wine or two because it hasn't been such a great day.[5] All of these actions, while they are understandable responses to feeling off, are unhelpful to natural sleep. So the side effects of sleeping pills and usual responses to them can perpetuate the cycle of poor sleep, reinforcing the perceived need for sleeping pills. It can feel like a trap, as it erodes confidence in the medication and faith in your ability to sleep.

Tolerance

Sleeping pills tend to only be helpful for around four weeks. Beyond this, they lose their effectiveness. So, after a month on the same nightly dose, the user is unlikely to experience the same improvement in their sleep. In frustration, they might be tempted to try a higher dose to get the result achieved previously. This kind of self-prescribing is a slippery slope. With higher doses, the side effects can be more significant even if the sleep benefits aren't.

Withdrawal

On and on it can go, until the person has had enough and decides to throw in the towel with sleeping pills. The pills may not be working, or may seem to be making things worse, or they may not feel like a good option long term. When someone stops taking sleeping pills (especially if they go cold turkey), they can encounter unpleasant withdrawal symptoms: irritability, anxiety, headaches, difficulty concentrating, sweating, dizziness, pounding heart. The symptoms can be more dramatic if the person has been taking higher doses or has been on sleeping pills for a long time. The list of horrible withdrawal symptoms (including seizures) continues, but here's the real kicker: when you stop taking sleeping pills, one of the withdrawal symptoms is *insomnia*.

Insomnia is a *withdrawal symptom* of sleeping pills.

Dependence

Stopping sleeping pills, especially if you have been taking them for more than several weeks or if they are stopped abruptly, is likely to create *rebound insomnia*. This can be as bad as, if not worse than, the insomnia experienced before taking the medication. Restarting the sleeping pills when experiencing rebound insomnia (and other withdrawal symptoms) resolves these ghastly problems, which tends to reinforce the perception that the sleeping pills are needed, and a vicious cycle of physical and psychological dependence takes hold. Dr Charles Morin captures this familiar pattern of behaviour in his diagram of life in the sleeping-pill vortex.

THE CYCLE OF HYPNOTIC-DEPENDENT INSOMNIA

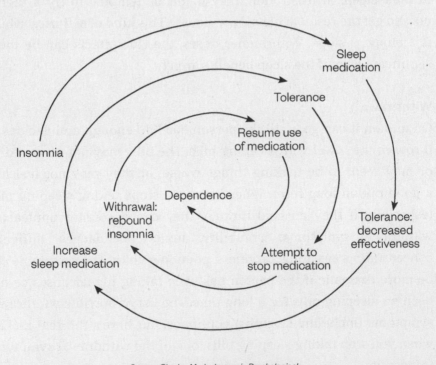

Source: Charles Morin, *Insomnia Psychological Assessment and Management*, Guildford Press.

When sleeping pills may be appropriate

Given the low-key benefits of sleeping pills, the side effects, and the likelihood of tolerance, withdrawal, or dependence issues, it's not surprising that sleeping pills must be prescribed by a healthcare professional. The most effective long-term therapies for insomnia are non-drug treatments (namely CBTi), but sleeping pills may be prescribed alongside. The general guideline is to use sleeping pills as a last resort and to recommend the minimum dosage for the shortest time (generally under four weeks).

There are undoubtedly many factors that your doctor must consider, but trust them when they are reticent about prescribing sleeping pills or are labouring the precautions. If they are resistant to writing the script, or restrict the number of pills they permit you, know that they ultimately have your best interests at heart.

If your insomnia symptoms are severe, and they're impacting your life, there are some critical times when sleeping pills may be worth discussing with your doctor.

- **Addressing acute short-term insomnia:** the situation is extreme and you feel you can't self-manage with non-drug strategies like exercise, relaxation, meditation and sleep hygiene.
- **A temporary reprieve from chronic insomnia:** you've reached your threshold and need a rest from the experience of persistent insomnia. This can enable you to recalibrate before or while embarking on a CBTi-based approach to sleep improvement to learn to sleep naturally once more.
- **Stuck between a rock and a hard place:** the risks posed to you (or others) by your extreme insomnia outweigh the risks associated with taking sleeping medication.

If you are having these conversations with your doctor, be sure to discuss:

- clinically proven sleep benefits offered by the medication (so you have realistic expectations of the drug)
- side effects

- the risks of tolerance, withdrawal and dependence
- the safest way to use the medication for your insomnia, while mitigating the risks (dosage, frequency of use)
- an exit strategy (when and how to come off the medication).

Sleeping pills and CBTi

If you are currently taking sleeping pills, you probably want to know how to manage them as you embark on your CBTi-based sleep-improvement programme. There are two options to think through, and each has pros and cons. It's best to explore the options with your doctor and figure out which one suits your situation.

1. **Stop before you start CBTi:** come off your sleeping pills before you begin the CBTi sleep-improvement programme. This will allow you to work out where things really are with your sleep before you start. This option may be appropriate if you haven't been taking sleeping pills for very long, they're at a low dose, or you've been taking them very intermittently. If you have been taking sleeping pills for less than a month, your stopping plan can be relatively brief and can be conducted while you carry out your two-week baseline sleep diary. Read the guideline overleaf about stopping gradually, and contact your doctor to tailor a plan for your circumstances (if this wasn't discussed when the pills were prescribed).

2. **Start CBTi before you stop:** continue with sleeping pills alongside the CBTi programme. This way, you can improve your sleep as well as your knowledge, skills and sleep confidence before beginning to come off the medication little by little. This approach is advisable if you have been taking sleeping pills for a long time, they're higher dose, or you're feeling reliant on them. Inevitably, as you come off sleeping pills, there is risk of withdrawal symptoms and rebound insomnia, so it helps to be feeling more confident about sleeping so that you can anticipate and work through this phase of your sleep-improvement journey.

A combined approach of CBTi and sleeping pills can be a good option. Dr Charles Morin's view is that it's best for a person with chronic insomnia to be entirely off their sleep medication by the time they reach the maintenance phase of the sleep-improvement programme.[6] Discuss how best to manage this with your doctor, so that you can be off your sleeping pills within the six weeks of the CBTi programme. (If you need more time than this to taper off your medication, consider delaying the start, or stretching the programme out a few additional weeks.)

Coming off sleeping pills can be a tough experience physically and psychologically, so it's essential to have a workable plan. While stopping sleeping pills may cause a setback in your sleep progress, know that you are ultimately heading in the right direction.

Generally, the longer you have been taking sleep medication, the longer it will take to come off it. Check the guideline provided overleaf by Sleepwell, an initiative from Dalhousie University in Canada. Get a sense of what to expect, then discuss a plan with your doctor to make sure you come off sleeping pills as safely and kindly as possible. You know it's going to be a bit rough, so you need a plan that is doable.

Guidelines for tapering off sleeping pills

According to Sleepwell, the time it takes to reduce and stop sleeping pills varies a lot depending on how long you've been taking them and how sensitive you are to withdrawal symptoms. They have prepared a helpful reference tool that indicates what tends to be appropriate based on how long you've been using sleeping pills.[7]

Reducing your medication takes planning—each time you lower the dose, there's a possibility your sleep will be disrupted from the withdrawal effect.[8] It's essential to be prepared and know that your sleep might be wobbly for a few days as your body adjusts to the lower dose.

It's strongly advised that you taper off sleeping pills very gradually. This is a weaning process, where the dosage is decreased little by little over time. This approach reduces the intensity of side effects and is safer. It's important to work out your plan with your doctor. Be kind and patient with yourself as you reduce the dose. Coming off sleeping pills takes time. You will get there—think tortoise, not hare.

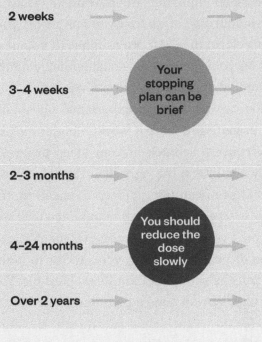

SLEEPING PILLS TAPERING GUIDE

You have used sleeping pills for:

2 weeks		No taper required. Increase your sleep drive – rise 15–30 minutes earlier than usual the morning after your last dose.
3–4 weeks	*Your stopping plan can be brief*	Reduce your dose by half for 2–5 days before stopping it. Increase your sleep drive – rise 15–30 minutes earlier than usual the morning after your last dose.
2–3 months		Reduce your dose by half for 1–2 weeks. Optional: then ¼ dose for 1 week. Increase your sleep drive – rise 15–30 minutes earlier than usual the morning after your last dose.
4–24 months	*You should reduce the dose slowly*	Plan to gradually reduce your dose over 6–12 weeks. Use CBTi to treat insomnia.
Over 2 years		Plan to gradually reduce your dose over 6–52 weeks. Use CBTI to treat insomnia.

• Use CBTI to help you manage insomnia.

• Develop your dose reduction (taper) plan with your doctor and pharmacist. Check in with them often.

• Aim to reduce your dose on the same day of the week every 1 or 2 weeks.

• You can reduce your dose the same amount each time until stopped. Or, you can slow things down, especially near the end, by making smaller dose reductions, lengthening the interval between dose reductions, or both.

• Your plan should be flexible. Make adjustments based on how you are feeling.

Each stopping plan should be personalised to suit your needs. Source: Gardner and Murphy, mysleepwell.ca

What about melatonin?

Melatonin is a bit different from other sleeping medications. It's a synthetic version of the body's natural sleep hormone—the Dracula hormone that is released as daylight fades and makes you feel sleepy at night, helping you get to sleep and stay asleep.

According to SleepHub, supplementary melatonin as a sleep aid for insomnia may make you feel sleepier, get you to sleep more quickly, make you stay asleep longer and enable you to feel like you've had better-quality sleep.[9] However, as is the case with conventional sleeping pills, these improvements aren't radically impressive. A

2013 summary of research into melatonin showed that, on average, melatonin got people to sleep 7 minutes faster, allowed them to sleep 8 minutes longer, and improved the quality of their sleep.[10] So the potential benefits of melatonin don't seem to be as generous as sleeping pills, but the side effects aren't as bad either. Rates of side effects—which include headaches, dizziness, nausea and drowsiness—are lower.

But melatonin doesn't work for everyone, and response to it is highly variable. The best evidence for this drug as a sleeping tablet is when it's used for people 55 years and older.[11] (Melatonin does have other uses and can be a valuable option when dealing with jet lag or delayed sleep phase disorder.)

In Australia and New Zealand, melatonin is available only on prescription. When used as prescribed it's generally safe, it seems to have fewer side effects than other sleeping pills, and there's less chance of building a tolerance or becoming dependent on it.[12] If you're taking or considering taking melatonin, discuss with your doctor whether you need a rapid-release or a slow-release option. Talk through the recommended dosage (2 milligrams is common), when to take it before bed (usually one hour), and how long to stay on it (it's generally only recommended for short-term use).

If you are taking melatonin, keep in mind that this chemical is signalling to your body that it's dark outside and that bedtime is on the horizon. So be careful about your exposure to light after taking it—dim the lights, turn off phones and screens. You're trying to help the body prepare for bed, so giving it mixed signals is confusing.

Melatonin is not a silver-bullet solution for insomnia, but it may have value in supporting you in your journey learning to sleep. There's a role for medication when a reprieve from extreme symptoms is needed to gather the strength to put in place a sustainable sleep-improvement plan. This is how I used melatonin. I needed the slow-release version to experience any benefit, and, even then, the effectiveness was relatively short-lived. But it gave me a much-needed break from insomnia. Most importantly, it reminded me how truly remarkable sleep is for my body and soul, which put me in a much stronger position to embark on my totally natural sleep-improvement journey.

Cannabis and medicinal cannabinoids

Recreational cannabis is a commonly used illicit drug, with typically 12 per cent of Australians (fourteen years and older)[13] and 11 per cent of New Zealanders (fifteen years and over)[14] having used it in the past year. Some people use recreational cannabis to wind down and to help with sleep.[15] A 2017 review of the research on cannabis and sleep reported that findings are mixed—sometimes showing that people may fall asleep more quickly, or have less disrupted sleep.[16] Other studies have shown that when used for sleep it may induce a deep-sleep state after initial consumption, yet it may not increase total sleep time. Controlled studies are lacking, so the jury is still out on its exact sleep effects, but the signs are that it can help with some aspects of sleep in the short term. Anecdotally there are firm believers in the use of cannabis for sleep. But with considerable variation in the quality and levels of active cannabinoids in street cannabis, it's not surprising that there can be real discrepancies in the drug's effect on sleep. Relying on cannabis for sleep can be a bit hit and miss.

The research is clear, however, that the sleep-inducing effects of cannabis can vanish with repeated use as tolerance builds, resulting in shallow, non-restorative sleep.[17] Over time this can lead to the need to take more in an attempt to get better sleep. As this habituation continues, it increases the risk of dependence.

If there's cannabis dependence, coming off tends to have withdrawal effects on sleep. As is the case with sleeping pills, insomnia is a key withdrawal symptom of cannabis. When quitting cannabis, a person may experience difficulties falling asleep or reduced sleep duration.[18] Withdrawal can also manifest as sleep disturbances or vivid dreams.[19] These withdrawal effects can be horrible and last much longer than you'd expect, which makes it hard to stop.

If you decide to stop using cannabis, know that, if you go cold turkey, your sleep is likely to be disrupted for a while. Accept this as part of the process of cessation, rather than a problem with your innate ability to sleep. It's temporary. Not a good time, but temporary. You may prefer to taper off the drug more gradually (warm turkey!), so your sleep is likely to be less affected. Consider contacting your local Community Alcohol and Drug Services (CADS) in New Zealand or your local Alcohol & Drug Information Service (ADIS) in Australia for information and advice on your circumstances.

While recreational cannabis has limitations in its value for sleep, especially long term, medicinal cannabis can have value in some situations. Medicinal cannabis is available only on prescription in New Zealand and Australia, and quality and cannabinoid concentrations are stringently controlled. The key cannabinoids within cannabis— cannabidiol (CBD) and tetrahydrocannabinol (THC)—differ in the way they affect the body. Among many other actions, THC is the component responsible for a euphoric high and can be sedating. CBD, on the other hand, is non-intoxicating and can be stimulating or sedating to the body depending on the dosage. The two cannabinoids vary in their ability to relieve pain, sedate, reduce anxiety, ease nausea and relax tense muscles.

While research on the therapeutic use of medicinal cannabis for insomnia is limited at this stage, indications are promising, especially in cases where insomnia is related to chronic pain. Emerging research suggests that cannabinoid concentrations, ratios (CBD:THC) and dosage, and how the drug is administered, influence the effect medicinal cannabis has on sleep quality and insomnia symptoms.[20]

In his Auckland clinic, Dr Graham Gulbransen, GP, addiction specialist and cannabis consultant, has seen encouraging sleep improvements with cannabis among patients suffering insomnia as a result of challenging conditions such as chronic pain, high anxiety, or nausea from chemotherapy treatment.

The efficacy of medicinal cannabinoids on insomnia is an emerging field of research, so time will tell. In the meantime, under medical supervision, it seems that cannabinoids may well have therapeutic potential in the treatment of insomnia.

Over-the-counter (OTC) medication

In 2017 the AASM recommended that common over-the-counter antihistamine and antihistamine-analgesic sleep aids are not used for chronic insomnia. There is insufficient evidence that these products, primarily formulated for alleviating allergy symptoms or relieving pain, are effective or safe for use with insomnia.[21]

Being able to buy these products pretty cheaply at the local chemist can make you feel like they are harmless and more permissible than prescribed sleeping pills. But you're kidding yourself. They aren't designed for the task at hand. At best, they will be useless at addressing the core problem, and they come with inherent risks. Short-term problems, especially at higher doses, include carry-over sedation resulting in daytime sleepiness, grogginess and even falls. Long-term use comes with risks. Many of these medications come under a drug category (anticholinergics) that has been linked with dementia and Alzheimer's. (Given that the possibility of losing my mind is so frightening to me, thank heavens I didn't persist with my sneaky Blue Oblivion behaviour.)

*Everyone does what they do for what
they believe are the right reasons.*
—UNKNOWN

Herbal remedies

The AASM isn't keen on herbal remedies as a treatment for ongoing sleep difficulties. Again, it's the lack of evidence of their effectiveness and safety that makes the AASM cautious. The Sleep Health Foundation also has reservations. While a lot of people use all sorts of herbal options in the quest for better sleep—valerian, kava, hops, chamomile, passionflower, etc.—there is wariness because, so far, there's little proof that these substances work well for improving sleep.

The following table from the Sleep Health Foundation provides some insight into current levels of confidence with different herbal medicines.[22] These conclusions are based on how well the remedy performs in randomised controlled trials for insomnia compared with a placebo treatment. (*Low* evidence means that most of the research is inconclusive or unsupportive of the remedy being better than a placebo in research trials of acceptable quality. *More research needed* means that the research trials aren't of sufficient quality to make a fair call on the remedy's effectiveness compared to a placebo at this stage.)

Herbal medicine	Evidence level for helping insomnia
valerian (*Valeriana officinalis*)	low
kava (*Piper methysticum*)	low
hops (*Humulus lupulus*)	low
chamomile (*Matricaria recutita*)	more research needed
passionflower (*Passiflora spp.*)	more research needed
valerian–hops combination	more research needed
St John's wort (*Hypericum perforatum*)	more research needed

While the Sleep Health Foundation is not saying that these herbal remedies have no effect on insomnia, they are saying that they don't have much of an impact compared to a placebo, or that more robust research is needed to make a call on the remedy's effectiveness. There isn't yet hard-hitting clinical proof that these remedies improve sleep significantly or in a sustained way.

I like my herbal and natural remedies and use them happily for some aspects of my health and well-being. But, when it comes to turning around chronic insomnia, it's unlikely that herbal remedies alone will provide sustainable improvement. I don't know about you, but I got fed up with all of the half-empty bottles of herbs and supplements that cost me a bomb and failed to deliver significant change in my ability to sleep.

If you do decide to try a herbal remedy to support your sleep, have realistic expectations about what it can do and make sure you give it a decent chance. Most studies that review the effectiveness of herbal remedies are based on people using the herbs for several weeks. Valerian, in particular, is thought to take time to start working. So take your remedy most nights for two or three weeks before you make a call on how it's working for you. (Lots of people take them and, as is the case with sleeping pills, expect them to have an effect overnight.) If you feel that you are on to a herbal remedy that provides some relief or improvement, you may like to use it alongside the CBTi programme. As you progress and build confidence in your ability to sleep, experiment and decide for yourself if the remedy makes a difference.

Even for those of you who, like me, have traditionally held the high-horse view about sleeping pills, it's worth keeping in mind that there's a time and place for everything. While my natural inclination is to be anti sleep medication, there is no way I would have coped with the physically and emotionally harrowing aftermath of extensive surgery and reconstruction without the support of sleeping pills. My meditation skills and natural sleep potions were laughable in the face of pain levels that were fifteen on the one-to-ten scale.

Later, when I reached my personal tipping point with sleep difficulties and decided I couldn't tolerate my zombie life any longer, it was sleeping medication (melatonin) that gave me a temporary reprieve. It was the lifeline I needed to recalibrate and find a different, natural and sustainable way to improve my sleep.

On the matter of sleeping pills, I respect Dr Tony Fernando's open-minded view on holistic medicine. He believes that, to be truly holistic in your approach, you need to consider all of the sleep-management options available to a person—that includes complementary, integrative and alternative healing modalities *as well as* traditional Western medicine.

Chapter recap: what you can do

1. If you're already taking sleeping pills, book a consultation with your doctor. Decide whether to go off the medication before you start the programme or to take it alongside. If you decide to come off sleeping pills, work out a gradual tapering plan that is feasible for your situation—when to begin, how to decrease the dosage slowly, what to do if rebound insomnia is too harsh or if you need some flexibility.

2. If you're considering medication, book a consultation with your doctor to discuss the CBTi programme and whether a short course of sleeping medication may be appropriate to give you a reprieve as or before you get your sleep improvement under way.

3. Review the value of recreational cannabis, over-the-counter medication and herbal remedies. If you are currently taking any of these products, decide whether to continue with them throughout the CBTi programme or go au naturel.

4. Be non-judgemental and kind to yourself about your use or misuse of sleep medication to date. Your choices and behaviour are based on the knowledge you have at the time. Learning about sleeping medication provides you with the insight to make helpful choices for your future; it's not to fuel judgement and criticism of previous decisions.

5. Keep reading, keep learning and stay curious about your sleep.

Supporting your sleep-improvement journey

SUSPEND YOUR TENDENCY TO JUDGE YOUR SLEEP

As humans, we automatically evaluate and judge things—like or dislike, good or bad, positive or negative. It's what we do. It's a super-quick way for the brain to assess a situation or experience, a mental shortcut that makes you think you have the jump on what you're dealing with. However, it's useful to suspend your judgement while you are learning about your sleep and exploring new ways to approach sleep.

Pausing and allowing things to be as they are, without judgement, gives you the opportunity to acknowledge what you are experiencing, reflect on it and wisely choose what, if anything, is required. It creates space from the reactive automatic responses that may not be serving you so well.

For instance, if you think being awake in bed is negative, bad, terrible, dreadful or catastrophic, this creates anxiety that's less conducive to sleep. Consider being awake as simply resting in bed—neither good nor bad. Just a state of being where you lie still with your eyes closed, feeling warm, comfortable and supported by your bed, with nothing required of you. When you relate to your experience non-judgementally, it's easier to accept and be with things as they are.

LEARN TO TRUST AGAIN

After many months or years with insomnia, it's common to have severe doubts about your ability to sleep. You may have misgivings about whether your body even knows how to sleep any more. Indeed, your trust may be in tatters.

As you gain a better understanding of what healthy sleep looks like, how sleep works and how insomnia evolves, feel reassured in your biology. Changing your thoughts and behaviours allows you to sleep easier, and knowing this helps to build trust again. Be confident your mind and body have the capacity to self-regulate sleep given the right conditions. Be reassured that CBTi is a validated treatment for insomnia.

CHAPTER 9

Set meaningful sleep goals

In a gentle way, you can shake the world.
—MAHATMA GANDHI

The usual practice when setting goals is to apply the SMART management tool: make the goal specific, measurable, achievable, realistic and time-bound. This creates hard goals, ones that are fixed and concrete. They make you get your act together and apply yourself fully. They've been proven to help clarify ideas, focus efforts, make productive use of time and resources, and increase the chances of achievement. Management loves this kind of goal-setting, and many of us have been indoctrinated to adopt it in some shape or form.

The problem is, the last thing you need if you are undersleeping is to put additional pressure on yourself with rigid sleep goals. The added stress of a time-bound, specific goal sabotages your ability to attain what you most want—easy sleep. Failure to achieve that goal will most likely have you feeling disillusioned, disempowered and judgemental towards yourself. Again, not helpful. If you do this, you are likely to give up. So to hell with hard goals.

A gentle and kind approach to goal-setting is far more likely to support you in your sleep-improvement journey. The purpose of these goals is simply to keep you on the journey—they are not fixed destinations to strive vigorously towards, they are an inner pull that helps you continue to be open to the process, even when you'd like to walk away. It is very much a 'set and forget' approach. Welcome to the world of soft goal-setting.

Before our daughter was born, I was quite the goal-setter. My ambitions were broken down into annual goals, monthly plans and weekly, even daily, to-do lists. Without meaning to, I had adopted some Type A tendencies (though I am not naturally that kind of person!). Goals helped me get shit done and I pretty much lived by them. When I became a mum and my time was no longer my own, this kind of goal-setting was disastrous and frequently ended with me in tears. In those confronting early months with so much to learn and focus on in loving and caring for Lily, I was unable to achieve even my most basic goals. I'm talking about really simple goals, like getting out of my PJs, having a shower and putting mascara on. It was confronting and stressful. I felt inadequate and useless compared to what I had envisaged life as a new mum to be.

Everything changed when I adjusted my thinking on what I wanted to achieve. I still desired the same outcomes, but I changed the way I positioned my goals in my mind. My to-do list became my fantasy list. While I still wanted to get out of my PJs, have a shower and put on mascara, I was less attached to the outcome. I wasn't under time pressure and I cut myself a lot of slack if things didn't come together. I had faith that tomorrow was another day, and maybe things would align better then. By being kinder to myself and more patient with my new circumstances, life became more manageable. I felt more at ease, and surprisingly my little goals were attained more often.

It's beautiful if fantasies happen in real life, but we don't get shitty if they don't. There's no sense of failure if a fantasy doesn't play out, and this takes the pressure off. You can breathe and move at your own pace, and you can handle any zigzags and detours. By being less attached to the result, you stop pushing, and the outcome is more likely to unfold as you gently do what needs to be done to get there.

When a fantasy comes to fruition, it feels like a miracle has happened, whereas completing something on a to-do list only provides satisfaction that something that should've been done is done. Having a fantasy come true feels incredible—you're more likely to celebrate your win, give yourself an inner high-five, and tell yourself you rock. Acknowledging success and revelling in the positive emotions that accompany it boosts your morale, motivation and confidence, making it more likely you'll continue your progress and growth.

So, it's time to get on with some soft goal-setting and create a fantasy list of how you'd like your sleep to be. While you've been reading, you've been thinking about what is meaningful for you in terms of sleep onset, duration, continuity and depth. Plus, you know how sleep works, so you can set sleep goals that are biologically feasible.

It's crucial that you set goals that matter to you. Err on the conservative side—you want your goals to move you in the right direction without creating pressure or setting yourself up for failure and frustration. As you progress and see improvement, you can adjust your goals towards the sleep of your dreams. Or, as your sleep gradually improves, you may begin to trust the process and let go of the need to set any sleep goals at all.

Make sure you frame your sleep goals positively. You want to take the focus off the problem or issue, and turn your attention to the sleep you aspire towards. Mentioning the problem in your goal-setting will create negative connotations that unconsciously stir up self-criticism and judgement. If you frame things positively, your attention turns to where you want to go, triggering a sense of optimism, hope and possibility. These feelings are much more conducive to feeling good about yourself and making progress.

When I set my sleep goals, my main one was to sleep right through the night. I was struggling with that hateful wakeful period in the early hours of the morning. However, rather than state my goal as 'Stop waking for ages in the night', I flipped it: 'Sleep easily through the night.' Play around with the language to reposition the issue in your mind.

Having clarity on your aspirations will give you a sense of intention. Allow yourself to look positively towards the future that you desire for yourself as your sleep improves. By articulating this vision and having it in your mind, you can let go of some of the struggle and negativity that may be surrounding your sleep. Think about sleep with more openness, kindness and with a sense of possibility: 'What if . . .' or 'Imagine if . . .' comes into play, as you consider a different outcome.

While it helps to have your vision clearly in mind, make sure you position your sleep and daytime goals gently as 'soft' goals. Keep them as your aspirations, your fantasies, to avoid creating performance anxiety. It's a subtle and important distinction to make. (That said, it's imperative that you respect and honour your vision as a destination that you're heading towards in time—operate in the realm of 'soft' goals, not 'flaky never going to get there' goals.)

Set a main sleep goal

What's the one improvement to your sleep that would be most meaningful for you? Be clear with yourself about what matters and what you want your sleep to be like eventually. You may want to fall asleep more easily, stay asleep throughout the night, sleep all the way through till your nominated wake-time, or sleep more deeply. Or your goals may be more gradual than this—settling yourself easily at bedtime, staying calm if you wake in the night, being accepting of what healthy sleep is actually like. Whatever your main goal, clarify it and get it written on the page. Be sure to keep it aligned with the realities of how sleep works.

My main sleep goal is _____

_____

Set a daytime goal

The propensity to sleep is a 24-hour affair. What happens in the daylight hours affects sleep at night and vice versa. The sleep impacts you are likely to be experiencing most profoundly are in your daytime functioning and your moods. Jot down the improvements that you'd like to see for yourself by day as your struggles with sleep fall away. It may be about your energy levels, focus and concentration, productivity, motivation, or relationships. (Just keep in mind that sleep isn't the only factor that affects daytime functioning.)

My daytime goal is _____

_____

Set an emotional or mood goal

Think about how you're likely to feel as sleep becomes easier. What difference would you like to see in your mood and emotions? You may want to feel calmer, kinder or more patient, or perhaps more positive, confident and optimistic. Your goal could be about feeling more relaxed, happy or more open and loving. You will know what really matters to you, and how you'd like to feel.

My emotional or mood goal is _____

_____

Set a sleep-efficiency goal

One goal where the softly, softly approach doesn't apply is sleep efficiency. This is a very tangible and necessary measure to track your progress throughout the programme. Sleep efficiency is the percentage of time that you are asleep while you are in your bed, and a more useful measurement than sleep duration. By now, you will have a week or two of information gathered, and you will have done a few calculations. If you haven't done a weekly review, now's a great time.

Sleep efficiency = total sleep time ÷ total time in bed × 100

Look at your sleep-efficiency percentages from the previous week or two and jot down how things are currently looking. They may be all over the place at the moment, so choose an indicative average. Write it in the space below as your baseline sleep efficiency. The goal that you will be working towards is a handsome 85 per cent—you are aiming high (even if this feels like a fantasy right now). Once sleep efficiency is getting up to 80 to 85 per cent, things start feeling *very* satisfying.

Baseline sleep efficiency: _____ %

Goal sleep efficiency: _____85_____ %

The journey ahead

By now, you have prioritised your sleep, you have set realistic, meaningful and aspirational goals for your nights and your days, you have a sleep-diary habit in place, and you have gathered your baseline sleep data. You've done a fair bit of reading and you're better educated about sleep. Your perceptions of sleep will already be shifting and opening up to other possibilities. You're in an excellent space to get under way with the core programme.

Before you proceed, it's important to be honest: the journey ahead is vital to your quality of life, your well-being and your future, but it's no picnic. There are parts of the sleep-improvement journey that will be frustrating, challenging or counterintuitive. There will be times when you feel like you're not making progress or even that things are getting worse. You will make headway, then you will slip backwards or sideways before making progress again. It's essential to go in knowing that sleep improvement is a non-linear journey. While the overall direction is positive, the process takes a zigzagging route and unfolds on its own time. You must have realistic expectations of the process and how your progress will evolve.

Sleep improvement is non-linear.

This darling chart depicts how we expect and hope and pray the sleep-improvement journey will play out, from night to night, week to week.

SLEEP IMPROVEMENT EXPECTATIONS

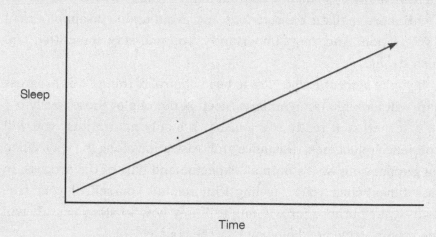

Sleep

Time

Sorry, it's not going to be like that. Here is an example of how the sleep-improvement journey is likely to actually occur.

SLEEP IMPROVEMENT REALITY

Sleep

Time

Naturally, because everyone is an individual with their own particular sleep challenges and responses to behaviour-change initiatives, you will have your own version of this crazy-looking chart. Don't get hung up on the hiccups and glitches along the way. Keep your attention on the overall upward trajectory. Knowing the path will have many ups and downs from night to night means that you go in with more realistic expectations and avoid undue disappointment or frustration. And, most importantly, you will stay committed and finish strong!

If you're someone who likes to be in control of things, this progress chart will look like a nightmare. Sleep is not one of those lovely $a + b = c$ scenarios. It really is a journey. It's only natural that you will experience reluctance, resistance and frustration along the way. When that happens, know it's normal, expected and part of the process. In those times when you're feeling lost, remind yourself of your true north—your purpose for wanting to know how to sleep easy. It will give you direction and help you stay the course.

While the weeks ahead will feel tough at times, think of them as short-term pain for long-term salvation. Humans sleep for approximately a third of their lives. For an average person, that's about 25 years. Think about how many years of life you have ahead and divide that by three—that's about how much sleep you still have to experience. According to my super-rough calculations, I still have about ten years of sleeping to do (if I live till I'm in my eighties like my nana), and there is no way I'm prepared to do ten years of lousy sleep. If you take the big-picture view, six weeks seems not only doable, but worth it.

Keep in mind, too, that you're strong and tenacious. You've endured months or years of sleep deficiency—you are built of powerful stuff. (Let's not forget that sleep deprivation is used as a form of torture.) Having lived through years of insomnia, I know how resilient you have to be to get through the days after relentless nights of dreadful sleep. It takes courage, mettle and resolve to live with sleep debt. And here you are. You've got yourself together enough to pick up this book and read up to here. You're primed, prepped and ready to use those character strengths to apply yourself to discovering a new and sustainable approach to sleep.

CBTi has been around for decades. It's clinically proven to be highly effective for improving the sleep of people experiencing chronic insomnia, and it's recommended internationally as a first-line treatment. It's grounded in the science of behavioural change, psychology and sleep. It is highly likely that it will work for you. But it's also challenging, especially in the first few weeks. Significant behavioural change is tough—just ask anyone who's tried to get fit, lose 5 kilograms or give up smoking or drinking. Implementing CBTi will take commitment and cooperation—don't go into the programme half-hearted. You need to be all in. You've made it this far, which is a good sign—you're open to new ideas and destined to progress well.

But here's the proviso: CBTi, especially self-directed CBTi, does not work for everyone. The DIY approach takes greater commitment and resolve than a programme supported by a CBTi-trained psychologist or sleep specialist. If you like the CBTi approach but, at any point in the programme, find that you are really struggling to stick with it solo, don't give up on your sleep. It's too important. Instead, use the resources in Appendix II to find a supported CBTi option. You will go into that programme better prepared than most, with higher chances of success.

For some, the direct approach of CBTi just doesn't gel. The process puts too much focus on sleep and creates more anxiety and stress. This programme tempers that propensity by integrating principles from MBTI and mindful self-compassion (MSC). There is increasing evidence of the merit of mindfulness when used alongside CBTi. Some of you may find the gentler, less direct method of MBTI better suited to your personal learning style. If so, A Mindful Way, developed by Dr Giselle Withers, a clinical psychologist in Melbourne, is one example of an online mindfulness and CBTi programme for sleep you could explore.

Whatever you choose to do, stay committed to your sleep-improvement journey.

Be prepared that some parts of CBTi can make things worse initially. I will let you know when a specific CBTi technique is challenging for some people, and I'll provide suggestions for support.

Remember, if you have or suspect that you have severe anxiety or depression, it's better to carry out your sleep-improvement programme under the supervision of a healthcare professional who understands the broader context of your situation.

Now that you have set meaningful 'soft' goals and you have realistic expectations of the journey ahead, let's keep up the momentum and get on with it. Do you recall Donna, who was keen to sleep better to be the happy, wholehearted mum she knew she could be? Here's what she had to say about her experience using this six-week programme to improve her sleep.

It's so worth investing in your sleep

This programme offered me some very powerful tools to get my sleep back on track. I kept a sleep diary and, from that starting point, I was able to gain an understanding of my sleeping behaviours and my low sleep-efficiency percentage. Several contributing factors were identified, and I learned about and implemented techniques that worked.

I am amazed and delighted that, from this programme, my sleep has improved so much that I feel I am completely transformed. It's hard to express exactly how getting a good night's sleep can make you feel like a new person. I now go to sleep easily, have a healthy and deep sleep, and wake up happy. What more could I ask for? I am happy again. Life is not just good—it's fantastic.

—Donna (44, creative assistant)

Chapter recap: what you can do

1. Summarise your preparation. Complete the worksheet on the next page to put your purpose and goals together in one place before heading into Week One of the core programme.

2. Complete your baseline sleep information. Use this opportunity to catch up on reviewing your sleep diary. Make sure you have worked out your sleep-efficiency scores. They will be the primary reference for monitoring your progress throughout the programme.

3. Make an appointment with yourself. Decide which day will be day one of the programme. Choose a day of the week that will be easy for you to read the week's chapter. Put appointments on this day in your calendar for the next six weeks.

4. Work out a plan B. Write down a backup option in case self-directed CBTi doesn't suit your needs. Know that you have options, and that you're not going to give up on your sleep.

5. Congratulate yourself. Take a moment to acknowledge what you have achieved in the last week or two. You've opened your mind to a new approach to sleep improvement, you've done a lot of learning, you're well prepared, you're committed to this journey, and you're ready to give it a decent go.

MY COMMITMENT TO IMPROVING MY SLEEP

I, _____ , commit to my journey towards sleeping better.

Purpose

Improving my sleep matters deeply to me because . . .

_____

_____

Soft goals

I aspire to the following goals, and I will patiently move towards them without getting uptight or stressed.

My main sleep goal: _____

My daytime goal: _____

My emotional or mood goal: _____

My sleep-efficiency goal: To be asleep 85% of the time I spend in bed.

Progress expectations

- ☐ I understand that progress towards my sleep goals will be non-linear and it will unfold in its own way and time.

Responsibilities

- ☐ I'm committed to reading the material each week for the next six weeks.
- ☐ I will implement the weekly plans appropriately for my life.
- ☐ I will monitor my experiences daily with my sleep diary.
- ☐ I will review and learn from my experiences and progress each week.
- ☐ I will take responsibility for my own well-being and take any precautions seriously.
- ☐ I will draw on my inner strength and the reserves that have enabled me to get to here.
- ☐ I accept that it's normal to encounter frustration, reluctance and resistance at times.
- ☐ I will be calm, kind and patient with myself and the process.

☐ If I have setbacks, I will be resilient and keep things in perspective.

☐ I will seek the help of a healthcare professional if I am concerned at any point.

☐ If I decide that the self-directed approach using CBTi is not for me, I will try this alternative approach to improving my sleep:

_____

(If needed, refer to the options in Appendix II for your plan B.)

I acknowledge that sleep difficulties are common, but they defy our biology. I know living with ongoing sleeping difficulties has been hard on me. I promise that I'll allow myself to discover new ways to improve my sleep, for my well-being and health now and in the future.

Signature _____

Date _____

CHAPTER 10

Sleep—the inside job

Nature does not hurry, yet everything is accomplished.

—LAO TZU

F alling asleep is a passive process—it comes to you if conditions prevail. Your relationship with sleep plays a central role in creating conditions that are conducive to sleep. How you feel about your sleep, your thoughts about your ability to sleep, even how you approach sleep improvement, all affect (and are affected by) your inner state. This state influences whether sleep is likely to occur or elude you. It can seem mysterious, even fickle, until you understand more about what's going on behind the scenes. Once you comprehend the process at play, you have the freedom to make choices to support your journey towards sleeping with ease.

The autonomic nervous system plays a big part in how easily

sleep will occur. This system responds to the thoughts, emotions and sensations being experienced. If you are experiencing (or believe you are experiencing) some kind of threat or potential danger, your body responds with a **stress response** via the sympathetic nervous system. This system revs you up so you can fight, freeze or flee to save or protect yourself. Your heart beats faster, your breathing becomes rapid and shallow, blood rushes to your muscles in readiness for action, and you get a boost of stress hormones (including adrenaline and cortisol) so you can do whatever is required to rescue yourself from the threat. The focus is on doing what needs to be done to fix or escape from the problem.

In contrast, when your thoughts, emotions and sensations are reassuring the body that all is well, there's nothing to worry about and it is safe, your body responds with a **relaxation response** via the parasympathetic nervous system. This system calms you so that you can rest, digest and restore yourself. Your heart beats slowly, your breathing is deep and slow, blood flows to the gut and lungs, stress-hormone levels abate, and you slow down and relax. You're better able to accept things as they are and just be, knowing that all is okay as it is (there's nothing to fear).

Stress response	Relaxation response
Sympathetic nervous system	Parasympathetic nervous system
Revs you up so you can fight, freeze or flee	Calms you down so you can rest, digest and restore
Heart beats faster Breathing is fast and shallow Blood rushes to muscles for action Gut is less active—digestion difficult Stress hormones (adrenaline and cortisol) increase Expends or depletes energy	Heart beats slowly and rhythmically Breathing is deep and slow Blood flows to the gut and lungs Gut is active—digests, absorbs nutrients Levels of adrenaline and cortisol lower Conserves energy

These two systems are made to work in harmony. The stress-response system kicks into gear when there's a threat, and once the threat is resolved or seems manageable the body calms once more and remains in a relaxation response until there's next a sense of danger.

It doesn't take a rocket scientist to identify which system needs to be operational for a decent chance of falling asleep—the relaxation response.

When sleep has become a battleground

Often, for those with chronic insomnia, thoughts, feelings and sensations related to sleep trigger the stress response. You may have worries about whether you will sleep or not; you may feel irritated, frustrated or annoyed at being awake at night; you may be tossing and turning in bed; you may be fearful of the implications for tomorrow. These kinds of thoughts, feelings and physical sensations trigger warning sirens, and your stress response gets well and truly switched on. Sleep starts to seem like a battle. It worries you, or it may frustrate and anger you. So you make efforts to improve it. Yet, the more you try, the more wakefulness you experience. Your stress response remains firmly stuck on, leaving you feeling burnt out, wired, vigilant and desperate to fix your sleep. Not only do you suffer the experience of sleep difficulty, but your reaction to it (your struggle against it or your resistance) creates further suffering that perpetuates the problem.

> *What you resist not only persists,*
> *but will grow in size.*
> —CARL JUNG

Mindfulness: changing your relationship with sleep

It's all very well to understand the cycle conceptually, but what can you do about it? How do you learn to be okay about something that is so clearly not okay? How do you stop worrying when you're genuinely worried? How do you try without really trying? These sorts of paradoxical questions drove me around the twist initially.

Fortunately, there's a highly effective way to be with yourself, even when sleep is difficult. It's called mindfulness.

Mindfulness is not about clearing your mind and thinking of

nothing, or sitting cross-legged for hours on end, or pretending all is well when it isn't. It's a useful, learnable practice that will support you on your journey towards sleeping with ease. With mindfulness, you can change your relationship with sleep. Dr Tony Fernando, a true advocate of living mindfully, encouraged me to explore mindfulness when I was on my journey to sleeping easy. He, like many others, is convinced of the value of this practice for people struggling with sleep.

With its origins mainly in Buddhism, mindfulness has been around for centuries. In the 1970s Jon Kabat-Zinn, founder of the Stress Reduction Clinic and the Center for Mindfulness in Medicine, Health Care, and Society at the University of Massachusetts Medical School, developed a secular programme of mindfulness, pioneering its value for stress reduction within medicine, health and society in the West. Over the last decade, mindfulness has been shown to help people with a whole range of health conditions, including anxiety, depression, post-traumatic stress disorder and chronic pain. Jason Ong, associate professor at Northwestern Feinberg School of Medicine, has advocated for its use in the treatment of chronic insomnia, and its value as a therapy is now well established.[1]

What is mindfulness?

Mindfulness is the awareness that arises from paying attention to the present moment in a non-judgemental way.

Why it matters

When you practise mindfulness, you become more aware of the thoughts, feelings and sensations you are experiencing in the here and now. You become conscious of the content, intensity and frequency of your thoughts, feelings and sensations. You notice whether you're inclined to get attached to or fixated on them, and how your body responds when you do.

You also gain an understanding of how you experience these

thoughts, feelings and sensations if you don't judge or get caught up in them. When you notice them—even the difficult ones—with curiosity, kindness and openness, you're better able to gently accept them as they are and know they're part of being human. When you acknowledge your thoughts, feelings and sensations in this way, you discover they are transitory and temporary. If you accept them as they are, they are more likely to pass.

This knowledge and these skills require practice to develop, but they are incredibly liberating. Mindfulness gives you the ability to be with whatever you are experiencing, even if it's difficult, knowing it too shall pass.

By being intentionally aware of your experiences around sleep, you can clock even difficult thoughts and feelings as they happen. Instead of rushing to judgement or reacting in an instinctive, unhelpful way, being mindful gives you the ability to pause. From there, you can make helpful, supportive choices. You get the chance to respond, rather than react.

When you are caught up in thoughts and feelings, especially when they are unpleasant, uncomfortable or difficult, it is easy to react impulsively to avoid the experience or to try in earnest to fix or stop it. Alternatively, you can overidentify with the experience, causing you to extrapolate it and exacerbating your difficulties. While it's natural to want to change what you don't like, your responses need to genuinely support you. Mindfulness shifts you from being on autopilot (oblivious, fixated or impulsively reactive) to being more aware of your experience. It creates space, which allows you to be grounded, centred and wise in your responses.

Mindfulness is built on seven fundamental principles: beginner's mind, trust, non-judgement, patience, non-striving, acceptance and letting go. These ideas are seeded throughout the book to help you be more at ease with your current sleep difficulties, and to support you in developing a mindset that's more conducive to sleep improvement. Jason Ong's book, *Mindfulness-Based Therapy for Insomnia*, is helpful in understanding these principles.[2]

- **Beginner's mind.** Be willing to see everything as though for the first time.
  - Approach each bedtime with thoughts that are unrelated to past nights.
  - Each night is a fresh opportunity; nothing is exactly the same as it was yesterday.
  - How you slept last night will not define your sleep tonight.
  - Keep an open mind about how your sleep will be tonight—it's a new canvas.
- **Trust.** Develop trust in yourself, your body and its wisdom.
  - Know that your body can self-regulate sleep with the conditions.
  - Your sleep isn't 'broken'.
  - Knowledge about the thoughts and behaviours that support sleep builds confidence.
  - Understanding how sleep works and insomnia evolves is reassuring.
  - CBTi and mindfulness are proven to help with chronic insomnia.
- **Non-judgement.** Be an impartial witness to what you're experiencing—awareness without preference.
  - Being awake in bed is not negative.
  - If you are awake in bed, remind yourself that you are resting.
  - Sleep is not a performance—there's no success or failure.
  - This is an opportunity for your body to take the sleep it's able to in these conditions.
- **Patience.** Accept that things unfold in their own time.
  - Be patient about the process.
  - Improved sleep takes time.
  - You can't hurry sleep.
- **Non-striving.** Pay attention to whatever is happening, rather than trying for a result.
  - Know that you can't force sleep. Falling asleep is not the result of effort.

- Find a balance between desire for sleep and allowing sleep to unfold in its own way.
- Accept that falling asleep or back to sleep just happens.
- **Acceptance.** Accept things as they are rather than denying or resisting them.
  - Accept that you can't control sleep.
  - Acknowledge that sometimes you will sleep, and sometimes you'll be awake.
  - Know that acceptance is not giving up; it's about allowing things to be as they are for now.
- **Letting go.** Let go of experiences rather than holding on to them or pushing them away.
  - Let go of the sense that sleep is a problem to be fixed.
  - Avoid labelling yourself as an insomniac.
  - Let go of the notion that sleep difficulties are permanent.

You've already taken steps to inform yourself about sleep and you've committed to using the proven techniques of CBTi to help yourself on your sleep-improvement journey. CBTi will provide the map, compass, backpack and boots for the journey, so you're well equipped with the gear you'll need, but CBTi doesn't ready you on the inside for an at times challenging journey. Mindfulness does the inside job. It helps create headspace that makes being on the journey easier, even when the going is rough.

Cultivating mindfulness

Recently, mindfulness has become a bit of a buzzword. This popularity has spawned a lot of versions and varieties, ranging from authentic, validated programmes to commercialised 'get fixed quick' schemes. The 'McMindfulness' versions tend not to deliver the health and well-being benefits of authentic programmes taught under the guidance of qualified instructors. As a result, the meaning and perceived value of mindfulness can be diluted in the commercial wash.

As you proceed with the programme, you may be interested in further exploring mindfulness. If you do decide that you would like to develop your mindfulness practice, seek out a reputable mindfulness programme. Mindfulness is cultivated through a type of meditation, which can be taught in a weekly course (usually six to eight weeks), under the guidance of a qualified mindfulness instructor. In-person training, online training, books and apps on mindfulness are all available, which can provide a strong foundation for building your own practice. Some suggestions for further study are included in Appendix III. Cultivating mindfulness takes practice and dedication, but the gains made along the way are well worth the patience and persistence.

When I was on my own sleep-improvement journey, I understood a little about mindfulness conceptually, but I didn't have anything that resembled a daily practice. I dabbled with some guided meditations on apps, explored a bit of mindfulness through movement with sporadic yoga sessions, and did the odd breathing meditation, but I wasn't committed. I was exhausted, unfocused, forgetful and disorganised. Knowing what I do now about the value of mindfulness, I strongly recommend being open to it on this journey. It will make it easier.

> *Many people don't know how to stop worrying or how to relax the mind and body. Mindfulness can teach them this.*
> —DR GISELLE WITHERS

While this book is not a training manual for mindfulness, it does use the principles of mindfulness to support you on your sleep-improvement journey. Understanding these ideas can help you make some adjustments to your approach to sleep and the programme.

Below are some entry-level mindfulness practices, which you can use to get a sense of how mindfulness might support you. Think of them as a starter kit to explore mindfulness practices. The purpose of mindfulness practice is to support you in becoming more aware of your experience, by bringing your attention to the present moment without judgement. It's not about fixing or changing anything or putting you to sleep. It's not recommended that you practise any of these at bedtime or in bed during the night—keep your mindfulness practice to daytime for now.

A pause for breath

This mindfulness exercise is so gloriously quick and straightforward to put in place that it's hard to find a decent reason not to do it, even when you're tired or busy. In this practice, from *Mindfulness for Insomnia*, just be aware of what you're experiencing.[3] There's no need to assess, critique or change anything. Let everything be as it is.

1. Pause and take a breath.
2. Notice the sensations in your body.
3. Observe any thoughts in your mind (notice whether they are of the past, the future or now).
4. Notice any emotions that are with you right now.
5. Take another breath—a deep one.
6. Go on your way.

Create a habit of doing this a few times each day by associating it with a particular moment or setting—arriving home at the end of the workday, after the dishes are done or before you greet the kids home from school. You could put reminders up around the house or in your workspace to prompt yourself to 'pause for breath', or put a notification on your phone for certain times of the day.

Pausing for breath can be a reminder of how unaware you often are about your experience. I find it a reassuring way of casually checking in on myself throughout the day. When I paused for breath just now, I realised I was thirsty and had a bit of a headache! Yet, before my pause, I was oblivious to my body and focused on my word count.

Breath is a great place to start when exploring mindfulness. It's our life force—always there with us, a fundamental part of who we are, as much a part of the outside world as it is of our inner world. It's always coming and going, moving and changing, just like life. When you are aware of your breath, you are able to adjust it, if you choose. You can use it to help your body shift to a different mode of being. By slowing down, lengthening and deepening your breath, you call on your parasympathetic nervous system and help to calm your body.

A basic mindfulness meditation

Allow yourself some uninterrupted time in a quiet place during the daytime or early evening (away from bedtime) to practise this one. Focus on cultivating your practice of mindfulness—it's not about relaxing you or making you sleepy. Try to stay open, kind and curious—you're here to explore. When you've been in a state of overthinking, stress or anxiety, it's natural for your mind to be all over the show. Remember: you're not here to make it any different from what it is. Your intention is to be more aware of how things are for you, moment to moment.

1. **Sit quietly** on a chair, upright with your posture aligned, hands resting in your lap or on your thighs.

2. **Ground yourself** by feeling both feet on the floor and the support of the chair beneath you.

3. **Be still**, taking a moment to be softly aware of where you are, before gently closing your eyes.

4. **Breathe naturally.** Focus on your breath, being aware of your inhalations and exhalations.

5. **Be aware of your senses**, noticing any sights, sounds, smells, tastes and touches. Name them as you observe them—'sight', 'sound', 'smell', 'taste' and 'touch'—without judgement and let them go.

6. **Become aware of your body**. Gently scan your body from head to toe. Observe any physical sensations, such as warmth, heaviness, tightness or tingling. Without judgement, let the sensations pass.

7. **Notice any thoughts** that occur. Imagine each thought as a cloud drifting across the sky. Observe the shape, nature and size of the cloud without judgement. Simply label each cloud as a 'thought' and let it pass by. Notice the spaces between the thoughts.

8. **Allow emotions** to occur without judgement. Notice how they feel in your body. If you can, name the emotion—'sadness', 'joy', 'irritation' or 'impatience'. As best you can, allow yourself to feel what is there (even if the feeling is difficult), trusting it will soon pass.

9. **Return to your breath.** Focus on your breathing. Be aware of your inhalations and exhalations.
10. **Be still.** Take a moment to just be, then gently open your eyes.
11. **Sit quietly.** Notice where you are, and allow yourself to be with your experience of this moment.

Use this meditation as a guide to explore mindfulness in your own way. There are no fixed rules that you must adhere to for it to be 'right'. Nor are you after any particular results. Your role is to be with everything, just as it is, right now. You are exploring and discovering for yourself, to cultivate a practice that feels doable. Start small and get used to the process.

The meditation outlined above can take around twenty minutes, to bring your awareness to each aspect of your experience—breath, senses, body sensations, thoughts and emotions. But your mindfulness meditation doesn't need to take this long—dedicating ten minutes a day to practising mindfulness will help you develop your ability to be mindfully aware in other areas of your daily life.

If you prefer to meditate for a shorter time, focus your attention on one of the key aspects of your experience—either your body sensations, thoughts or emotions. Follow the meditation guideline, but allow one of those three elements to be in the foreground of your attention. Observe it thoroughly, and take your time to experience it. Other elements in the background may come into your awareness from time to time and that's no biggie. Just acknowledge them for what they are—'thought', 'emotion' or 'sensation'—and let them pass, then gently escort your attention to where you intended it to be.

When cultivating an authentic mindfulness practice, meditate daily if you can. Developing mindful awareness takes practice. Do what you can—aim for progress, not perfection. You are gradually creating a shift from operating on autopilot, where you're unaware of what you're experiencing in the present moment or you're aware and upset by it, to being conscious of your experience, with kindness, curiosity and non-judgement. By uncovering what's going on in your mind, body and mood, you can become more understanding of yourself. You create space between what you experience and how you respond to it.

Mindfulness through movement

Another way into mindfulness is through movement. Ancient practices such as yoga and tai chi combine awareness of the breath and body with gentle movement. In slowing things down, turning your attention inwards and intentionally moving the body, these practices can bring your awareness to what you are experiencing in the present. They're another way to tune in to yourself and create space between yourself and difficult thoughts, emotions and sensations.

If you're interested in exploring mindfulness through movement, know that there's yoga and there's *yoga*. It's best to learn from qualified instructors, starting with a foundation course to ease yourself in gently—always listen to your body. If you're not up to attending or forking out for local classes, there are some decent options online to try at home. My pick is the YouTube channel 'Yoga with Adriene'. Adriene combines quality yoga practice with mindfulness, offers free and subscription courses with practices to suit all levels, and brings incredible warmth and compassion to your yoga mat each day. I find it a pleasure to invite her into my home.

Mindfulness, however you chose to explore it, will support you in understanding your relationship with sleep and the way you approach your sleep-improvement journey. Do what you can to adopt the principles of mindfulness and start cultivating a mindfulness practice for yourself, even in a low-key way. It will serve you well.

Let self-compassion be your new best friend

Mindfulness and self-compassion are often described as two wings of the same bird. With mindfulness, you become aware of what you are experiencing. Self-compassion provides you with a way to take care of yourself in the face of these experiences. It's another practice you can use to support yourself on your sleep-improvement journey.

Living with persistent, often unpredictable sleep difficulties takes its toll. It's easy to fall into a bit of a hole, where things feel grim. While sleep deprived, I spent time pinballing between difficult emotions like frustration, anger, resentment, despair, shame and sadness. My body felt depleted. When you're chronically sleep deficient, you may start giving yourself a hard time or experience self-pity. You may think that the situation is unfair, that life's a struggle, that you're alone or somehow flawed because of your inability to sleep as well as you think you should. All of this exacerbates your stress response, unintentionally perpetuating your insomnia.

When sleep difficulties endure, this internalised negativity is disheartening, disempowering and sometimes debilitating. When you are hard on yourself, the physiological effect is the same as if you were being criticised and put down by someone else. You may not be fully aware that you're doing this to yourself, but there is often a pervasive sense that your sleeplessness is causing you a lot of suffering. As you cultivate mindfulness, you'll become more attuned to what you're experiencing, as it exists, and you will need to take good care of yourself.

Self-compassion is choosing to be kind and caring for yourself in times when you're going through difficult experiences, or feeling inadequate or like a failure in some way. Dr Kristin Neff, a pioneer of the empirically supported mindful self-compassion programme, describes it as being a good friend to yourself.

What is self-compassion?

Self-compassion is the tendency to soothe oneself with kindness and non-judgemental understanding in times of difficulty and suffering.

To be honest, when I first learned about self-compassion, I thought it was a bit naive. It sounded pretty airy-fairy—be nice, be kind and everything will be okay. My views changed once I understood more about it and learned that there is solid science behind its effectiveness.[4]

In a nutshell, self-compassion is composed of three core components.

1. **Mindfulness.** Be aware and take an open, balanced, non-judgemental view of the struggles and pain you're experiencing. Accept them as they are rather than becoming caught up in how terrible everything is (overidentifying) or, conversely, trying to deny or suppress the experience.
2. **Common humanity.** Recognise that you're not alone. Know that these experiences are shared with others and are part of being human, instead of feeling isolated or like an outlier.
3. **Self-kindness.** Be kind to yourself when you're suffering or feeling inadequate or flawed, instead of being harsh, judgemental or critical.

Self-compassion is a type of inner strength that can be learned and developed. It will enable you to acknowledge how tough insomnia can be at times, and understand and accept without judgement how it came to be and how you feel. Most importantly, you will learn how to make the changes necessary to improve your sleep with a spirit of genuine self-care.

> *With self-compassion, we give*
> *ourselves the same kindness and*
> *care we'd give a good friend.*
> —DR KRISTIN NEFF

Self-kindness can manifest in a passive or active way. Neff describes this as the yin and yang of self-compassion.[5] Both types of self-kindness can be incredibly valuable on your sleep-improvement journey.

Yin compassion, the passive kind of self-compassion, involves accepting things as they are right now, allowing yourself to be with the difficulties you're experiencing, and looking after yourself in a kind, caring and nurturing way. You do this not to change the situation but simply because you are in this situation. Your discomfort is acknowledged, and you tend to yourself with love and kindness because you're feeling miserable or distressed. For instance, when you have had a rough night, you may choose to lower your expectations for yourself the next day, giving yourself permission to have a slow day. If you wake in the night, you may choose to soothe yourself by feeling reassured that your body has had some sleep, and now you have an opportunity to rest quietly in your warm and comfortable bed and listen to the rain a while. (Importantly, when you practise self-compassion, you are being kind to yourself not to make yourself sleep, but *because you are awake*.)

Yang compassion, on the other hand, has a bit more fire and energy (in fact, it's a wee bit stroppy). It's the active self-compassion that gets you standing up for yourself, saying, 'Enough is enough.' It's a type of kindness empowered by clarity and confidence. Yang compassion decides what's needed, then motivates you to take the action that has your best interests at heart, even if it can be challenging. You'll be calling on yang compassion when you do the more challenging CBTi techniques. (Imagine you're going 'mother tiger' on yourself, getting stuck in to do what needs to be done for your own ultimate good.)

Dr Anna Friis, an Auckland-based health psychologist and MSC teacher, says it's essential to understand that you practise self-compassion *because* you are suffering, not to make the suffering go away. By looking after yourself, you will feel more supported regardless of the nature of the suffering. This has the effect of reducing the stress involved, which, from a sleep perspective, is a good thing. It's a bit like soothing a child who has the flu. You comfort the child not to make the flu go away, but because they are suffering. You support them until it passes and they feel better.

Friis suggests that, when you wake in the night and feel stressed about not being asleep, you give yourself a self-compassion break. This simple exercise is based on the practical tools provided on Dr Kristin Neff's website, self-compassion.org. It makes use of several elements that trigger the experience of compassion: you feel warmth and safety, you hear kind words expressed with a gentle voice, and you experience a soothing touch. This will help you feel safer, and more connected and at ease. Your inner alarm bells quieten down, and your parasympathetic nervous system is more inclined to come into play.

Self-compassion break

When you're in a difficult situation (for example, you're awake in the night) and it's causing stress, see if you can actually feel the stress and emotional discomfort in your body. Now, say to yourself:

- 'This is a moment of suffering.'
  - In your own words, say what the experience is—name it.
  - For example: 'This is anxiety.' (Or frustration, annoyance, fear, tension, restlessness, etc.)
- 'Suffering is a part of life.'
  - Remind yourself that you're not alone in your sleep difficulties. For example, about one in three adults struggle with their sleep.
  - Place your hands over your heart, and feel the warmth of your touch on your chest.
- 'May I be kind to myself.'
  - Ask yourself, 'What do I need to hear right now to express kindness to myself?'
  - For example, you might answer: 'May I be patient,' 'May I be calm' or 'May I rest easy.'

If you are often hard on yourself, this exercise can seem odd, different, even confronting initially. Self-compassion might feel clunky and paint-by-numbers when you start, but keep an open mind and allow yourself to experiment. Tune in to how your body responds to self-care and kindness. (It can be very different to the effect of harsh self-talk, criticism and judgement.)

Dr Kristin Neff's website is an excellent resource to explore if you're interested in reconnecting with your innate skills in self-compassion. It has guided meditations and practical exercises. A couple with real value for those struggling with sleep are outlined below.

How would you treat a friend?

Reflect on how you would treat someone you care about if they were in this difficult situation, struggling with insomnia. Think about what you would say to your friend and the tone of voice you would use as you extended your support. Then contemplate how you treat yourself in the same difficult situation. What words do you use? What tone of voice? Notice if there is a discrepancy. Next time you're experiencing a difficult sleep-related situation, consider treating yourself as you would a good friend. See what happens.

Changing your critical self-talk

This is an ongoing exercise, to be worked on over time if changing the way you treat yourself in difficult situations is of interest to you.

- Start noticing when you're being self-critical, and get a clear sense of how you talk to yourself.
  - Take note of what you actually say—keep tabs on any specific words or recurring phrases verbatim.
  - Notice your tone of voice—is it severe, cold, angry, disappointed?
  - Be aware of what sets off your inner critic.
- Explore softening your self-critical voice.
  - Acknowledge that this voice has been trying to help, but is actually causing unnecessary stress.
  - Try finding a more compassionate inner voice, and allow it to talk.
  - Explore using self-talk that's supportive, understanding and kind—experiment with the words you choose and your tone of voice.
  - You can even add physical gestures of warmth, like stroking your arm or putting a palm to your cheek.

The practice of self-compassion has struggled over the years—it has an image problem in a culture filled with 'toughen up' messaging. When you're surrounded by phrases like 'pull your socks up', 'man up', 'harden up', 'suck it up, princess' and 'don't be a sook', choosing self-kindness may make you cringe at first.

However, I made some interesting discoveries when I explored self-compassion. My inner critic could be a right bitch to me about my lack of sleep. She was nothing shy of savage in what she said and how she said it. Once I became aware of this and the impact it was having on me, I simply couldn't allow it to continue. Things changed a lot. My inner self-talk is now very warm, good-natured and light-hearted—she calls me 'darling' when she notices I've got myself into a bit of a pickle. She's more like a kind sister than a wicked stepmother.

In the context of sleep problems, self-compassion means recognising and accepting that things are tough for you right now instead of harshly judging and criticising yourself. From a place of kindness and understanding, take care of yourself as you experience the suffering that your sleeplessness is causing and do what's genuinely needed for your well-being.

It would be great to be able to apply a whole lot of effort and hard work to just fix your sleep problems, once and for all, but that's not how sleep works. Falling asleep is a passive process, and it needs to be approached indirectly. While CBTi provides you with the equipment needed for your sleep-improvement journey, there are shifts that you need to make internally to further encourage the conditions for sleep. You are responsible for taking care of your own inside job.

Chapter recap: what you can do

1. Reflect on the nervous system's role in sleep. Consider how an activated stress response makes sleep more difficult, yet insomnia (and anxiety around it) keeps this nervous system stuck on. Think about how the relaxation response could support you in sleep improvement.

2. Revisit the principles of mindfulness. Consider how they compare to your approach to sleep. Think about how you might bring mindfulness to your sleep-improvement journey.

3. Explore mindfulness. Reflect on how you could begin to cultivate mindfulness in your life.

4. Develop self-compassion. Explore some self-compassion exercises, to experience how kindness and care affect you when you're having sleep difficulties.

5. Keep reading, keep learning and stay curious about your sleep.

PART 2

The Six-week Programme

A consistent sleep schedule and permission to wind down

Storms make trees take deeper roots.

—DOLLY PARTON

You've called time on endlessly weathering the storm of sleep difficulties. It's time to act.

Sleep improvement requires a strong foundation. Establishing and honouring a consistent sleep schedule gives you this foundation. From your sleep diary, you'll know how regular or erratic you've been in the times you go to bed at night and get out of bed in the morning. You'll know whether there are discrepancies in your behaviour throughout the week versus on the weekends. Plus, you'll know whether your current schedule (or anti-schedule) delivers the quality and quantity of sleep you need to feel awesome, or even just okay.

This week you're going to revise your bedtime and wake-time plan. You'll prescribe yourself a new sleep–wake schedule—one that's consistent, workable and more conducive to sleep improvement throughout the programme.

There's a tendency among people with persistent sleep difficulties to spend too long in bed. It's done with the best intentions—to give yourself plenty of opportunity to sleep—but the sleep science makes clear that this is unhelpful. Going to bed too early or staying in bed too late (or napping too much) works against sleep improvement. Instead, you need to realign the time you spend in bed with the time actually required for sleep.

Schedule your wake-up time

Throughout the six-week programme, you need to keep a fixed wake-up time. This will be the anchor as you build towards a consistent sleep schedule. Having a variable wake-up time makes it difficult for your body to know what it's supposed to be doing, when. Help support your body clock to get back to a natural rhythm by setting a very predictable and consistent wake-up time. This is the time that you will wake up and get out of bed each morning—weekday or weekend, rain or shine.

Your wake-up time will become a habit. We are creatures of habit—what's repeated is learned. You are retraining your brain and your body because what you do currently is not working for you. By getting up at the *same* time each day, you're providing a predictable daily rhythm, which is conducive to sleep improvement. You are trying to get back in sync with your biology—bodies work best when there is a regular rhythm. Being consistent while improving your sleep puts in place behavioural patterns that support progress.

Select a wake-up time that's workable in your life both during the weekdays and on the weekend. It's tempting to cut yourself some slack and have a bit of a sleep-in on the weekends; however, this only slows down your progress by making it more difficult for your body to sense a pattern. Throughout the programme, you need to be regular, regular, regular. It's not going to be forever, but, for now, consistency is your friend.

The wake-up time I can commit to on weekdays and weekends is _____ a.m.

Schedule your total time in bed

It's time to review and adjust how much time you are spending in bed. Obviously you need to be in bed long enough to allow yourself some core sleep, but you don't want to spend more time in bed than is helpful. If you are in bed much longer than you are asleep, your sleep-efficiency figures will be low. Low sleep-efficiency scores generally mean more time staring at the ceiling, tossing and turning, or fretting about the day ahead. By reducing your time in bed, your figures are likely to start improving.

People who sleep well (those skitey-pants) tend to have sleep-efficiency scores hovering up around 90 per cent, which is why their sleep feels stellar and they crow on about it. The average sleep efficiency of people with sleep difficulties is around 65 per cent.[1] While that is the average for troubled sleepers, in reality they tend to experience a crazy compendium of good nights and hell nights, so there are usually some nights when sleep-efficiency scores are higher and some when they hit rock bottom. At an average of 65 per cent, those with sleep difficulties spend about a third of the night awake. (And we know all too well how loathsome that feels!)

People with persistent sleep difficulties have a tendency to gradually spend longer and longer in bed, trying to catch up on their sleep. They may go to bed earlier and earlier, or stay in bed later on mornings when they can (like on the weekend), or they may start napping whenever they get the chance to slope off to the bedroom during the day or nod off in a comfy chair. Whichever route they take, the end result is often spending much longer in bed than what the body needs for healthy sleep.

Sleep science describes this as a strategy of extending time in bed, and it *perpetuates* insomnia. When I first learned this, I felt a bit indignant. For someone experiencing sleep debt, spending more time in bed makes perfect sense. You are trying to get more sleep, so it's logical to try to maximise your opportunity to sleep. However, the problem with extending my time in bed (with increasingly early bedtimes) was that my sleep became shallower and more fragmented.

To understand how this works, imagine the body needs 7 hours of high-grade sleep to perform optimally. If your sleep was water, you'd need 7 litres. You can choose the size of container for your water: too small; just right; too big; or a disappointing waste of time. If you put your 7 litres of water in a tiny bucket, it overflows and you miss out on sleep. If you put it in the right-size bucket, you'll have a full, deep, satisfying sleep. If you pour that same 7 litres of water into a wide basin, your sleep will be shallow. And, if you pour your 7 litres into a paddling pool, the water will be so shallow that there'll be dry patches—no fun for anyone. Similarly, if you want deeper, more continuous, more satisfying sleep, you are going to need to decrease the amount of time you spend in bed.

So how much time do you need to start with? The National Sleep Foundation chart in Chapter 1 outlines the amount of sleep recommended for different age groups: around 7 to 9 hours for adults and 7 to 8 hours for older people. It also says that, for adults, 6 hours and, for older people, 5–6 hours may sometimes be appropriate (but this isn't the case for many).

Given that you are most likely operating on an average sleep duration considerably lower than this, build your sleep–wake schedule on the National Sleep Foundation's lower sleep-duration figures to begin with—that's a sleep schedule based on 6 hours of potential sleep. However, given that you likely also take time to fall asleep, wake in the night or wake early in the morning, add a one-hour buffer to give yourself some wiggle room in your initial sleep schedule.

The total time in bed that I'll work with this week is 7 hours.

By scheduling a realistic amount of time in bed, you are moving towards *compressing* your sleep.

(If you are up for compressing your sleep more than this, feel free to adjust your time in bed down to 6 hours. Some of you will be itching to get on with it at this stage, while others will prefer to ease into the protocols more slowly.)

Schedule your earliest bedtime

Based on the figures you've chosen above—your wake-up time and your time in bed—work out what your new bedtime will be.

My earliest bedtime (6 to 7 hours before wake-up time) is _____ p.m./a.m.

Your new bedtime is the *earliest* time that you can go to bed this week. By all means, stay up later if you aren't feeling sleepy at that hour, but remember your wake-up time remains unchanged. Your new bedtime is probably later than you usually go to bed—your challenge will be staying up till bedtime rather than trying to sleep!

Staying up later and reducing your time in bed might seem to defy logic, but trust the process. I too pushed back on this approach initially, as it went against everything I knew and had grown up with. (My mother's voice resounded in my head: 'Go to bed early and catch up on your sleep.') I believed I needed more time in bed, not less. My sleep schedule had been variable, and my bedtimes were reflective of how good or bad my sleep had been the previous night. But here's the thing: when I got consistent with my sleep schedule and reduced the amount of time I spent in bed, my sleep progressed. It didn't happen overnight, but I was on my way to better sleep.

Schedule time to prepare for bed

Set yourself up to get into bed at your earliest bedtime by including the inevitable time it takes to get ready for bed in your sleep schedule. This includes all the end-of-day rituals and responsibilities that must be attended to before lights out: put the cat out (or, if it's like mine, bring the cat in), lock the door, take your make-up off, put on your anti-wrinkle potions and super-radiance cream, brush your teeth, get naked or put your sleepwear on, etc. Somehow I twiddle around for about twenty minutes doing all this. (Blokes might have it easier in this department and get the job done in five!) Regardless of the specifics of your regimen, factor in some time. Fifteen minutes should do the trick, but adjust as needed to suit your habits.

I will prepare for bedtime in _____ minutes.

Schedule time to wind down

Do what you can to allow yourself 60 to 90 minutes of wind-down time before getting ready for bed. For some of you, this will sound extraordinary, decadent or even impossible. But if you're committed to improving your sleep, and you have already made this commitment to yourself, time to wind down needs to be valued and integrated into your programme. (Once you start doing it and reap the benefits, it becomes pretty damned hard to relinquish!)

When you're struggling with sleep debt, the evenings can get chewed up while you're in catch-up mode after a slow, inefficient or scattered day. You might be burdened by relentless household chores or work responsibilities, or you might be putting everyone else's needs before your own. Many of you will be beating yourself up and feeling undeserving because your self-esteem has been eroded by months and months of undersleeping. If any of these scenarios sound familiar, and it feels hard to justify some space for yourself, please give yourself permission to wind down at the end of the day. Don't let yourself skip this. You matter; self-care matters. Try it—once the guilt passes, you'll like it.

Try not to skimp on your wind-down time. Allocate as much time as you can—60 minutes at the minimum, if you can swing it. Ideally it will be longer, as relaxation can't be hurried, but the reality is that you are juggling priorities—work, family, chores, responsibilities. There is no point in allotting a period that makes you stressed about what you're not getting done! If wind-down time longer than an hour is simply not possible within your life, there's no point forcing it. Pressure defeats the purpose. Stick with an hour minimum, and make it longer on the days when the gods of time smile on you.

I will wind down for _____ minutes (preferably 60–90 minutes).

This week you'll get into the swing of always getting up on time and going to bed at an appropriate time once you're sleepy. This might sound a bit boring and low key, but it helps. Your new sleep–wake schedule will provide consistency for your body clock, and it will set things up for your sleep efficiency to improve. Your schedule will allow you to be asleep for more of the time that you are in bed. By only having as much time as you need in bed, you are training your body to be more efficient with the time available for sleep. Eventually, this will mean less time awake in the night.

To summarise your plan, write the specific times in your schedule below.

My sleep–wake schedule for Week One

Wind down (60–90 minutes): _____ p.m.

Prepare for bed (15 minutes): _____ p.m.

Earliest bedtime: _____ p.m./a.m.

Morning wake-up time: _____ a.m.

A note of caution: keep yourself safe during your sleep improvement

I mentioned earlier that I'd give you a heads-up when a part of the programme potentially poses risks and needs to be avoided by some people. This is one of those moments. Reducing your time in bed can cause additional sleepiness, especially initially as your body adjusts. If you need to be alert and on to it, or if there is risk of serious accident for yourself or others in your job or daily life, you need to take responsibility and decide if it is appropriate to try this approach. If it seems unsafe or unwise, then trust your judgement and don't proceed with this approach on your own. Instead, explore doing it under the guidance of a healthcare professional.

Others who need to be cautious of this technique are people with epilepsy and pregnant women, and it also applies to people with conditions that are made worse by less sleep, including mental disorders (e.g., bipolar disorder, schizophrenia, other psychotic spectrum disorders) or other sleep disorders (e.g., obstructive sleep apnoea, parasomnias). Individuals who have unstable illnesses, degenerative diseases or are at risk of falls are also advised not to try this on their own. Trust your instincts on this and err on the side of caution. Remember you are committing to this programme to improve your health and well-being, not to put yourself at risk. Look after yourself.

If you are unsure about the wisdom of this approach for you, consult your doctor, specialist or mental-health professional.

Implementing a consistent sleep schedule

With your new sleep–wake schedule worked out for Week One, the challenge will be implementing these new times and behaviours consistently. Let's talk through each part of the schedule, covering off any pointers to help you stick with your intentions and any other considerations for the week.

Revise your sleeping environment

In preparation for the six-week programme, check and review your bedroom. Sleep hygiene was introduced in Chapter 4, and now is the time to make adjustments if needed. The goal is to create an environment that's helpful for sleep.

Check your bedroom basics

Temperature. Keep your room around 18 degrees Celsius. The body struggles to fall and stay asleep if it's too hot or too cold. If you're unable to make adjustments to the room temperature, do what you can with your sleepwear and bedding to warm things up or cool them down. (If the summer heat is extreme check Chapter 12 for options, or if menopause is messing with your personal thermostat check Appendix I for some cool-down ideas.)

Ventilation. If it's safe and not too noisy, latch a window open overnight for fresh air to circulate.

Darkness. Dim the lighting in your bedroom before heading to bed, to cue that it's nearly bedtime. When it's bedtime, make sure all lights are off and the curtains or blinds block out as much light as possible. The darker the room, the better. (Use a comfortable eye mask if you must.)

Quiet. Keep your bedroom quiet. Ask others to turn down the music or television if it's playing elsewhere in the house. Close doors to muffle any sounds. (Use comfortable earplugs or consider using white noise if you must.)

Technology. Keep all technology, screens, devices, clocks and, most importantly, phones out of the bedroom, especially while you are learning to sleep well again. It's not just about the light and sound they emit, it's about avoiding the mental stimulation they create with their content and endless options.

Bed and bedding. Make sure your mattress and pillow are adequately comfortable and supportive for your body, neck and head. Ensure your sheets and bedding are inviting and give you good temperature-control options if you get hot or cold in the night.

You may need to relearn how to wind down

When you've been living with sleep difficulties for a long time, it's easy to feel wound up or like you're falling behind on what you hoped to get done in the day. This can make winding down physically or psychologically tricky.

For some, extreme sleep deficit manifests as a state of hyperarousal, where you feel both tired and wired. You may feel very alert, on edge or anxious. Your mind may be agitated and your body restless. Your heart rate may be elevated, your breathing shallow, and so you keep pushing, driving ever onward even though it feels like there's little left in the tank. One woman I know who'd struggled with insomnia for years described herself as a 'high-functioning zombie', an expression that captures the lived experience of hyperarousal. If 'high-functioning zombie' sounds like you, you know that it can be difficult to slow down and take time out at the end of the day. It's like your on switch won't ever turn off.

Other people feel like they are always behind the eight ball. They may think that their exhaustion makes them slow, that everything is difficult and a bit fraught. It's that 'running through wet sand' feeling— as hard as you try, the going is achingly slow. If this is you, you may feel that you are continually trying to catch up with where you think you should be in your day, your week, your life. You believe you must press on regardless of how you're feeling, or how slow the headway actually is. Often you will give yourself a hard time about your lack of progress (regardless of how difficult daytime functioning can be when a body and mind is depleted).

After years of being one of the tired and wired, I fell into the latter camp and became worn out. I was regularly cruel to myself about how 'slow' and 'useless' I was on days after dreadful sleep. If I'd had a friend in that situation, I'd have showered them with compassion and reassurance, encouraging them to take time out to get some rest. We can have unreasonably high expectations of ourselves when we are tired.

Whether you're wired or feeling like you're lagging behind, many of you will be pushing yourself right till the finish line of the day. Then you might panic about how late it is, freak out about how little time there is for sleep and race to bed, where you clamp your eyes shut and *try* to go to sleep. Or, if you're a bit more informed about the importance of relaxation before sleep, you might be trying to *hurry up and relax!* (There's a subtle aggression in trying to relax.)

The body just doesn't work this way. Going to bed in this state means your body and brain are energised and alert. Have you ever tried to put a child to bed when it's overtired, overstimulated or out of sorts? It's like trying to settle a jack-in-the-box. There's a reason that parents have wind-down and settling routines for babies, toddlers and children. If you look online, there are plenty of charts and how-to guides on this for youngsters. But, for adults, you're expected to know and do this instinctively.

Yet that's not always the case. Some of you, in your struggles with sleep and the impact it has on your waking time, may have let your personal interests slide and fall away or may have even lost touch with some of the little things that you find relaxing or that bring you joy. You no longer know the gentle art of winding down and 'settling' yourself before bed. In some respects, many of us have forgotten how to relax.

For some, the default is staring mindlessly at the TV. With so much on offer, it's easy for an exhausted person to park up on the couch and channel surf or binge-watch at the end of the day. It requires so little of you. However, staring at the screen for hours on end, bathed in blue light and mental stimulation, is not the ideal wind-down option for someone with persistent sleep difficulties. While a bit of TV is okay, it's better to keep it to a minimum during your wind-down time while you're working on improving your sleep. Instead, lean towards non-screen-based activities.

Allocating 60 to 90 minutes to unplugging and unwinding in the evenings provides an opportunity to get reacquainted with things you find relaxing and that bring you joy. This is helpful self-care to create inner conditions that are more conducive to sleep. You have to consciously slow down and un-busy your evenings.

While winding down, you are allowing your body to switch over to the parasympathetic nervous system. When you do this, you feel calmer, your shoulders drop, your forehead unfurrows, your breathing deepens, your heart rate slows, and you go into a more restful state of being. Once you have mastered this art and your body knows that wind-down time can be trusted, it's infinitely easier to feel relaxed at bedtime.

So what do you do to wind down? After consciously allocating time to winding down, make it a priority—a valued part of your day as you improve your relationship with sleep. Scheduling your wind-down at a particular time of day for a certain period makes you more likely to keep the appointment with yourself. Set a reminder on your phone for when wind-down time begins. (While you are at it, change the settings on your phone so that the screen is dimmed from this time of the evening onward to minimise the blue light emitted.) Then, sweet, gentle quiet time begins.

As a qualitative researcher, I've had the privilege of listening to literally thousands of people open up about all sorts of personal details in the context of whatever product, service or social issue I was investigating. Regardless of the category, the common denominator is always that people are busy, and this creates pressure. Collectively, we're crying out for more personal time and an opportunity to take time out. This desire usually manifests as much-revered and longed-for 'me time'—a deep inner yearning to be allowed to slow down. Your wind-down time is for this.

During your wind-down time, consciously slow down. Do little, do it slowly, and only do things that you enjoy. This is the time for passive relaxation. Read a book or magazine. Listen to music that you love. If you choose to do exercise, go with slower, gentler options—a stroll, hatha yoga, tai chi, etc. Spend time with people you enjoy being with, keeping conversations positive and low key—no heated debates. If you watch TV choose some light, easy viewing (avoid shows that are confronting, exhilarating or scary) and keep it to a minimum—don't let autoplay lure you into the next episode. You may have arts, crafts or hobby projects that you find relaxing or a musical instrument that you enjoy playing. If it's mild outside, you might want to be in nature or watch the night sky. You may choose to take a leisurely bath or paint your toenails. Choose things that you genuinely look forward to doing.

When you haven't been allowing yourself time to unwind, or have been hypnotised in front of the telly night after night, it's easy to lose touch with what you genuinely enjoy doing in the evenings. Make a note of things that you'd like to do with this precious time.

The activities I'll enjoy in my wind-down time are:

_____

_____

_____

_____

_____

_____

_____

In preparation for your evening wind-down time, make use of what you've learned about encouraging habit formation. Earlier in the day, set up a visual cue or make it super easy and convenient to start winding down. Have a book or magazine that you're longing to read set out somewhere comfy and inviting. Locate the bath crystals, find a plush towel and set up a lovely candle in the bathroom. Make your wind-down time truly yours—something you look forward to and relish. (If you're a parent or caregiver, let your family know that you're off duty and unavailable at this time. You need to look after you. As someone once said to me, 'The mothership cannot go down!')

Add meditation to the mix (even a tiny one)

Meditation is an excellent aid to winding down. If you already have a practice, go with what works well for you. If you haven't explored meditation yet, haven't been able to get the hang of it (which is common) or are a bit resistant to it (that was me), it's worth considering or reconsidering. Learning to check in with yourself and become aware of how you truly are is a helpful resource on this journey.

We covered the principles of mindfulness as they apply to insomnia and sleep improvement in Chapter 10, along with some meditation options to consider. Your wind-down time might provide an opportunity to explore some of these practices. If you're still feeling a bit iffy, experiment with a one-minute meditation. It's a chance to connect with your breath and have a brief check-in with yourself. Yup, it's only 60 seconds. Hard to argue with that.

Learn how to stay up until or past your new bedtime

Your new earliest bedtime is likely to be a bit later than what you're used to, so you may need to make a plan to avoid falling asleep before then. By staying up later, you are consciously building sleep pressure so that, when it is time to go to bed, you will feel ready for sleep to come. With increased sleep pressure, you may be tempted to go to bed earlier than scheduled or to have forty winks on the couch. If at all possible, don't do this. You want to use this pressure to allow yourself to fall asleep more easily and quickly in your own bed, at your prescribed bedtime.

To keep from nodding off before bedtime, anticipate that this might happen and have a few tricks up your sleeve. The objective is to temporarily stave off falling asleep, not to thoroughly energise and wake yourself up. The sleepy feeling—characterised by itchy eyes, yawning, your eyes wanting to close and your head nodding—can be quite overwhelming and make it a struggle to stay awake. Sleepiness comes as a wave of symptoms.

Getting up and moving around the house will help, as will doing easy, mindless physical activities. Try saving a few no-brainer chores for later in the evening—for instance, emptying the dishwasher, folding washing, prepping lunch boxes. With each wave of sleepy symptoms, just get moving till it passes. Your bedtime will be getting closer. Meanwhile, have a laugh at the irony of it—you're having to apply yourself to stay awake for longer to improve your sleep!

Know the difference between tired and sleepy

We tend to use the terms tired and sleepy interchangeably. Yet, from the point of view of understanding and improving sleep, they are very different signals. It's vital to learn the difference and become discerning about what your body is telling you. Throughout the programme, only go to bed (at or after your prescribed bedtime) when your body is showing signs that it is *sleepy*. You may feel tired throughout the evening, but it's the sleepy feeling that tells you it's time for bed.

Tired versus sleepy

Being tired is not the same as being sleepy. Learn how to make the distinction.

Tiredness relates to exhaustion and fatigue. This may occur from overexertion (mental or physical) or from insufficient sleep. You can be tired but not sleepy. When you are depleted, it is possible to still feel alert and unable to fall asleep.

Sleepiness is what you experience when sleep pressure is high. You'll have itchy eyes (that's why you rub them), your eyelids will be heavy or closing, you'll be yawning or nodding your head. Sleepiness is your body telling you it's time to go to bed because it's ready for sleep.

Streamline preparation for bed

Getting ready for bed can be a faff when you're exhausted and sleepy. You've got a schedule to keep and you'll likely be staying up later than usual, so make sure that preparing for bed doesn't pose a barrier to getting you into bed once you're sleepy and you've reached (or passed) your earliest bedtime.

For a long time, I couldn't work out why it took me forever to make the transition from the lounge to the bedroom. Even when I was really tired, really sleepy and really wanting to be snuggled up in bed, I delayed. *What is my problem!* I thought. Then I realised that I actually loathed certain little jobs at the end of the night. Yes, I was being unreasonable and irrational, but the prospect of flossing and dealing with panda eyes seemed insurmountable! Plus, I hated getting into a cold bed.

Once I understood this, I removed these little barriers. I flossed and removed my make-up earlier in the evening. My bed was warmed in advance, the curtains were drawn, and the bedding was folded back invitingly. All that was left before I retired for the evening were the easy jobs and lovely rituals (pat the cat, kiss the child, climb between warm sheets).

You may be more reasonable and pragmatic about getting into bed than me, but if you dilly-dally despite best intentions, consider that some tasks might be acting as roadblocks. Do them in advance or make them easier to smooth your transition into bed.

Go clock-free and phone-free from bedtime to wake-time

If you haven't done so already, now is the time to get those time-telling, distracting, light-producing, alertness-invoking, stress-inducing, toxic-to-sleep devices out of your bedroom. (If you *must* have a phone for emergencies, keep it well away from you, at least out of arm's reach from your bed, and adjust your settings to minimise intrusions, e.g., switch it to silent, flight mode, or emergency calls only; set the screen to its dim, night-time option.)

Placing your clock or phone outside the bedroom or at least beyond reach works in your favour. It prevents you from checking the time overnight (and doing distressing sleep duration calculations) and it allows you to relax knowing that it will be there when you rise. Plus, it forces you to get up straight away in the morning, getting your wake-up system operational.

Start developing (even faking) a rise-and-shine mentality

When your alarm calls out to you in the morning, it's time to take action. Get up and turn it off. What you do during the day helps set you up for sleep at night—remember, it's a 24-hour sleep–wake cycle that you are working with. Even if your natural tendency is not bright-eyed and bushy-tailed first thing in the morning, get your eyes open and yourself moving. Your job is to support your body in getting its circadian rhythm back on track. You want to synchronise your body clock with the day so that wakefulness gets under way as soon as possible, sleep pressure begins its gradual build, and you feel sleepy come bedtime.

Remember, getting your eyes exposed to daylight is the key to making this happen—light triggers alertness, increases body temperature to get you moving, and pauses the secretion of melatonin. So get the curtains open and get outside into the daylight. Ideally, it's good to get at least fifteen minutes of exposure to natural light as early as you can in the day. Consider taking a walk outside, and, even if it's bright out, don't wear your sunglasses—you need the light to work its magic on your biology.

The other upside of getting out of bed pronto is that it boosts your sleep-efficiency score—less time in bed will improve that sleep time to time in bed ratio!

Avoid napping

While you are on your sleep-improvement journey, avoid napping unless it's absolutely necessary for your or others' safety. This week, with the changes that you're making to your habits, you are likely to experience more sleep pressure during the day. This will help make you feel more sleepy at night. If you nap, you release some of this pressure, which can cause sleep to be more elusive at night. If possible, avoid taking a nap this week.

However, if you are really struggling to stay awake during the day, be responsible and look after yourself. This is especially important if you need to drive or operate machinery. You may be able to boost your alertness temporarily with a brisk walk or some fresh air. (Don't fall into the trap of jacking yourself up with loads of caffeine as that only makes sleep more tenuous at night.) If the temporary fixes just aren't going to cut it, consider taking a nap. If you do opt for a nap, apply the advice from the World Sleep Society—keep it early and keep it brief. Try setting a timer for a maximum of 45 minutes; this will allow up to 30 minutes of sleep. Be sure that your nap is completed before 4 p.m.

What to expect from the programme

In your journey towards better sleep, keep in mind that the path will zigzag. You are changing behaviours and learning new skills. You're experimenting with your sleep to find out what improves it. It does take time, so be patient and keep an open mind. Having set expectations can lead to exerting effort to try to attain specific results. Because of the way sleep works, this sets you up for frustration and disappointment.

That said, it's understandable to want a sense of how things usually unfold. Generally, if CBTi is going to work, a person will experience sufficient progress within three to four weeks to know that it's worth continuing.

When I talk with people with sleep difficulties, they inevitably ask what they need to do to improve their sleep. Reading between the lines, they're often asking for a quick-fix one-night-wonder answer that will give them brilliant sleep *tonight*. If only it were that simple. Improving sleep is a lot like building your fitness or losing weight. There is no quick-fix 'go for a run' or 'eat a lettuce leaf' solution. It takes motivation, commitment, openness to learning new ways and trying different things, resilience when things aren't progressing or go backwards, and persistence and patience to find out what works for you and your body.

The schedule changes that you've worked out here will take some getting used to. That is the intention this week—to get used to a different sleep–wake schedule and observe what, if any, difference it makes to your sleep. The outcome will be what it is. It's early days. There's no need to be disheartened or disillusioned—there won't be a miraculous transformation. This is Week One of the programme, and there are many strands of CBTi to learn and experiment with. Have faith that, along the way, you'll find what's helpful for your sleep.

As you implement changes in your sleep schedule and introduce new and different behaviours, anticipate that there will be changes to your sleeping patterns. These changes may be improvements, but sleep can also slide sideways or go backwards. This can be alarming if you aren't aware of this possibility in advance. It's impossible to predict how your body is going to respond initially. So, if your sleep is upset by the changes, don't panic. Your body takes time to adjust. If your muscles were screaming after the first couple of sessions of a new fitness programme, you wouldn't stop working out. It's just a signal that your body isn't accustomed to the exercise yet. So stay with it, and do your best to follow your new sleep schedule this week, giving your body seven days to get familiar with a new approach.

This week, adhere to the regular schedule to the best of your ability—aim for daily adherence. If you are more free-range and loose by nature, you are at risk of being a bit non-compliant or even rebellious. You will need to focus on honouring your schedule so that you boost your chances of making progress. If you have an innate tendency to be orderly and organised, you'll likely be less resistant to implementing the new schedule.

Some of you will get really stressed by the schedule, or feel the need to rigidly comply with it, fearing consequences for your sleep. If you are in this latter group, please go easier on yourself—anxiety makes sleep more elusive. So be kind, cut yourself some slack and head in the direction of your schedule most of the time. If it doesn't quite come together every night, it's okay. For you guys, near enough is good enough. Try following it for at least four out of the seven days, and explore how it affects your sleep. (Hey, free-rangers—don't be thinking that this note applies to you. Your job is to adhere to the schedule *more* consistently.)

This week you have the opportunity to lay the groundwork for improved sleep by implementing a consistent schedule and anchoring your wake-up time. You are giving yourself permission to wind down at the end of the day, and you're honouring some key aspects of the World Sleep Society's commandments of sleep hygiene by getting devices out of the bedroom, and using napping appropriately if it's needed. You are slowly but surely on your journey towards better sleep. When you start out, there are a lot of changes to make and this can feel overwhelming. Dr Bronwyn Sweeney, a Wellington-based clinical psychologist and sleep researcher working with CBTi, encourages balance while implementing these new learnings. You don't want to be strict with yourself, but you do need to find a way to make some changes.

Go easy on your sleep and yourself. Consistent behaviours applied with flexibility and care are a powerful approach to finding sleep in our twenty-first century world.
—DR BRONWYN SWEENEY

Week One recap: what you can do

1. Summarise your Week One plan on the next page. Writing your sleep–wake schedule out again helps reinforce it in your mind, building engagement and commitment.

2. Carry out the new sleep schedule as best you can. You're looking for progress, not perfection.

3. Complete your sleep diary for Week One. Be sure to update your sleep diary each morning. At the end of the week, work out your sleep-efficiency scores and make some observations about what's working and any progress.

4. Be patient and open-minded about the outcomes. Learning and progress come from experimenting with different CBTi tools. You can't know which aspects will ease sleep for you until you explore them for a while. Remember, sleep improvement is non-linear.

5. Focus on and celebrate any positive changes that occur. This may be your sleep efficiency, your sleep quality, how you feel during the day. It may be your commitment to the schedule, your resilience, or the sense of agency fostered by proactively taking care of your sleep. Look for the upside in what you are doing. Notice how you feel about making time for yourself in the evening.

6. Keep reading, keep learning and stay curious about your sleep.

WEEK ONE GUIDE

My sleep–wake schedule for Week One

Wind down (60–90 minutes): _____ p.m.

Prepare for bed (15 minutes): _____ p.m.

Earliest bedtime: _____ p.m./a.m.

Morning wake-up time: _____ a.m.

- Set reminders for each element of your new sleep-wake schedule.
- Prepare and plan enjoyable activities to do during wind-down time.
- Include a mindfulness meditation each day while winding down (even if it's just a one-minute meditation or a pause for breath).
- Make a plan for how to stay awake until bedtime.
- Know the difference between being tired and being sleepy.
- Go to bed at the new earliest bedtime or later (when sleepy).
- Streamline preparation for bed.
- Remove your clock, phone and devices from the bedroom.
- Get up at wake-time.
- Fill out your sleep diary.
- Expose your eyes to daylight for fifteen minutes at the start of the day. Ideally go for a walk.
- If it's essential, take a brief nap before 4 p.m. (set a timer for 45 minutes maximum).

SLEEP DIARY

Fill out your sleep diary every morning. Guess the approximate times, there's no need for clock-watching. On the next page, note any factors that helped with sleep or may have been unhelpful for your sleep. You're looking for clues and patterns . . .

Week One	Night 1	Night 2	Night 3	Night 4	Night 5	Night 6	Night 7
Start Date ____							
Day of Week							
What time did you go to bed?							
What time did you first try to go to sleep?							
What time did you fall asleep?							
How many times did you wake in the night?							
How long did these awakenings last in total?							
What time did you wake for the final time this morning?							
What time did you get out of bed for the day?							
How would you rate the quality of your sleep? *(1 Terrible, 2 Bad, 3 OK, 4 Good, 5 Great)*							
Total Sleep Time In total, how many hours' sleep did you get?							
Total Time in Bed In total, how long were you in bed?							
Sleep Efficiency % (Total Sleep Time ÷ Total Time in Bed X 100 = %)	%	%	%	%	%	%	%

SLEEP DIARY

Week One	Night 1	Night 2	Night 3	Night 4	Night 5	Night 6	Night 7
Start Date _____ Day of Week							
Any factors that may have been unhelpful for your sleep last night?							
Any factors that may have helped with sleep last night?							

Observations & Insights:

Sleep consolidation —less, but better

What the caterpillar calls the end of the world, the master calls a butterfly.

—RICHARD BACH

ongratulations, you made it through Week One of the programme. You're here, ready to embrace the next stage of the journey, full credit to you. Having made it this far, you have a good base to build on, and I'm confident that you have the commitment needed to take on this week's plan. Week Two takes your consistent sleep schedule to the next level. It's one of the most challenging tools in the CBTi toolbox, but it can be one of the most effective: sleep consolidation.

Sleep consolidation is one of the most challenging tools in the CBTi toolbox, but it can be one of the most effective.

You'll need to dig deep, put resistance aside and have faith that sleep scientists wouldn't recommend this unless they were confident it worked.[1] If you were dieting, this would be the detox week where you'd only be allowed a few carrot sticks and a stalk of celery; if it was a fitness programme, this would be bootcamp. I kid you not, this week is going to be tough. Know what you're in for. But, most importantly, know that it can help move your sleep patterns in the direction you're after. Sleep consolidation builds on what you learned last week, moving from a consistent sleep schedule to a consolidated schedule with reduced time in bed. It's temporary, and it's doable.

What is sleep consolidation?

Sleep consolidation involves restricting the amount of time you spend in bed. The aim of this process is to consolidate your sleep, reducing the number of awakenings and the length of time you are awake throughout the night. It works towards more continuous, less fragmented sleep and improved sleep efficiency.[2] Once sleep has consolidated fairly consistently, time in bed is gradually increased.

Week One review

Before getting started with sleep consolidation, let's review Week One. If you haven't done so already, review last week's sleep diary. Work out your sleep-efficiency figures and look over your week for *little wins*. Keep an eye out for any positive signs—maybe you were falling asleep a little more easily some nights, had fewer awakenings in the night, weren't waking ages ahead of your scheduled wake-time, or your sleep-efficiency score crept upward some nights. At this stage, you're looking for incremental shifts forward. If these signs aren't emerging so far, that's all good—it's early days. Some of you may have found that your sleep was topsy-turvy last week as you changed your regimen. This can happen, and there's no need to be alarmed. Your body is adjusting to a different pattern, and it may take some time to settle into a new rhythm. Progress will unfold in its own way and time.

It's worth being honest with yourself about how thoroughly you implemented the new sleep-promoting behaviours that you planned last week. If you were reasonably consistent with it, give yourself a high-five regardless of whether you're reaping the rewards yet. If your new schedule habits were sketchy, acknowledge the inroads that you did make but encourage yourself to up your game this week, as persistent sleep difficulties are persistent—they don't tend to sort themselves out. Give yourself a helping hand—you'll know the areas you need to continue to take care of.

Plan Week Two

In Week One, you consciously reduced the hours you spent in bed to be more closely aligned with what you actually needed. Week Two continues this work. Last week you compressed your sleep into a smaller sleep window; this week, you will restrict that window further, if required, to consolidate your sleep. The goal of sleep consolidation is to increase your sleep efficiency, so you're asleep for more of the time you are in bed. It also helps to build sleep pressure, as you will be staying up for a longer time. Increased sleep pressure works in your favour by enabling you to fall asleep more easily.

Let's work out a sleep-consolidation plan that's appropriate for you.

Schedule your total time in bed

In Week Two, the length of time you get in bed will be determined by how much sleep your body has actually got last week. Look at your sleep diary from last week, and find the row capturing the total time that you were asleep each night—your total sleep time. We'll use this to calculate your average total sleep time. Jot down Week One's figures below, then tally them up to provide a total for the week.

Night 1: _____

Night 2: _____

Night 3: _____

Night 4: _____

Night 5: _____

Night 6: _____

Night 7: _____

Week One TOTAL SLEEP TIME: _____

Now, take your Week One total and divide it by the number of nights for which you have data, to get your average total sleep time. Write this number below, including any half or quarter hours.

Week One average total sleep time: _____ hours

NOTE: If your average total sleep time is below 5 hours, base your sleep consolidation on 5 hours. (Less than this is brutal, especially when you've opted for the self-help route and you're not supported by a healthcare professional.)

The figure above is the average amount of sleep you had each night last week. This quantity probably hasn't felt great for you, but you've demonstrated that it's manageable. Not great, but doable. You'll build your new sleep–wake schedule using this number—it will become your allocated total time-in-bed figure. It's okay, you can do this. The amount will likely be less than it was last week, and there will be no one-hour buffer this time around. You are giving your sleep opportunity a good squeeze!

Now, let's build this week's sleep–wake schedule around this new information, using your average nightly sleep duration for the past week as your new total time-in-bed figure.

The total time in bed that I'll work with this week is _____ hours.

Schedule your wake-up time

Keep this the same as last week to maintain consistency. Your morning wake-up time is the anchor for your weekly schedules throughout the programme. Remember, this is a constant every day of the week. Don't be tempted to sleep in on the weekends as this tends to unravel any progress you've made during the week.

The morning wake-up time I'm still committed to is _____ a.m.

Schedule your earliest bedtime

Using your average total sleep time (or 5 hours if your average is lower than this), work out what time you need to go to bed. For example, if your wake-up time is 6 a.m., and your average total sleep time is 5.5 hours, your new bedtime is 12.30 a.m. Radical. But, give it a go. You're on the journey towards better sleep, and you will only learn what works for you if you are prepared to experiment with this well-researched technique. (If it helps, remind yourself that what you were doing previously wasn't working so well.)

My new earliest bedtime is _____ p.m./a.m.

This is the earliest time you can go to bed this week. If you're anything like I was during sleep consolidation, it will take everything you have to stay awake till your prescribed bedtime—there was no way I was staying up later! As your sleep consolidates—becomes deeper, and less broken—you will gradually make your bedtime earlier, in 30-minute increments, until you reach a total sleep time that works well for you. Remember, the aim is not to restrict the amount of time you sleep—it is to restrict the amount of time that you spend in bed so that your time in bed more closely matches the amount of time you sleep.

Schedule time to prepare for bed

Continue to allow yourself around fifteen minutes to prepare for bedtime. You're not changing the components of your schedule, you're adjusting the time at which they occur.

Schedule time to wind down

Continue to allow 60 to 90 minutes to wind down each night.

Summarise your schedule for this week in the box below.

My sleep–wake schedule for Week Two

Wind down (60–90 minutes): _____ p.m.

Prepare for bed (15 minutes): _____ p.m.

Earliest bedtime: _____ p.m./a.m.

Morning wake-up time: _____ a.m.

A note of caution: keep yourself safe during sleep improvement

As was the case in Week One, there is a risk of sleep reduction and additional sleepiness when undertaking sleep consolidation. Take responsibility for yourself and decide if it's safe to proceed in a self-directed way, or whether you need guidance from a healthcare professional. Potentially at-risk groups include: those at risk of serious accident in their work or daily lives, pregnant women, people with epilepsy, people with other sleep disorders or mental health issues, people with unstable illnesses, people with degenerative diseases or those at risk of falls.

If your new scheduled earliest bedtime is much later than what you're accustomed to, make sure you plan relaxing things to do during your wind-down time. Also, have options available to keep you moving, occupied or distracted as the evening wears on in case you struggle to stay awake till your threshold bedtime. It's a great time to attend to simple chores—get that washing folded. In my experience, overwhelming feelings of sleepiness tend to come in waves. While they are intense, they are temporary. Knowing that they pass will help you to prepare and deal with them when sleep threatens to envelop you before curfew.

It's likely that you will initially experience some mild to moderate sleep loss (in terms of the time you spend asleep) this week, but the sleep that you do get is likely to be better quality. While you may get less sleep, it's more consolidated—less waking in the night and longer stretches of sleep. Even so, as your body switches over to a different approach to sleep, there may be some tough days. Generally, the first few nights are the hardest.

You may want to work out the best time to start this regimen. Choose a day of the week when poor sleep may be easier to manage. If there are days when less is required of you, begin your sleep consolidation the night before. This will help remove some pressure as you get your new protocol under way.

Over the first week or two of sleep consolidation, sleep efficiency starts to improve. As it does, you will gradually increase the amount of time you spend in bed. In time, your sleep duration and continuity will build back up, improving your daytime functioning and energy levels.

Initially, sleep consolidation can be challenging, so be incredibly kind and compassionate with yourself throughout this week. Acknowledge that what you're doing is tough. This is not the time to be harsh, critical or judgemental about your sleep or about yourself. (Something people with sleep difficulties are prone to do.) If you have an inner voice that tends to give you a hard time, ask it to be quiet and patient with you this week. Even better, encourage your inner voice to speak softly and to be understanding, gentle and encouraging as you work through this week. If you are kind and patient with yourself, you're more likely to cope with the week and remain committed to trusting the process.

It's also worth letting someone close to you know what you're doing so that you have a bit of extra support and compassion as you make your way through this challenging stage of the programme. Keep in mind that it's just a phase, and have faith that any rocky bits will pass. There's little doubt that this week can be a tough one, but it's short-term pain for long-term gain.

For those of you rising to the challenge of trying a week of sleep consolidation, I salute you. Be brave, be strong, you've got this. As we say in New Zealand, kia kaha.

Can't face sleep consolidation?

If you are simply not up for sleep consolidation at this stage, that's okay. You may feel like you can't risk less sleep, even temporarily. Life may be too demanding at the moment, or you may feel like you can't face another challenge just now. Know that you can slow the programme down and do it at your own pace. Keep following the sleep–wake schedule you worked out for last week and give your body more time to adjust to those changes. From there, you can decide whether to do sleep consolidation or to move on to Week Three instead. You know your own circumstances best and you need to proceed at a pace that feels manageable and safe. There are extra sleep diaries in Appendix IV if you prefer to take things a bit slower. Let progress unfold at its own pace.

Week Two recap: what you can do

1. Summarise your Week Two plan on the next page. Writing out your sleep–wake schedule again helps reinforce it in your mind, building engagement and commitment.

2. Carry out your new sleep–wake schedule as best you can. Aim for progress, not perfection.

3. Complete Week Two of your sleep diary. Write down your sleep info daily. At the end of the week, work out your sleep-efficiency calculations and make observations about your experience.

4. Be kind with yourself, especially on tough days—as your body adjusts to a reduced opportunity to sleep, there'll be some bumpy nights, and the following days may be challenging. Be gentle with yourself on these days, and know this is a process that you're moving through.

5. Congratulate yourself at the end of the week. Celebrate that you have implemented sleep consolidation, to the best of your abilities, and were compassionate with yourself along the way.

6. Keep reading, keep learning and stay curious about your sleep.

WEEK TWO GUIDE

My sleep–wake schedule for Week Two

Wind down (60–90 minutes): _____ p.m.

Prepare for bed (15 minutes): _____ p.m.

Earliest bedtime: _____ p.m./a.m.

Morning wake-up time: _____ a.m.

- Set new reminders for each element of your revised sleep–wake schedule.
- Continue with your enjoyable wind-down activities.
- Do a meditation when you wind down each evening—a one-minute meditation, a pause for breath, or a mindfulness meditation—to check in with yourself (not to induce sleep).
- Plan for how to keep sleepiness at bay till your new earliest bedtime.
- Keep training yourself to know the difference between tiredness and sleepiness.
- Go to bed at or after your earliest bedtime, once you are sleepy.
- Keep clocks, phones and devices out of the bedroom overnight.
- Get up at your wake-up time.
- Fill out your sleep diary.
- Expose your eyes to daylight in the mornings—fifteen minutes, combined with a walk.
- If you must, take a brief nap before 4 p.m. (set a timer for 45 minutes maximum).
- Be kind and understanding with yourself.

SLEEP DIARY

Fill out your sleep diary every morning. Guess the approximate times, there's no need for clock-watching. On the next page, note any factors that helped with sleep or may have been unhelpful for your sleep. You're looking for clues and patterns . . .

Week Two	Night 1	Night 2	Night 3	Night 4	Night 5	Night 6	Night 7
Start Date _____ Day of Week							
What time did you go to bed?							
What time did you first try to go to sleep?							
What time did you fall asleep?							
How many times did you wake in the night?							
How long did these awakenings last in total?							
What time did you wake for the final time this morning?							
What time did you get out of bed for the day?							
How would you rate the quality of your sleep? (1 Terrible, 2 Bad, 3 OK, 4 Good, 5 Great)							
Total Sleep Time In total, how many hours' sleep did you get?							
Total Time in Bed In total, how long were you in bed?							
Sleep Efficiency % (Total Sleep Time ÷ Total Time in Bed X 100 = %)	%	%	%	%	%	%	%

SLEEP DIARY

Week Two		Night 1	Night 2	Night 3	Night 4	Night 5	Night 6	Night 7
Start Date _____	Day of Week							
Any factors that may have been unhelpful for your sleep last night?								
Any factors that may have helped with sleep last night?								

Observations & Insights:

Your bed as a cue for sleep

I've learned that I still have a lot to learn.
—MAYA ANGELOU

o you dread your bed or subconsciously harbour bad feelings towards your bedroom? Throughout your sleep difficulties, you've probably spent a lot of time lying awake at night in your bedroom. In the 'comfort' of your own bed, your mind has churned for hours—fretting about how long it's taking to get to sleep, how little time you've slept, how often you've woken and how long you've been awake. You've most likely ruminated or catastrophised about the impending horrors of the day ahead, or you may have been riddled with resentment towards your partner, fully zonked-out beside you. From such thoughts come stress and physical agitation. Your bed has probably been the site of tossing, turning and many deep sighs. Chances are, over time you have unknowingly built up an unhelpful association with your bed.

You may have invested in a lovely mattress, feather pillows and a beautiful duvet, but your bed has become the site of too many nights of crappy sleep. So much so that the bed itself, as stylishly *House & Garden* as it may look, has become a cue for fretful wakefulness and lousy sleep. These associations are spontaneous, automatic and super unhelpful in the quest for better sleep. In Week Three you're going to expose these associations and explore a process for retraining the way you feel towards your bed so that your bed (and bedroom) once again become a valuable cue for sleep. But first, let's acknowledge the week that you've just made it through.

Week Two review

Congratulations, you did it! A week of sleep consolidation is done. That's champion. I hope you were one of the minority who get through sleep consolidation relatively unscathed with just a few wonky nights. But it's likely it's been a rough one—things tend to get worse before they get better. So big ups to you for having survived it and for being back here, continuing the journey. That takes impressive resilience and tenacity, and highlights your commitment to making way for the sleep of your dreams. Sleep consolidation really is the bootcamp of the programme. Lots of you will be wanting to throw in the towel—don't be in too much of a rush to quit.

If you're starting to see *any* shifts in the right direction, be encouraged. You may notice your sleep-efficiency scores beginning to increase, you're falling asleep more easily, you're waking less often in the night, you're awake for a shorter time overnight, or your sleep quality is improving. These are signs to keep going. Progress may only be incremental at this stage, so be patient. If you're not yet making headway but feel up for persevering, go for it. For some people, sleep difficulties take a bit longer to start improving. Keep at it.

If you found sleep consolidation just too damned hard, that's okay. It's tough, and it absolutely doesn't suit everyone. Acknowledge that you gave it a go, be kind with yourself about the outcome, and consider your options moving forward. You can go back to the schedule you used in Week One if that feels more doable and use this alongside what you'll be learning in this chapter. Or, if you're really feeling like the approach in this book doesn't fit with your circumstances or your learning style, please see Appendix II for alternative options to improve your sleep. A self-help CBTi approach is only one option and it's probably the most demanding. You could try CBTi with professional support, explore MBTI, or check out other protocols available through sleep clinics, psychologists with insomnia training or online programmes. Keep experimenting with sleep-improvement options until you find one that works for you—learning to sleep really is worth it.

If you're sticking with it, let's discover how to retrain your body and mind so that your bed becomes a trigger for sleep.

Stimulus-control training: using your bed as a cue for sleep

Through a process of unconscious learning, it's easy for your bed (or even your bedroom) to become a cue for wakefulness and frustration.[1] Endless experiences of poor sleep condition you to associate your bed with being awake or annoyed, rather than being asleep. Sometimes you might lie in bed *trying* to sleep and getting wound up, other times you'll consciously *try* to rest and relax, *waiting* (and hoping) for sleep to arrive. Still other times you'll give up on these efforts and distract yourself with other activities to kill time while you remain awake in your bed. You'll read, listen to podcasts, watch something online, work, scroll through your Facebook and Instagram feeds, check something random online and fall down the rabbit hole of the World Wide Wonderland. All of these behaviours, as well-intentioned as they are, reinforce your association with your bed and being awake. This association can make you wary about your chances of slumber in your bed, even when you know your body needs sleep.

Later in the evening, I think, 'Oh god, I've got to go upstairs and do a night.' Some nights I can't even be bothered trying to sleep.

—MEGAN (51, PRODUCT DEVELOPER)

Others (like me) take things even further and abandon the bedroom in despair to set up camp elsewhere in the house. Here, you might amuse yourself for a while until you get sleepy and then fall asleep in this temporary nest—a nest that is not your own bed. The problem with this strategy is that not only are you learning to associate your own bed with wakefulness, you're also programming yourself to believe that you sleep better elsewhere.

The daybed in the dining room was my place of refuge on those hideous nights of broken sleep. After what felt like hours of mental gymnastics, clockwatching and midnight maths, I'd conclude that attempts to fall asleep in my bed were futile. I knew if I stayed there any longer, I'd get really ratty and end up accidentally waking my husband. So, I'd get up, make a cup of tea (herbal if I was being responsible, gumboot if I was feeling defiant), wrap myself in a blanket on the daybed, sip tea and read a book. This felt so much better than trying to fall asleep in my bed. When drowsiness finally overcame me, I'd stretch out on the daybed and sleep till the morning light woke me. I did this fairly regularly, until it became a bit of a ritual and falling asleep on the daybed was more reliable than falling asleep in my bed. It got to the point where I preferred to go to bed on the daybed—despite how narrow and hard the daybed was compared to my actual bed!

Some people get drowsy and nod off in the comfy chair in front of the TV, but as soon as they transition to their bed (even if they do this in a streamlined, low-key way), they find that sleep defies them. They know they're tired and sleepy, yet, once in their own bed, they feel alert, even wired.

Dreading your bed or preferring to fall asleep elsewhere are indicators that you have unknowingly formed associations with your bed that are counterproductive to sleep. The late Richard Bootzin, an American psychologist and pioneer in the field of behavioural sleep medicine, discovered this 'conditioned arousal' among people with insomnia and developed helpful pathways to overcome it. His approach continues to be part of the backbone of CBTi. His stimulus-control regimen is designed to strengthen the bed as a cue for sleep and weaken it as a cue for wakefulness. This can be useful for encouraging sleep initiation (falling asleep) and for sleep maintenance (falling back to sleep). It's recognised as an empirically supported treatment for insomnia.[2]

Over the last few weeks, some of you will have already integrated habit changes into your sleep-improvement regimen that are part of stimulus-control training—you'll be ahead of the curve on reconditioning what your bed means to you. But let's go over the fundamentals so everyone can get up to speed. These guidelines lay the foundations for a stronger association between bed and sleep.

Reserve your bedroom for sleep (and sex) only

Until your bed is once more associated with great sleep, don't use your bed or your bedroom for anything other than sleeping or sex. Remove all potential distractions and diversions, so there's nothing else to do in there. Your bedroom should no longer be the home of phones, TVs, screens, laptops or any other digital devices. There will be no work or study, no watching movies, no talking on the phone, no eating—nothing that encourages wakefulness. And, of course, you've already removed the clock. Eventually your bedroom is to become your sleep sanctuary. For now, just strip it bare of anything that might tempt you towards wakefulness. (The strict approach is no books, so ideally you'll do your reading elsewhere in the house. If you can't cope with that, make a sensible concession—if you go to bed when you're sleepy, you'll only manage a few pages before your eyelids get too heavy. Keep reading in bed to a minimum throughout this process.)

Maintain a consistent sleep schedule

You have been working diligently on this for the last two weeks. You have a non-negotiable wake-up time firmly in place that is helping to anchor your body clock each day. This helps you to be consistent in the time that you expose your eyes to daylight and switch off your melatonin. At this stage of your sleep-improvement journey, your wake-up time is the most stable part of your schedule. No matter what, get up at your scheduled wake-time, regardless of how many times you got up overnight, how long you have been awake or how dreadful you feel. Keep reinforcing the wake-up time as a daily constant to help your body establish a sleep–wake rhythm that supports a good night's sleep.

When you wake and get up at your scheduled time in the morning, sleep pressure starts gradually building early in the day, and your sleepy signals will be strong by your scheduled earliest bedtime. Even if your body and mind resist getting up when your morning alert sounds, get your eyes open, get your feet on the floor, and throw back those curtains. Think of it as an essential investment in your sleep tonight.

Go to bed when you are sleepy, not just tired

You've endured persistent sleep difficulties and you've done a couple of weeks with a new, more consolidated sleep–wake schedule, so you will likely be feeling tired. Even so, it's imperative that you only go to bed at or after your scheduled earliest bedtime, and only when you are actually sleepy. Remember the telltale signs of sleepiness—itchy eyes, rubbing your eyes, eyelids lowering, yawning or head nodding.

Minimise daytime napping

Try not to nap while you are building a robust and helpful connection between your bed and sleep. However, for some of you, it may sometimes feel impossible to safely get through the day without a nap. If this is you, taking care of yourself is the priority. If you must nap, keep it brief (set the timer for 45 minutes, so you'll get a maximum of 30 minutes) and make sure you've finished your nap by 4 p.m.

Retrain your brain: bed = sleep

You must unlearn the association that bed means unrest and wakefulness, and learn to associate your bed with sleep.

The 'out of bed' protocol

The most crucial element of stimulus-control training to introduce this week is likely to inspire a wild string of cussing and obscenities. If you thought sleep consolidation was bad, wait till you hear Mr Bootzin's brilliant idea. (I wish some of these sleep researchers could experience what their protocols are actually like to live through. I imagine it would have inspired them to keep researching and come up with more user-friendly methods. Until then, this is what we've got to work with.) There's no sugar-coating it—this regimen sucks. However, it's clinically proven to work, and it's temporary. I've road-tested it and I can vouch for its ability to improve your sleep continuity. Have faith that it can be done. It's ghastly, but doable.

Here it is: *If sleep hasn't come to you within fifteen minutes, get up and go to another room until you're sleepy.*

Once you've gone to bed, if you don't fall asleep or fall back to sleep within what feels like fifteen minutes, get up and go to a different room, stay up till you're really sleepy, then return to bed. (Don't allow yourself to fall asleep in the other room.) Once you're back in your own bed, if sleep *still* doesn't come within fifteen minutes, get out of bed again and repeat the process until you fall asleep rapidly in your own bed.[3] Dr Tony Fernando calls this the 'out of bed' protocol.

As rugged as it sounds, this new behaviour conditions you to associate your bed with falling asleep quickly and easily (not with frustration, stress, effort and wakefulness). With repetition of this behaviour, you'll begin to automatically associate your bed with a helpful, relaxed and more immediate sleep response.

What to expect

First of all, it's natural to be experiencing some gritty resistance to the 'out of bed' protocol. My initial response was along the lines of: 'You've got to be f**king kidding.' It felt like the absolute last thing I needed. It was as though the sleep gurus were intent on taunting and torturing me further—'Hey, sleep-deprived woman, why don't you get out of bed like a yo-yo for a few nights!'

Once I understood the rationale of conditioned behaviour and unhelpful cues, it made sense to retrain my brain to create useful sleep associations with my bed. But I certainly tried to wriggle out of it for a while.

At that time, I avoided this approach for as long as I could. My theory was that surely it was better to get some sleep somewhere in the house than to get hardly any sleep in my own bed. However, doing this was further conditioning me to associate falling asleep with the 'bad for my back, great for my chiropractor' daybed, and further reinforcing that my bed was not a great place to fall asleep. So while my theory worked as a temporary Band-Aid to my difficulties, it wasn't moving me towards a sustainable solution. I did actually want to be able to sleep well in my own bed.

Some people oppose the out-of-bed method, claiming they remain calm while they lie awake in bed. They believe it's better to wait in their bed in case falling asleep is imminent. In truth, the process of 'waiting and hoping' can be a subtle form of trying to sleep. It's a clandestine effort, a quiet wanting that can make sleep more elusive. While this may work sometimes, the reason that you're here reading this book is that your experience and your sleep diaries are telling you that your current approach (including deluding your sleep-deficient self that you're relaxed while you wait for sleep to hurry up and arrive) is not delivering the sleep that you want.

Some will argue that resting is better than getting up because it conserves energy. While that's true, conserving energy doesn't build sleep pressure—the very pressure that you need to fall asleep. Nor does rest allow your body to get on with genuinely restorative sleep, which is important for your physical well-being and brain function. Plus, resting doesn't break that unhelpful cycle of associating bed with wakefulness instead of sleep. Resting is a short-term tactic rather than a long-term solution. (When you have your sleep difficulties resolved, resting quietly as you fall asleep or fall back to sleep is fine, but while you're addressing your conditioning it's less helpful than getting out of bed.)

Debates aside, it's important to have realistic expectations of the experience. According to the late Dr Peter Hauri, a past director of the

Mayo Sleep Disorders Center, it's common to be in and out of bed many times on the first night of this protocol, but, over the next few nights, it becomes easier to fall asleep.[4] My experience with Bootcamp Bootzin's technique mirrored this. The first few nights were surreal. I felt like I was up every hour, sometimes multiple times. But it got easier more quickly than I'd anticipated. Seeing progress over consecutive nights spurred me on, and I gained confidence in my ability to fall asleep in my own bed. (Because getting up repeatedly was so horrible—Pavlov's dog was learning quickly!)

> *The first few nights were surreal. I felt like I was up every hour, sometimes multiple times. But it got easier more quickly than I'd anticipated.*

There's no doubt that it takes considerable willpower (and genuine understanding of and belief in the principles) to implement Bootzin's technique to change your associations with your bed. It is dreadful but doable, and completely worthwhile. The key to getting through this part of the programme is to be prepared—plan ahead. Support yourself through this 'character-building' experience.

How to support yourself this week

Timing matters
Decide which days of the week are best suited to start implementing these changes to your sleep regimen. Often people prefer to kick off on a Friday night, so they have a few days to get through the initial tumult that the Bootzin technique is likely to bring. If you need to delay a few days, just continue with the sleep–wake schedule that we'll work out below and start the 'out of bed' protocol when you are ready.

Reconnect with your true north
To stay motivated, remind yourself why you committed to improving your sleep. Double back to the last page of Chapter 7, where you wrote down why you are prioritising your sleep and why you're staunchly

dedicated to doing what it takes to improve it. Connect with this again to gather your resolve. Your true north was something that deeply mattered to you—keep it in mind as you ask even more from yourself this week.

Remind yourself it's temporary

Yes, it's going to be bad before it gets good, but remember the ghastly stage is temporary. When you're in the midst of it, your mind will play tricks on you. It might feel like time has dropped into eternal slo-mo (it hasn't) and your suffering will go on forever (it won't). This is a temporary process as you retrain your brain to associate your bed with the relief of sleep, not the anguish and dread of nocturnal wakefulness. Stay open-minded and accept that it's a measure to help you towards what you want. As you haul yourself out of bed in the night, quietly repeat to yourself, 'This too shall pass.'

Prepare a night haven

In advance, set up somewhere to go when you get out of bed during the night. It needs to be warm, comfortable and relaxing, but not so toasty or borderline horizontal that you'll be tempted to nod off. (Think of your night haven as a personal transit lounge.)

When I was implementing the 'out of bed' protocol, I used to go to my favourite corner—my treasured daybed. I set it up with comfy cushions, a blanket and a book. I'd make a herb tea on the way, and I'd keep the lights quite low. It was winter, so I'd put the heater on or fill a hot-water bottle to keep warm. It felt relaxed and, so long as I didn't lie down, I was able to read quietly until the telltale signs of sleepiness emerged.

Prepare something to do when you are out of bed

Make sure you prepare something to do while you are up. It may be a relaxing wind-down activity—reading, listening to music or listening to an audiobook are probably the easiest activities to have on hand. Make sure you choose something suitably benign—it needs to be passively relaxing without requiring too much of you. It's a balancing act: you don't want anything too engaging or stimulating that will keep you awake, but you don't want it to be so dull and tedious that you nod off in situ.

One night I made the mistake of leaving an excellent crime thriller out for myself. Doh. I've never been so eager to get out of bed during the night, and once I was up there was no way I was going back to bed till I'd burned through my page-turner! Stick to things that won't put your 'bed as a cue for sleep' initiative in jeopardy.

Let others know

If you live with others, it's worth letting them know what you're exploring this week. If you have a bed-partner, talk them through the rationale for this approach and reassure them that it's temporary while you retrain yourself to associate your bed with sleep. They may choose to sleep elsewhere over those first few nights. (Fair enough.)

It's also good to let others know that your sleep may go a bit haywire for a few nights, and there's the potential of daytime fallout from lost sleep. Having people close to you show support, understanding and respect as you continue through the programme will help you to maintain commitment. However, ask them not to continually check in on your progress or to offer advice. You don't want to dwell on interim difficulties or be disillusioned by other people's ease of sleeping!

No clock required in the bedroom

Even though you need to get up if you haven't fallen asleep or back to sleep in fifteen minutes, you still don't need a clock, watch or time-telling device in your bedroom. Trust your instincts and go by what feels like a quarter of an hour. A guesstimate is all that's needed. (Those luminous numbers are entirely unhelpful for your cause.)

Keep being kind to yourself

Acknowledge that this process will be gnarly and remind yourself that you're doing it because you value yourself and care about your long-term ability to sleep well. Be super compassionate with yourself on the hard nights and following days. Expect a bit less of yourself and ask for a bit more support—go gently, and make life a little easier through this time.

A note of caution: keep yourself safe during sleep improvement

The stimulus-control training that you are implementing this week is another form of sleep restriction, so the same cautions and exclusions apply as outlined in the first two weeks of the programme. Be careful about if and when you choose to do this if you need to be alert in your work or daily life, especially if there is risk of serious accident to yourself or others. Pregnant women, people with epilepsy, people with mental-health or sleep disorders made worse by sleep loss, people with unstable illnesses or degenerative diseases, and people who are at risk of falls should not attempt the 'out of bed' protocol without the support of a healthcare professional.

If the above cautions mean that stimulus-control training is not for you, continue with the sleep–wake schedule you plan for this week and implement the elements that feel more manageable. This means: reserve your bedroom for sleep and sex (you know the drill—no non-sleep activities, no phones, clocks, screens, devices, work, etc.); go to bed at or after your scheduled earliest bedtime when you are sleepy; and if you absolutely must nap, keep it to a minimum (with a timer set for 45 minutes, and your nap completed by 4 p.m.).

Plan Week Three

If your sleep-efficiency scores are the same or lower than they were, or if they are improving but still under 85 per cent on most nights of the week, stay with last week's sleep–wake schedule. (If you didn't do sleep consolidation last week but you're now ready to give it a shot, double back to Week Two, and work out a revised sleep–wake schedule for the week to come.) It's still early days to see improvements in your sleep, so keep the faith and keep going. Generally, only after three or four weeks of CBTi do people feel like they are experiencing substantial improvements. You've only just finished Week Two, so trust the process and give yourself time.

If your sleep-efficiency scores were 85 per cent or higher on at least four nights last week, do a victory dance. Celebrating your wins helps embed your new behaviours and will keep you motivated. You're in the minority of people who see fast improvements, so bathe in the glory of your excellent results.

Once your scores are at this heady level, it's time to reward yourself with a little more time in bed! Because you have demonstrated that you can now sleep for most of the time that you're in bed (on most nights), start very gradually building up the amount of time that you are asleep. You do this by incrementally increasing your total time in bed. Increase your total time in bed by 30 minutes this week, bringing your earliest bedtime back by half an hour. (Don't be tempted to rush the process by going to bed earlier than this—it risks fragmenting your sleep.) Implement this schedule for the whole week.

Even though this is only a 30-minute adjustment, be open-minded about how your sleep might respond. Allow your sleep to resist the change on some nights and accept the additional sleep opportunity on other nights. Suspend judgement and let your sleep progress unfold in its own higgledy-piggledy way in its own sweet time.

Tailor your Week Three sleep–wake schedule based on how things evolved last week.

Schedule your wake-up time

Keep this the same as last week—your wake-up time is the anchor for your weekly schedules throughout the programme. It's the same on weekdays and weekends.

The morning wake-up time I'm still committed to is _____ a.m.

Schedule your earliest bedtime

If your sleep-efficiency scores were lower than 85 per cent most nights of last week, keep your scheduled earliest bedtime the same as last week. If you are one of the few whose sleep-efficiency scores were 85 per cent or above on most nights of the week, then make your bedtime 30 minutes earlier than last week.

This is the earliest time that you can go to bed this week. If you're not feeling physically *sleepy* at bedtime, stay up a while until those signs appear—yawning, head nodding, rubbing your eyes, eyelids closing, etc.

My earliest bedtime is _____ p.m./a.m.

Schedule time to prepare for bed

Continue to allow fifteen minutes to prepare for bedtime. The components of your schedule remain the same, you're just adjusting the timing of things (if needed) based on how your sleep has responded so far.

Schedule time to wind down

Continue to allow 60 to 90 minutes to wind down each evening.

Summarise your schedule for this week in the box below.

My sleep-wake schedule for Week Three

Wind down (60–90 minutes): _____ p.m.

Prepare for bed (15 minutes): _____ p.m.

Earliest bedtime: _____ p.m./a.m.

Morning wake-up time: _____ a.m.

Okay, you're set to go. Another week of possible sleep improvement awaits. I wish you well. Remember that doing challenging and difficult things can be an act of self-compassion, if those things ultimately move your life in a direction that nourishes your well-being for years to come. Sometimes you have to go through temporary suffering to reach what you truly need. This week, keep the wise words of Zen master Thich Nhat Hanh with you: *No mud, no lotus.*

Week Three recap: what you can do

1. **Summarise your Week Three plan on the next page.** Writing your schedule out again might feel repetitive, but it reinforces your commitment and helps with motivation.

2. **Carry out your new sleep–wake schedule as best you can.** Progress, not perfection.

3. **Complete Week Three of your sleep diary.** Jot down your daily sleep info, including which bits of the plan you managed. After seven days, calculate your sleep-efficiency scores. Note and celebrate any improvements you've experienced.

4. **Prepare a night haven.** Make sure it's comfortable (warm in winter and cool in summer) and keep the lights dim. Have something low key, even a bit boring, to do until you feel sleepy.

5. **Be realistic, prepare for the week and be kind with yourself.** It won't be an easy one. Know that you'll experience some sleep loss as you retrain your brain to associate your bed with sleep, not suffering. Remind yourself it's temporary and have faith that new neural pathways are forming (*bed = sleep*). Make it easy on yourself by being prepared, and be compassionate with yourself throughout the process.

6. **Congratulate yourself at the end of the week.** Acknowledge that you've implemented another week of sleep consolidation, as well as stimulus-control training (making your bed a cue for sleep)—the two toughest protocols in CBTi.

7. **Keep reading, keep learning and stay curious about your sleep.**

WEEK THREE GUIDE

My sleep-wake schedule for Week Three

Wind down (60–90 minutes): _____ p.m.

Prepare for bed (15 minutes): _____ p.m.

Earliest bedtime: _____ p.m.

Morning wake-up time: _____ a.m.

- Continue building helpful habits from last week.
- Continue cultivating your mindfulness practice: one-minute meditation, a pause for breath, or mindfulness meditation to regularly check in with yourself.
- Implement this week's sleep-wake schedule.
- Implement the 'out of bed' protocol.
  - If you're still awake after fifteen minutes, get up.
  - Relax in your night haven.
  - Go back to bed only when you are sleepy.
  - If you don't fall asleep in bed within fifteen minutes, get up again.
  - Repeat this process till you easily fall asleep in your bed.
- Be very patient and kind with yourself this week.

SLEEP DIARY

Fill out your sleep diary every morning. Guess the approximate times, there's no need for clock-watching. On the next page, note any factors that helped with sleep or may have been unhelpful for your sleep. You're looking for clues and patterns . . .

Week Three _____	Night 1	Night 2	Night 3	Night 4	Night 5	Night 6	Night 7
Start Date _____ Day of Week							
What time did you go to bed?							
What time did you first try to go to sleep?							
What time did you fall asleep?							
How many times did you wake in the night?							
How long did these awakenings last in total?							
What time did you wake for the final time this morning?							
What time did you get out of bed for the day?							
How would you rate the quality of your sleep? (1 Terrible, 2 Bad, 3 OK, 4 Good, 5 Great)							
Total Sleep Time In total, how many hours' sleep did you get?							
Total Time in Bed In total, how long were you in bed?							
Sleep Efficiency % (Total Sleep Time ÷ Total Time in Bed X 100 = %)	%	%	%	%	%	%	%

SLEEP DIARY

Week Three	Night 1	Night 2	Night 3	Night 4	Night 5	Night 6	Night 7
Start Date _____ Day of Week							
Any factors that may have been unhelpful for your sleep last night?							
Any factors that may have helped with sleep last night?							

Observations & Insights:

Operation mind shift— dispel your sleep myths

We all have that possibility, that potential and that promise of seeing beyond the seeming.
—MAYA ANGELOU

There's no gentle way to break this to you, but, given that you've endured many, many nights of difficult sleep, there's a good chance some funky thinking about sleep has formed deep in your brain. This unhelpful thinking does you and your sleep absolutely no favours. It keeps you locked in a cycle of poor sleep. It's almost inevitable that, after persistent sleepless nights and fuddled days, you interpret your sleep difficulties as a threat to your well-being.

To manage your sleep and protect yourself, you become vigilant, monitoring your sleep and worrying about the consequences of sleep deficiency. Even though you may pay a lot of attention to sleep, you start to lose confidence in your ability to sleep, and there's an alarming sense you no longer have control over your situation.[1]

To explain, make sense of and even 'protect' yourself from what's going on, you develop a multitude of thoughts—which may not altogether be based on fact or reality. Some of them will spring from misinformation or general misconceptions about sleep. Some will be the by-product of common distortions of thinking built around your sleep experiences and beliefs. You aren't making stuff up, yet some of the thoughts you've formed may be misaligned with the truth.

On inspection, while on my own sleep-improvement journey, I discovered I had a ragbag collection of unhelpful automatic sleep thoughts. While I didn't think these thoughts all at once, they were definitely alive and well in my repertoire. They included little gems like:

I'm a terrible sleeper.
I'm going to wake at 2 a.m. and be awake for hours.
If I don't sleep well tonight, I'll be useless tomorrow.
Work is going to be a disaster.
I had only four hours of sleep last night—
I'm going to feel like hell.
I must go to bed early to catch up.
I have to cancel meeting my friend
this evening. I'll be too tired.
I haven't got the energy to exercise.
I never get eight hours' sleep.
My sleep is so unpredictable and it's getting worse.
I've tried everything, nothing helps.
This has got to be bad for my health.

Sleep psychologists use clinical terms like 'dysfunctional cognitions' and 'negative sleep thoughts' to describe these thoughts, which is a bit mean given we're doing our best in pretty crinkly circumstances.

They're referring to the unhelpful beliefs and attitudes towards sleep that evolve as we experience and try—valiantly but in vain—to cope with persistent sleep difficulties.

Over time as you repeatedly think these thoughts your brain creates neural pathways that make it really easy, even automatic, for you to believe these unhelpful thoughts until they are etched into your brain, like well-trodden goat tracks. While these thoughts don't serve you, you continue to think and accept them without question. Like obedient little mountain goats, we follow these trails over familiar and precarious terrain.

With the help of neuroplasticity, you can retrain your brain. Neuroplasticity refers to the brain's malleability—its ability to create new mental shortcuts (new goat tracks). With awareness, education and intentional repetition, you can replace unhelpful thoughts about sleep with more accurate insights that are more conducive to a good night's sleep.

Your job this week is to forage through and root out any distorted sleep thoughts that are not serving you.

You can retrain your brain[2]

Thanks to neuroplasticity, old goats can be taught new trails! Neuroplasticity refers to the brain's ability to reorganise itself. This means it's able to continue learning—making new neural connections, strengthening those that are repeated, and weakening those that aren't used. However, the brain learns whatever is repeated—whether helpful or unhelpful thoughts, actions or habits. It doesn't discern on your behalf. The brain's job is to make the connections. Your job is to choose which connections the brain needs to make.

Therefore, with thoughts and behaviours about sleep, you need to be intentional about what you choose to learn (new neural connections), repeat (strengthening neural connections) and refrain from using (weakening neural connections).

Neuroplasticity is enhanced by paying attention, learning, trying new experiences, and meditation.

Week Three review

The eve of Week Four is an excellent time to acknowledge and give yourself credit for what you've completed and achieved already. This is the halfway mark of the programme. Your sleep education is well under way, and you now know more about sleep than most people. You've personally implemented two of the toughest protocols of CBTi (the gold-standard treatment for chronic insomnia, which most people don't even know about)—sleep consolidation and stimulus-control training. What's more, you've done it barehanded, without the one-on-one support of a psychologist or sleep clinician. You've kept the momentum up plus you're back for more. This is a champion effort.

It's likely that you haven't been able to implement everything, every day, and that is entirely understandable and predictable—remember, the sleep-improvement journey is about progress, not perfection. At a minimum, congratulate yourself wholeheartedly and allow yourself a moment of deep pride. Sometimes, when you have high standards for yourself and you're accustomed to giving yourself a hard time about sleep, accepting praise can feel a bit weird. It's a muscle: start building it up. It will help you stay committed to the sleep-improvement journey and your goal to sleep with ease.

> ## Your sleep-improvement journey is about progress, not perfection.

Last week, with continued sleep consolidation and the introduction of stimulus-control training, you may have started to see glimpses of progress with your sleep. Not huge or consistent improvements, but, by now, you can hope to see indications that your sleep is starting to respond to the changes in your habits and behaviour. You may be falling asleep a bit more easily sometimes, staying asleep a bit longer, waking in the night less often, or feeling like the quality of your sleep is on the mend. It may be that your sleep-efficiency score has risen on some nights. Even though progress is unlikely to be consistent, look 'for indications that these two CBTi techniques are *starting* to have some traction for you.

Use your sleep diary to check objectively for signs of progress, as it's easy to slip into that old habit of focusing on your sleep problems, like seeing what's not improving yet or aspects of sleep that remain stubborn. Observe and respond to your sleep progress as you would a toddler learning to walk. Acknowledge and admire each tiny bit of progress you see—staying upright a moment longer, taking one wobbly step, getting up after falling and having another go. It doesn't matter if your sleep progress is slow and shaky—it's progress.

These weeks can be tough going, especially as you juggle these radical changes to sleep behaviours around your daily life. Plus, it's easy to feel impatient and annoyed if sound sleep continues to be elusive. I hope that short walks in the morning sunlight, increased wind-down time in the evenings, micro-meditations, whānau support and self-compassion are providing some comfort as you progress through this stage. Remind yourself that each person's sleep-improvement journey is different. Some people's sleep responds to the behavioural changes in CBTi; for others, it's the cognitive work that provides the catalyst for improvement. Keep trusting the process and apply yourself to exploring and experimenting with your thoughts around sleep as you work on cultivating a better relationship with sleep. This week may hold the key for a wave of progress for you.

If possible, continue to use sleep consolidation and stimulus control this week, alongside the cognitive training. You'll work out an updated sleep–wake schedule for this week at the end of the chapter. If you found the behavioural aspects of CBTi (sleep consolidation and stimulus control) too brutal to implement in your life at this time, know that this happens to some people and it's okay. Return to what feels doable—a consistent sleep schedule, including sleep compression (Week One's sleep–wake schedule), and apply yourself to retraining your brain about sleep this week.

Cognitive training: changing your thinking about sleep

With persistent sleep difficulties, it's easy to become preoccupied with sleep, and, based on your experiences, your thoughts about sleep can become dark and desperate. You may have intrusive thoughts about how difficult sleep is, how badly you've slept, how unfair it is, how dreadful life is going to be the next day, how detrimental poor sleep is for your health, and on and on it goes. These repetitive thoughts can occur night and day. You might fret pre-sleep or wake in the moonlight and stew, or maybe you have an internal tirade when you rise in the morning. Throughout the day, as you experience fallout from a lousy night's sleep or anticipate the night ahead, your brain cycles through a series of negative thoughts. Most of you will know these thoughts intimately.

What's more, many people who struggle with sleep have a tendency towards **overthinking**. You might be frequently plagued by distressing sleep thoughts, and you tend to dwell on them for an unhealthy amount of time. Such thoughts feel very real, they're hard to get out of your head, and they leave you in a state of emotional anguish. These endless inner monologues tend to follow two key destructive patterns: rumination or worry.

Rumination is when you rehash the past, gnawing at it like a dog with a bone. You focus on the horrible symptoms you're experiencing and what you believe may have caused them. It's the woulda, shoulda, coulda scenarios that run on a loop—*If only I didn't have that second coffee*; *If only I'd gone to bed before I got overtired*; *If only I'd been born a good sleeper*. Ruminating tends to leave you feeling hopeless, helpless and like a failure. It's characterised by disempowering feelings like sadness, regret, guilt and self-pity.

Worry, on the other hand, is when you make pessimistic predictions about the future. You extrapolate forward from what you're currently experiencing and run through the what-if scenarios as though they will definitely happen—*I've just ruined my whole weekend*; *I'm going to look like hell today*; *I'm going to screw up the presentation this afternoon*. Worrying is about fear of the future—you're sensing or predicting that there'll be 'danger' ahead. It may not be life or death, but you're convinced something terrible is going to happen to you as a result of undersleeping.

Whether you're ruminating on your current misery and its causes or worrying about the consequences, these head states aren't helpful. As outlined in Chapter 6, thoughts inevitably trigger emotions. These emotions impact you biologically—your body responds to the feelings you have. With negative sleep thoughts, the tendency is to wind up in a place where you feel like your well-being is under threat or there's a sense of danger—though you may get there via feelings of sadness, guilt, anger, resentment, powerlessness, frustration or concern. Not being able to sleep makes you feel like your well-being is at risk, and you become afraid for yourself. On some deep level, you're dealing with *fear*.

Biologically, the body responds to fear with the production of adrenaline and cortisol—stress hormones. When there's a whiff of danger (real or imagined), these chemicals surge into your bloodstream, mobilising you to protect yourself from the perceived threat (not being able to sleep or a bad day ahead). Your heart rate and blood pressure go up, your breathing rate increases, your mind races. Your body becomes pumped and ready to defend you—either through fight, flight or freeze. Paradoxically, while these stress hormones and the resultant physical state are trying to help you, they are the opposite of what you require for sleep. Negative sleep thoughts biologically sabotage the possibility of sleep.

Negative sleep thoughts sabotage the possibility of sleep.

Thoughts are powerful, so you need to be aware of what your sleep thoughts are and determine whether they are helping you towards sleeping with ease or putting that possibility in jeopardy. Rumination and worry are the main categories of overthinking about sleep. But, within this, there are many ways that thoughts about sleep can be distorted in the mind.

Garden-variety distortions in thinking about sleep

We tend to trust our own brains and believe our views of the world. This is essential and generally serves us well. However, people with persistent sleep difficulties are susceptible to some common distortions in thinking about sleep.[3] These thought patterns tend to accidentally be based on false or inaccurate information, or may have a slightly biased spin. Over time, these thoughts become a regular feature, so we don't even recognise that they are keeping us awake at night and need to change.

- **Catastrophising:** envisaging and believing the worst-case scenario, e.g., 'My husband will leave me if I don't sort out my sleep' or 'I'm going to lose my job.'
- **All-or-nothing thinking:** seeing things as extremes with no shades of grey—things are perfect or disastrous, e.g., 'I didn't sleep a wink last night.'
- **Fortune telling:** anticipating things are going to turn out badly and being convinced that your prediction is accurate, e.g., 'I'm going to be awake till 4 a.m.' or 'Tomorrow is going to be harrowing.'
- **Labelling:** attaching a negative label to a situation or ourselves, e.g., 'Being awake in the night is unbearable' or 'I'm a terrible sleeper.'
- **'Should' statements:** comparing yourself to an idealised (or even unrealistic) goal or expectation, e.g., 'A person should have an uninterrupted night's sleep' or 'I should be able to get eight hours' sleep.'
- **Magnification or minimisation:** exaggerating the difficulties you're having—e.g., 'My sleep is the worst it's ever been'—or, alternatively, minimising or discounting any improvements, e.g., 'I might have slept a little better, but not much.'
- **Disqualifying the positive:** any progress is dismissed altogether, e.g., 'Yeah, I had a decent sleep, but that was a one-off.'
- **Personalisation:** blaming yourself for your difficulties and believing you are flawed in some way, e.g., 'There must be something wrong with me. I can't even sleep properly.'
- **Control fallacy:** believing that you have no control and you are a powerless victim of the situation, e.g., 'Nothing I do about my sleep makes any difference.'

Negativity bias adds to the impact of these common thinking distortions. This is a general tendency for people to focus on, dwell on, believe more acutely and respond more strongly to negative information or experiences.[4] These negative patterns of thinking are common, but they distort the truth and play havoc with your chances of getting a good night's sleep.

Dealing with negative sleep thoughts

Cognitive training is the conscious process of identifying negative sleep thoughts, examining them for their validity and replacing them with more helpful, accurate thoughts about sleep. By doing this, you reduce anxiety and a raft of other upsetting emotions that trigger the stress response, generating wakefulness and making sleep elusive. With repetition and practice, these helpful sleep thoughts become more potent and automatic, making it easier for the body to remain calm—a condition that we know is conducive to sleep.

Be reassured, cognitive training is not about bullshitting yourself. This is not about pretending you don't have a sleep problem that's affecting your life, nor is it simply a whitewash of 'positive thinking'. Rose-tinted spectacles and happy-camper nonsense will not work for you, given the severity of your sleep experiences. You need hard facts and reality checks that you can truly count on if your biology is to stay relaxed. You need some dependable truths if you are to allay your sleep concerns.

The focus for Week Four is on completing an inventory of your sleep attitudes and beliefs, reviewing them and replacing any that aren't serving you with more accurate and helpful thoughts. Cognitive-training worksheets are provided at the end of the chapter to write down the main negative sleep thoughts interfering with your sleep and holding you back from sleep improvement. You may know them already, or they may show up throughout the week now that you are being mindful of your sleep thoughts.

For each thought, follow this practice to work your way towards a more useful mindset for sleep. It draws on the inspired work of Tara

Brach, an American psychologist and an advocate of mindfulness and self-compassion. She uses the acronym RAIN[5] to outline a process to support yourself with thoughts and experiences that have you feeling upset, vulnerable and not okay. It's best to do this in a quiet, reflective place, where you can tune in to what's going on at a deeper level.

- **Recognise what's going on.** Identify the unhelpful sleep thought and capture the details of when the thought occurs, how the thought is expressed in words, and how it makes you feel emotionally or in your body. You can even add the intensity of the feeling it stirs up, by giving it a rating from one to ten. The higher the score, the more intense the feeling.
- **Accept the experience as it is.** Allow the thoughts and feelings to be there as they are. Know that the thought or belief exists because you're worried about your well-being, and education about sleep and insomnia has been lacking, and you're concerned about the consequences of poor sleep.
- **Investigate with interest and care.** Explore what's really going on with the thought. Be curious to see if there are distortions in your thinking. Is the thought based on inaccurate information? Are there other possibilities? Acknowledge that the thought may not be serving you in your journey towards better sleep
- **Nurture** yourself using self-compassion. With a spirit of kindness, find a more accurate and helpful way to revise or reframe this thought so that you feel reassured, calmer or more okay. You want your thinking about sleep to avoid any sense of anxiety and stress.

This week requires a fair bit of thinking and reflecting, and most people with sleep difficulties are overthinkers. To date, overthinking has contributed to your sleep problems, but now it's time to use it to your advantage. Choosing new and better sleep thoughts (that are better aligned with helpful emotions and sensations) will build new neural pathways (goat tracks), then your natural tendency to repeat thoughts will help you strengthen those new pathways. Be careful to keep your mind focused on the new tracks—don't let those goats go wandering down those old, unhelpful trails any more.

Step one: identify negative thoughts

The first step is to identify your negative sleep thoughts and home in on the ones giving you the most grief. Sleep thoughts can be sneaky little tricksters that are inconspicuous at first or seem innocuous, so you need to pay attention to find out what thoughts are actually worming into or racing through your sleep-deficient mind.

In *Insomnia: A clinical guide to assessment and treatment*, Dr Charles Morin and Dr Colin Espie identified several recurring themes in the content of people's negative sleep thoughts.[6] These themes, along with typical examples of negative beliefs,[7] are summarised below.

- **Misconceptions about the cause of insomnia:**
  - 'My insomnia is essentially the result of a chemical imbalance.'
  - 'My sleep problems are the result of ageing.'
- **Unrealistic expectations of sleep requirements:**
  - 'I need eight hours of sleep to feel refreshed and function well during the day.'
  - 'My partner falls asleep quickly and stays asleep through the night, so I should be able to, too.'
- **Distorted perceptions about the consequences of insomnia:**
  - 'I'm concerned that insomnia may have serious consequences for my physical health.'
  - 'I know that, if I have a poor night's sleep, it will interfere with my activities the next day.'
  - 'When I feel irritable, depressed, or anxious during the day, it's mostly because I didn't sleep well the night before.'
  - 'It usually shows in my appearance when I haven't slept well.'
  - 'When I sleep poorly one night, I know it'll disturb my sleep schedule for the rest of the week.'

- **Faulty beliefs about sleep-promoting practices:**
  - ○ 'A nightcap before bedtime is a good solution to my sleep problems.'
  - ○ 'When I have trouble getting to sleep at night, I should stay in bed and try harder.'
  - ○ 'When I don't get enough sleep, I need to catch up by napping the next day or sleeping longer the next night.'
  - ○ 'If I need to function well the next day, I'm better to have a sleeping pill than a poor night's sleep.'
- **Perceptions of powerlessness and lack of control over sleep:**
  - ○ 'I can't ever predict whether I'll have a good night's sleep.'
  - ○ 'I'm worried that I may lose control over my ability to sleep.'
  - ○ 'My sleep problem is getting worse, and I don't believe anyone can help.'
  - ○ 'I have little control over the consequences of disturbed sleep.'

These themes and examples may help you spot some of your own negative sleep thoughts. The ones above may be on the money, or they may prompt you to recall your own. You'll probably find that yours are some variation on these themes. Make a list below of the unhelpful sleep thoughts you're aware of already—these genuinely are the thoughts that keep you awake at night!

My negative sleep thoughts are:

_____

_____

_____

_____

_____

_____

_____

_____

_____

Having turned the spotlight on this negative sleep thought phenomenon, you can expect to start noticing other unhelpful attitudes and beliefs about sleep as they occur throughout the day and night. Keep adding them to the list.

Your negative sleep thoughts will vary in frequency, how intensely you feel them, and which emotions they provoke for you. As you start being mindful of your sleep thoughts, you'll notice that some negative thoughts are more problematic for your sleep than others. In the list on the previous page, put an asterisk beside these bad boys. They're the ones you need to focus on examining and restructuring first.

As you become aware of your negative sleep thoughts, be very kind to yourself. It's a weird feeling to know that your mind has been riddled with unhelpful beliefs while you've been wanting to help yourself with your sleep. Remind yourself that it's very normal for people with persistent sleep difficulties to have a barrage of these counterproductive thoughts. There is a lack of education about how sleep works and what constitutes healthy sleep in modern society, plus you've been fed some misinformation along the way. It's little wonder that you are at this crossroads. It's all part of the process; accept it for what it is.

Step two: check and challenge these thoughts

Once you've identified your negative thoughts about sleep, it's time to investigate. Check and challenge them based on facts, reality and objectivity. Rather than looking at sleep through a lens of anxiety and fear, look at it in a proactive, empowered way, using what you are learning about sleep and insomnia.

When reality-checking your sleep thoughts, follow in the footsteps of ancient Greek philosopher Socrates. He encouraged his students to explore the validity of their ideas and discover the truth for themselves by asking them insightful, thought-provoking questions. When you have a negative sleep thought, you need to take the time to investigate it. Ask yourself some probing questions—is it accurate? Is it valuable to what you are trying to achieve? Your immediate response is likely to be: 'Hell yes it's true, and what else am I supposed to think?' But is this really so? Step back, and take time to review and challenge it in the broad light of day. Helpful questions include:

- What evidence supports this idea?
- What evidence contradicts it?
- Is there a different explanation for this?
- What's the worst outcome, if this is true?
- Could I live through that scenario?
- How likely is it that the worst outcome will actually occur?
- What's the best-case scenario?
- Is there a chance this best-case scenario could occur?
- If it was someone else, would they interpret this scenario in the same way?
- If a close friend was thinking this thought, what would I say to them?

In the middle of the night, when these negative sleep thoughts are percolating, it's hard to adopt an objective, reasonable or rational frame of mind to do such analysis. (Besides, thinking about it in the night will only wind you up!) Try reviewing your negative sleep thoughts at a time of day when you're feeling pretty okay.

Step three: replace negative thoughts with helpful information

When you realise that a sleep thought is unhelpful or iffy, find out if there's a more accurate, helpful alternative thought available. You'll notice that when you think the helpful thought, the emotions that spontaneously occur are much easier to be with—you'll feel more relaxed, calm or positive (or at the very least less anxious). These emotions won't trigger your stress hormones the way the negative sleep thought did, and may even encourage your biology to help out with some chemicals—like gamma-aminobutyric acid (GABA) and adenosine—that are more conducive to sleep.

Throughout this book, you've read information and insights about sleep, insomnia and sleep improvement. Use this knowledge to challenge your negative sleep thoughts and create helpful, accurate views about the cause of your sleep problems, your expectations of sleep and your ability to improve your sleep. Take a bit of time to recalibrate your thoughts, de-escalate beliefs that have got away on you, and boost your chances of getting some much-needed sleep.

Use the cognitive-training worksheets at the end of this chapter to write down your negative sleep thoughts and the helpful thoughts you will use to replace them. To help you with this exercise, seven examples of the process are included below. Each example focuses on a sleep topic, recaps key information that you have learned in previous chapters, and shows how this information can be applied to an unhelpful sleep thought in order to restructure it and bring perspective.

Use these examples as a template for what to do with your own unhelpful sleep thoughts, but remember that they are just examples—you must find sleep thoughts that are meaningful to you. When wording your helpful thoughts, play around with the language to find a way of expressing the thought that really rings true for you (like you did when describing your true north).

Example 1: Be realistic about sleep expectations

Situation	Negative thought	Feeling	Helpful thought	Feeling
Struggling to fall asleep	'I *must* get eight hours of sleep to feel okay.'	Stressed	'Heaps of people thrive on less than eight hours of sleep.'	Less stressed
Awake in the night	'I *should* be able to sleep right through the night.'	Worried	'Surfacing throughout the night is a natural part of the sleep cycle.' *or* 'Sleeping in two segments, with a period of quiet wakefulness, can provide solace.'	Calmer

By now you know that sleep durations vary considerably from person to person and that 8 hours is only an average. Some people will thrive on shorter periods of sleep, others will need a bit longer. You also know that a person's sleep duration is not consistent every single night— people aren't machines. Some nights time asleep will be a bit longer, sometimes a bit shorter.

It's commonly believed that, once you fall asleep, you drift from light sleep through to deep sleep as the night progresses, then your sleep gradually gets lighter towards the morning when you wake. In reality, sleep is made up of a series of stages (light, deep, deepest NREM and REM), and the body cycles through these stages multiple times each night. As a result, there are periods of light sleep throughout the night. During the light stages of sleep, it can feel as though you are awake, even though you are sleeping.

If you've been worrying about being awake for a long stretch in the middle of the night, it's worth knowing about monophasic and biphasic sleep patterns. The norm that's generally aspired to is monophasic sleep—where sleep occurs in a long, single bout of sleep overnight. However, in some cultures and at various times throughout history, biphasic sleep has been revered. Biphasic sleep is when sleep occurs in two distinct periods, for example in a long period of sleep at night, followed by a shorter period of sleep in the afternoon (i.e., the siesta). Another example is when sleep occurs as two segments of sleep throughout the night, separated by a few hours of highly valued nocturnal wakefulness.[8] The secluded quiet time between the first sleep and the second sleep has been used for solace, self-reflection and spirituality.

Example 2: You may be getting more sleep than you think

Situation	Negative thought	Feeling	Helpful thought	Feeling
On waking	'I barely slept last night.'	Despairing	'Chances are I will have had more sleep than what it seems.'	Encouraged

If you fret about how little sleep you manage to get overnight, keep in mind that studies show that people experiencing insomnia aren't that accurate in their estimates of sleep duration.[9] They tend to overestimate how long it takes to fall asleep and how long they were awake throughout the night. Meanwhile, they underestimate how long they've been sleeping. So their perceptions of their sleep duration tend to be skewed. It's a bit annoying to discover, but the data shows that people tend to exaggerate the extent of the problem compared to what actually shows up in clinical sleep recordings. That doesn't mean you're falsifying the facts, it's just that those periods of being awake feel really long and the time asleep feels really short. (And this perception isn't helped by those periods of light sleep that don't really feel like sleep even though they are!)

Example 3: Reconsider the cause of sleep difficulties

Situation	Negative thought	Feeling	Helpful thought	Feeling
Before bed	'Older people always have sleep problems.'	Helpless	'There are several things I can do to improve my chance of sleeping well.'	Hopeful

It's common to attribute sleep problems to external factors that you have little control over—pain, menopause, ageing, some kind of chemical imbalance. Believing that something beyond your control is the sole cause means you feel powerless, even like a victim. While things beyond your control absolutely do have an impact on your sleep, numerous factors *within* your control can make a difference to your sleep, too. For example: your sleep schedule, the relationship you have with your bed, your thoughts and beliefs about sleep, your lifestyle habits. It's important to know that sleep difficulties are generally the result of numerous factors—there are many things you can do to support your sleep.

Example 4: Poor sleep isn't the only cause of impaired daytime functioning

Situation	Negative thought	Feeling	Helpful thought	Feeling
Daytime	'I always end up fighting with my husband after a bad night's sleep.'	Resigned	'My husband and I have different views on the kids' screen time, and we need to resolve this.'	Proactive

It's easy to blame shitty sleep for *everything* that goes wrong in the day. While insufficient sleep can impact your quality of life, it's not the only variable. Even on those days when you manage to get a good sleep, you can have an off day—good sleep doesn't guarantee a brilliant day. Really excellent sleepers can have terrible days. Challenging days are a completely normal part of life—everyone has days when they look like hell or argue with their spouse. Sometimes the kids will get on your nerves, or your workday won't be as productive or creative as you'd like. Be realistic, and remind yourself that there are a lot of other things that could be contributing to your 'suboptimal' daytime functioning.

Example 5: Keep catastrophising in check

Situation	Negative thought	Feeling	Helpful thought	Feeling
Awake in the night again	'Tomorrow will be a disaster. I'm going to get fired.'	Afraid	'Tomorrow won't be great, but I'll get through it. My boss hasn't commented on my performance before—even after a night of short sleep.'	Relieved
After several nights of poor sleep	'My bad sleep is going to give me Alzheimer's.'	Terrified	'While there are links, they are not causes. There are lots of other factors, and there are things I'm doing to improve my sleep.'	Reassured

When worrying is taken to the extreme, it's possible to conjure epic worst-case scenarios. For people with persistent sleep difficulties, catastrophic thinking can have a dodgy night's sleep causing severe health issues, disasters at work or relationship breakdowns. When you are freaking out in the middle of the night, these things can feel very real—even inevitable. It's essential to do a reality check: acknowledge that you may be exaggerating and talk yourself down off the ledge. While your thought may indeed be a worst-case scenario, check in on the actual likelihood of the outcome occurring after this particular night of poor sleep.

Example 6: Keep sleep in perspective

Situation	Negative thought	Feeling	Helpful thought	Feeling
Awake at 4 a.m. and unable to get back to sleep	'I'll have to cancel that movie with my friend tonight.'	Disappointed	'I'm really looking forward to seeing my friend and watching a film. I'll reschedule to the earlier time slot. It'll be fun.'	Happy
Struggling through the workday after a patchy sleep	'I just can't do the analysis on this project. My brain is fried.'	Defeated	'This is actually a really challenging project. Anyone would need more support on it. I'll ask my manager.'	Relieved

When sleep is not going the way you'd like, it's easy to become a bit obsessed by it. You might be super watchful about what you do and don't do to conserve energy during the day or improve your chances of sleep at night. This kind of vigilance can make you a bit uptight about sleep, to the point where a lot of your choices revolve around sleep. You may opt out of exercise, activities or socialising, start cancelling commitments or taking sick days. Your world gets smaller as you try to preserve yourself and sort out your sleep. In the process, your quality of life and sense of joy diminish.

Sleep occupies only a third of your life, and, while it's important, you mustn't let it take over your life. Instead, give your waking hours the attention they too deserve. Living well and enjoying your days plays a role in your ability to sleep well. Shifting your focus off sleep can help you to use up energy, have some fun, relax, make some progress in your endeavours, get you feeling better about yourself and distract you from worrying about your sleep.

As you'll know only too well, trying to push on when you're tired can be a challenge. Everything is that bit harder. However, you must build up a bit of resilience to being underslept so that you can continue to look after and enjoy your waking life. The quality of your daytime life can contribute to how well you sleep at night.

Some of you may also be attributing more power to sleep than it really has. You might feel that things aren't going well with work, relationships or your appearance, and believe that it's all because of poor sleep. On broader review, there might be lots of other factors that affect your performance at work, the harmony in your relationships and whether or not you're looking like a million bucks.

Example 7: Give up 'trying' to sleep

Situation	Negative thought	Feeling	Helpful thought	Feeling
Struggling to fall asleep	'I must fall asleep before 10 p.m. to get eight hours of sleep.'	Fretting	'I don't have any signs of sleepiness yet. My body will let me know when it's time to go to bed.' or 'A shorter stretch of consolidated sleep will feel better than a long stretch of broken sleep.'	Trusting

Effort is the enemy when it comes to falling asleep—the more you try (or even try not to try), the less likely you are to sleep. Unlike almost every other aspect of life, trying harder works against you. It generates wakefulness. Instead, sleep is about slowing down, doing less, letting go, trusting and allowing it to come. If you like to feel in control of things, this is damned annoying—you want to make it happen on your own schedule, on your command. You need to learn a very tricky life lesson: to gain control, you must lose control.

Beware: is there a hidden upside to your insomnia?

While working through your negative sleep thoughts, consider that there may be hidden upsides to your insomnia, called **secondary gains**, that are quietly undermining the good work you're doing towards improving your sleep. They need to be brought into the light of day, too.

This was something really icky that I discovered to be true for me. Without realising it, I'd found an upside to my sleep difficulties. After such a long time living with sleep deficiency, I'd learned that feeling exhausted meant I missed out on a lot of events, experiences, social gatherings and work opportunities that mattered to me. It was upsetting and frustrating.

However, what I didn't realise initially was that I'd also been using my sleep difficulties as an excuse to get out of things I didn't want to do! Oh yes, I'd been pulling the 'I'm too tired' card for quite a few things. It had become my semi-legitimate leave pass if a project sounded too gnarly, or if a social function would be tedious. While it had been handy to be able to get out of things without a fuss, the 'insomnia advantage' I'd unconsciously discovered was perpetuating my sleep problems.

There are other upsides to insomnia that may make you cringe if you find some truth in them. Do you use your sleep difficulties to set you apart from others or as a badge of honour? Has it become part of your identity or a way to garner sympathy? Have you been using it to compete with your partner—who's had the worst sleep, therefore who should do the heavy lifting on the home front today?

It can be really uncomfortable to acknowledge an unconscious benefit to your sleep issues. However, once you become aware of it, you can't unsee it. I felt better about myself once I'd owned up to my secondary gains, and I made different decisions going forward. If you discover that there's a squirm-worthy upside of insomnia that you've had in play, it's worth finding other ways to meet these needs. You will feel better about yourself, and it helps to improve your sleep.

Plan Week Four

If your sleep-efficiency scores were 85 per cent or higher on most nights (that means four or more) last week, celebrate and do some hollering and high-fiving! Reward yourself with a little more time in bed, and an opportunity for your body to increase its time asleep. Increase your time in bed by 30 minutes this week—bring your earliest bedtime back by half an hour. (Don't get cocky and rush this process. Too much, too soon risks fragmenting your sleep.) Implement this schedule for a whole week. Remember that your sleep might be unsettled by the changes, but continue with the plan and give it time to improve.

If your sleep-efficiency scores were under 85 per cent on most nights of the week, stay with the same sleep–wake schedule as last week. You've now completed three weeks of CBTi, and this next week will be instrumental in showing whether the self-help approach is going to make the difference for your sleep. Keep up your commitment to your sleep-improvement journey.

Continue with stimulus-control training, if you can. You want to keep building that association between your bed and sleep. It's tough, but remind yourself that it's temporary. You've already completed a week, so the cue between your bed and sleep must be strengthening night by night.

Let's map out your sleep–wake schedule for Week Four.

Schedule your wake-up time

Keep this anchor point the same every week.

My morning wake-up time I'm still committed to is _____ a.m.

Schedule your earliest bedtime

If your sleep-efficiency scores were 85 per cent or above on four or more nights last week, make your bedtime 30 minutes earlier than last week. Otherwise, keep it the same as last week.

This is the earliest time that you can go to bed this week. You're welcome to stay up later if you're not experiencing physical signs of being *sleepy*—yawning, head nods, rubbing your eyes, eyelids getting heavy, etc.

My new earliest bedtime is _____ p.m./a.m.

Schedule time to prepare for bed

Continue to allow fifteen minutes to prepare for bedtime.

Schedule time to wind down

Continue to allow 60 to 90 minutes to wind down each night.

Summarise your schedule for this week in the box below.

My sleep–wake schedule for Week Four

Wind down (60–90 minutes): _____ p.m.

Prepare for bed (15 minutes): _____ p.m.

Earliest bedtime: _____ p.m

Morning wake-up time: _____ a.m.

Week Four tends to be a decider. If CBTi is going to work for you, it will really start coming together this week. Once you've applied the CBTi protocols pretty consistently across four weeks, you'll know whether this approach is working for you. Some of you will have made progress from the behavioural changes of the last three weeks; others will find that it's this week's cognitive changes that provide the catalyst for improvement. Either way, after a month, most people will have experienced an encouraging shift in their sleep and they will have a sense of confidence in the process. For others, it might be time to explore alternative options. (Remember: at the end of Chapter 9, you jotted down your plan B to improve your sleep if it was needed.) This is the week to rally and apply yourself to yet more learning about how to improve your sleep. Go well with your brain retraining!

Week Four recap: what you can do

1. Summarise your Week Four plan on the next page. Writing it out again will reinforce your commitment.

2. Carry out the new sleep–wake schedule as best you can. Progress, not perfection.

3. Complete the cognitive-training worksheets. Focus on reviewing, challenging and reworking the unhelpful sleep thoughts that are holding you back. Be kind to yourself in the process.

4. Update Week Four of your sleep diary. Jot down your daily sleep info and, at the end of the week, work out your sleep-efficiency scores. Note and celebrate any progress you experience.

5. Keep reading, keep learning and stay curious about your sleep.

My sleep–wake schedule for Week Four

Wind down (60–90 minutes): _____ p.m.

Prepare for bed (15 minutes): _____ p.m.

Earliest bedtime: _____ p.m./a.m.

Morning wake-up time: _____ a.m.

- Continue building on your **sleep–wake schedule habits** from previous weeks.
  - Maintain a consistent sleep schedule.
  - Always give yourself time to wind down (include some meditation).
  - Go to bed when you're *sleepy* (at or after your scheduled earliest bedtime).
  - No clocks, phones or screens in the bedroom.
  - Get up at your wake-up time.
  - Get fifteen minutes of daylight and exercise ASAP in the morning.
  - Only nap if you genuinely have to (keep it brief and before 4 p.m.).
- Keep doing **stimulus control** (the 'out of bed' protocol) if possible and still needed.
  - Get up if you're not asleep within fifteen minutes.
  - Relax in your night haven.
  - Return to bed when you're sleepy.
  - Repeat the process until you fall asleep easily.
- Shift your attention to helpful sleep thoughts with **cognitive training**.
  - Identify negative sleep thoughts.
  - Accept the role they have played in your sleep challenges.
  - Question, challenge and revise them.
  - Replace them with more accurate, helpful sleep thoughts.

COGNITIVE-TRAINING WORKSHEET

In the following worksheet, jot down negative sleep thoughts you experience. Come up with alternative thoughts that are more helpful and accurate to use in the relevant situation.

Situation	Negative thought	Feeling
Struggling to fall asleep	'I must fall asleep before 10pm to get eight hours of sleep.'	Fretting, restless, agitated

Helpful thought	Feeling
'I don't have any signs of sleepiness yet; my body will let me know when it's time to go to bed.'	Trusting, calm

SLEEP DIARY

Fill out your sleep diary every morning. Guess the approximate times, there's no need for clock-watching. On the next page, note any factors that helped with sleep or may have been unhelpful for your sleep. You're looking for clues and patterns . . .

Week Four	Night 1	Night 2	Night 3	Night 4	Night 5	Night 6	Night 7
Start Date _____ Day of Week							
What time did you go to bed?							
What time did you first try to go to sleep?							
What time did you fall asleep?							
How many times did you wake in the night?							
How long did these awakenings last in total?							
What time did you wake for the final time this morning?							
What time did you get out of bed for the day?							
How would you rate the quality of your sleep? *(1 Terrible, 2 Bad, 3 OK, 4 Good, 5 Great)*							
Total Sleep Time In total, how many hours' sleep did you get?							
Total Time in Bed In total, how long were you in bed?							
Sleep Efficiency % (Total Sleep Time ÷ Total Time in Bed X 100 = %)	%	%	%	%	%	%	%

SLEEP DIARY

Week Four Start Date _____ Day of Week	Night 1	Night 2	Night 3	Night 4	Night 5	Night 6	Night 7
Any factors that may have been unhelpful for your sleep last night?							
Any factors that may have helped with sleep last night?							

Observations & Insights:

Use nutrition and exercise to your advantage

Freedom is choosing between what you want now, and what you want most.[1]

When it comes to food, caffeine, alcohol and exercise, I'm more likely to make healthy choices if I feel like I'm not being forced into anything. It has to be about what I want, and what my priorities are for the day, not what I'm supposed to do or what's right or wrong. The idea of discipline, self-control or restraint makes me feel controlled—I get uptight and more likely to rebel, even if that means sabotaging what's best for me.

Week Five is not about preaching to you about what you should or shouldn't do—it's about laying out relevant facts on how food, beverages, substances and movement can help or hinder your sleep. Once you're informed, you have scope to experiment and check out how different things work or don't work for your sleep. When you understand how these lifestyle factors affect you, based on your own experiences, you have genuine freedom of choice. That doesn't mean you won't have little internal battles some days, but at least you'll know the consequences—favourable or unfavourable—before you make a call.

Before embarking on how nutrition and exercise can bring sleep benefits, let's check in on last week's progress.

Week Four review

Week Four was essentially make or break for self-directed CBTi. You've done the hard yards with the behavioural changes and you've spent a week on cognitive training. If you've been able to adhere to the programme pretty well, you should see some noticeable improvements in your sleep at this stage. Some of you will have achieved real gains in your sleeping patterns and will be feeling the benefits in your energy levels, mental clarity, productivity, mood and optimism. Others will have experienced an encouraging shift, feel more empowered and know it's worth continuing with the programme.

If you haven't yet made the progress you'd like, know that this can happen. Some of you will be aware that you've been a bit loose in your implementation of the techniques. (In clinical terms this is referred to as 'non-compliance', which always makes the deviant in me laugh!) If this is you, you may choose to recommit and give the techniques a fair chance—just double back to wherever your commitment waned, and have another go. If you feel like the self-help CBTi approach just isn't your gig, remember that you've got your plan B to explore. Stay engaged with your intention to improve your sleep and check out an alternative approach. There are options in Appendix II.

If you're ready to move forward with the programme, here's the plan. You'll use your sleep-efficiency scores to determine your sleep–wake schedule for this week, you'll continue using stimulus control as needed, and cognitive training will be an ongoing process as you embed your helpful sleep thoughts. This week, your new learning will be to review and experiment with lifestyle habits that might be influencing your sleep.

Food: what you eat can help you sleep

There's a lot of information (and misinformation) about what you should and shouldn't eat for your health. It can be pretty confusing and hard to know which diet or regimen to follow. So far there is no clinically proven 'sleep diet' that will guarantee sleeping well every night. There are some dietary patterns (e.g., Mediterranean) that show promise in modulating sleep, but more research is yet to be done.

What is known from the research is that sleep deficiency makes people more prone to eating poorly. When you're shy on sleep, you're likely to eat more than usual, gravitate towards less-healthy options and snack more frequently—bring on the sugar, fat, carbs and processed foods. Chippies, anyone? Lack of sleep also makes it tricky to plan your foods well, go to the trouble of sourcing them, and take the time to create the nutritious meals that will nourish your tired soul. When you're feeling ragged, shortcuts make sense—even when you know they're not brilliant for you nutritionally.

Now that you're in a better position with your sleep, you'll be able to take a look at your eating habits and decide if you want to experiment with some modifications.

A 2016 review of the research on the role of food consumption in sleep provides some helpful general guidelines.[2] Indications are that diets high in saturated fat, carbohydrates and sugars are less helpful to sleep. (Annoyingly these are the foods you're pulled towards when you're short of sleep.) Diets that are higher in vegetables and fruit, high in fibre (think whole grains), and which favour vegetable oils (low in saturated fats) show signs of supporting better-quality sleep. So, while there is no need to adopt a radical sleep diet, making adjustments towards healthier general nutrition is likely to support your sleep.

Eating well can be complicated and challenging from a financial, logistical and emotional perspective. I've tried (and continue to explore) a raft of different approaches to find something that works for me and how I like to look, feel, and live my life. One of the most helpful little tools that I've adopted along the way is considering a simple question when I'm making a food choice: 'Will this make me more healthy or less healthy?' Distilling the decision down to its essence makes it so much easier.

Eating well supports better sleep, so the 'more healthy or less healthy' question can be handy on your sleep-improvement journey.

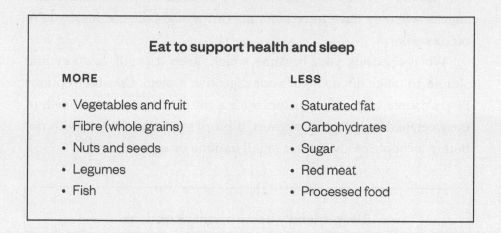

Eat to support health and sleep

MORE	LESS
• Vegetables and fruit	• Saturated fat
• Fibre (whole grains)	• Carbohydrates
• Nuts and seeds	• Sugar
• Legumes	• Red meat
• Fish	• Processed food

Of course, sometimes you'll choose to eat foods that are rich, heavy, spicy or high in sugar. While these can be fabulous options from a pleasure point of view, they play havoc with your sleep if you have them too close to bedtime. These foods are more taxing on the digestive system, because it has to kick into high gear to process them. When you sleep, the digestive system slows down, so if you've eaten this type of food in the evening, your digestive system is going to be activated to attend to its job overnight. This is not conducive to sleep, making it difficult to fall asleep and stay asleep. You may experience discomfort, heartburn or seemingly unspecified wakefulness. That doesn't mean these delicious feasts are forever off limits—remember the World Sleep Society's recommendation that challenging-to-digest foods be consumed at least four hours before bed, to give your body a chance to process it. Book that restaurant dinner early!

While overindulging before bed doesn't work, neither does being hungry. A growling stomach or edgy, peckish feeling makes it difficult to fall asleep. Ideally, we eat well throughout the day and don't need to snack before bed, but life is life. Sometimes a little something is needed before turning in.

Choose foods that have shown some indication of supporting slumber. Again, there's no hard evidence of sleep-guaranteeing bedtime snacks at this stage, but there are indications that some foods are more likely to help.[34] Several foods get the nod, including foods that contain tryptophan, magnesium, calcium or potassium. While snacks will only have trace amounts of these goodies, at least you're doing no harm.

When choosing your bedtime snack, keep it small, low key and simple, to make life easy for your digestive system. Consider options like a couple of grainy crackers with a bit of cheese, a small dish of unsweetened muesli with yoghurt, a bit of wholegrain toast with nut butter, a couple of kiwifruit, a small banana or a glass of milk.

Sleep-friendly bedtime snack options

- Dairy (milk, yoghurt, cheese)
- Whole grains (bread, crackers)
- Nuts (almonds, walnuts)
- Bananas
- Kiwifruit

You may want to consider bolstering your magnesium levels. Magnesium is one of those rock-star minerals that support hundreds of functions within the human body. It helps with stress reduction, mood stabilisation, muscle relaxation and sleep. Certain foods, such as brown rice, green leafy vegetables, nuts and seeds, and bananas are naturally high in magnesium.

However, insomnia, prolonged stress, lots of caffeine and alcohol, and poor food choices take a toll on the body's supply of magnesium. (And it doesn't help that soils in New Zealand and Australia are low in magnesium.) Not surprisingly, magnesium deficiencies are widespread, with about one in three people in Australia being low in this mineral. Symptoms of deficiency include agitation, irritability, anxiety and sleep disorders, including insomnia and restless-leg syndrome.

To support yourself, it's worth boosting your intake of magnesium-rich foods or talking with a pharmacist about an appropriate magnesium supplement. There are many different types of magnesium, so get advice about one that's specifically helpful for your sleep.

Water: stay hydrated throughout the day

The body is about 60 per cent water, so staying hydrated is vital for health and well-being—it helps with the transportation of nutrients throughout the body, aids digestion, regulates temperature, supports detoxification and elimination of waste, improves concentration and relieves fatigue. You need to make sure you drink enough water each day to keep your body running smoothly and feeling good. While research is ongoing as to the role of hydration in sleep, it makes sense to support your body with a decent supply of water.

According to the National Sleep Foundation in the US, if you go to bed even mildly dehydrated it can disrupt your sleep with snoring, leg cramps and awakenings. After a night disrupted by dehydration, you may wake a bit parched, with low energy and compromised alertness and cognitive function.[5] People with chronic insomnia often experience daytime fatigue (to put it mildly), and given the rugged nights experienced it's easy to put the blame entirely on a lack of sleep. However, sketchy hydration could also be playing a big part.

There is a lot of variation in opinion on how much water is needed to maintain optimum levels of hydration. I like the approach of Ben Warren, a New Zealand nutrition guru. His view is that 0.033 litres of water per kilogram of bodyweight is needed daily. This roughly works out as 2 litres if you're 60 kilograms, 2.5 litres if you're 75 kilograms, 3 litres if you're 90 kilograms and 3.5 litres if you're 105 kilograms.[6] Obviously the amount needed will increase in hot weather or if you're physically active. Only water and caffeine-free herbal teas count towards the water tally. (Tea and coffee increase dehydration—for each coffee, you need to drink two glasses of water to catch up!)

When improving sleep is the goal, it's not just about how much water you drink—it's also about when you choose to drink it. It's easy to forget or fall behind in drinking water during the day, despite best intentions. But catching up in the evening can make you a bit waterlogged and more likely to wake in the night to go to the bathroom. Minimise these awakenings by sorting out the timing of your water consumption. Do what you can to create water-drinking habits that pace your intake throughout the day.

As is the case with all habit-building, make it really easy and convenient for yourself. Make drinking water a no-brainer. Think about the timing of when to have a glass, or pair drinking water with existing habits. As a visual reminder, I used to keep a glass of water on my desk and on the windowsill in the kitchen. It was a great way to have hydration high profile and on hand. Of course, that was until I discovered our cat, Lucy, on the windowsill with her face plunged deep into my glass, whiskers squished back, lapping at pace. It's water bottles all the way now!

Caffeine: consider a quota and a curfew

Quality coffee is my good friend, so I won't tell you to ditch your dearest companion. Even though I delayed appraising my caffeine intake, I reached the point where it was clear that I needed to better understand the effect caffeine was having on my slumber. My wake-up call came when a fellow actor was at my house to rehearse a scene. I offered her a coffee, and after two sips of my usual brew she started sweating and thought she was having heart palpitations! My initial reaction was uncharitable—I decided she was a lightweight. Later I wondered just how strong my coffee actually was, and how much caffeine was okay for a human body.

As a stimulant, caffeine perks you up, providing a sense of mental alertness and a physical boost that can be bloody helpful for getting through the day. (Especially if you have a track record for undersleeping.) Caffeine gives you pep by blocking adenosine, the chemical that tries to build up during waking hours to create sleep pressure, so you can feel sleepy at night. In modern society, the use of caffeine is normalised, embraced, even revered, so it's not seen as a drug. It's merely part of daily life. Much of its use is habituated—it's often consumed automatically, without question.

While caffeine is highly valued by day, it can put sleep in jeopardy by night. Caffeine stays in your system for a long time, and if you have too much lurking in your body at bedtime, it works against you if you want to sleep well. It can make it more difficult to fall asleep, sleep can be lighter, and there can be more awakenings in the night. Obviously, these consequences run counter to your sleep aspirations.

In getting to grips with the impact of caffeine on your sleep, you need to consider which products contain caffeine, how much caffeine they contain, how much caffeine is okay, how the timing of consumption matters, and your own sensitivity to caffeine.

Sources of caffeine

The Sleep Health Foundation provides a summary of the most common sources of caffeine, along with a guide to how much caffeine these products tend to contain.[7] This information is outlined below. Of course, actual amounts vary depending on different brands, varieties, brewing techniques, etc. It's worth noting that black tea, the standard gumboot option, isn't as innocent on the caffeine front as most people think.

Product type	Caffeine content
coffee (250 ml, average cup)	
brewed	80–350 mg
instant	65–100 mg
decaffeinated	2–4 mg
tea (250 ml, average cup)	
black	50–70 mg
green	30–60 mg
herbal	0–30 mg
soft drinks (375 ml can)	
energy (V, Red Bull, Mother, etc.)	80–150 mg
cola (Coke, Pepsi, etc.)	35–50 mg

chocolate	
hot chocolate or ooooa	10–70 mg per cup
dark chocolate	20 mg per 50 g
milk chocolate	10 mg per 50 g
caffeine tablets No-Doz	100 mg per tablet

Caffeine levels

The European Food Safety Authority reviewed the safety of caffeine in 2015 and came to the conclusion that moderate caffeine consumption (up to 400 milligrams of caffeine per day) is okay as part of a balanced, healthy, active lifestyle.[8] This gives you an upper limit to consider. However, your lifestyle may be a bit less than balanced, healthy and active at this juncture, so less caffeine may be appropriate.

Because people vary in their sensitivity to caffeine, these figures provide a guideline only. (But don't get all gung-ho about it like I did, thinking for a long time that I was impervious to the effects of caffeine.)

Timing of caffeine

It takes a long time for your liver to break down caffeine and remove it from your system, so it's not just about how much caffeine you ingest throughout the day, it's also about the timing of consumption. The rate at which caffeine is broken down varies a lot from person to person, but it really does take a long time to process—almost 24 hours to leave your system altogether. The World Sleep Society recommends people quit consuming caffeine at least six hours before bed, but some may need to knock off much, much earlier.

Sensitivity to caffeine

Your sensitivity to caffeine and your body's ability to process it vary depending on many factors, including age, genetics, gender, weight and medications. Over time with routine use, people can build up a tolerance for caffeine. While you can 'handle' it, that doesn't necessarily mean it's doing your body or your sleep any favours. (I think I was in this group, feeling staunch and slightly superior because of my ability to down a potent brew unscathed, and refusing to see the relationship between caffeine and nights that were in tatters!)

Working out what's okay for you personally requires some good old trial and error. Use your sleep diary to establish if caffeine is hampering your sleep progress. Keep an eye on the amount of caffeine you have throughout the day and also what time you stop consuming it. Compare that with how you sleep that night. Over time, you may notice a pattern emerging. The amount of caffeine may need to be moderated, or you may find the timing requires some fine-tuning.

Shuffling your timing to an earlier finish is reasonably workable. But, if you want to reduce the amount of caffeine you're consuming or you're thinking about stopping altogether, there are a few things to consider. Often people who most need to cut back, myself included, have developed a strong dependence on caffeine—physically and emotionally.

Cold turkey can be harsh. With abrupt cessation or reduction (especially following prolonged daily caffeine use), there is likely to be horrible withdrawal symptoms—headaches, tiredness, anxiety, low mood, tremors, irritability and grumpiness. This kicks in 12–24 hours after stopping, and peaks around 20–24 hours. If your body's been accustomed to high levels of caffeine for a long time, it can take days to come right. The recommendation is not to do this to yourself, but some people want to get it over and done with—all or nothing. If you're going to do it this way, get your timing right so that not much is required of you over the brutal period. Perhaps dedicate a weekend to getting through the worst of it—drink heaps of water and have painkillers on hand for that specific 'caffeine withdrawal' headache. (Also, tell your nearest and dearest not to take your bad mood personally—it's just the caffeine detox.)

Gradual reduction or cessation takes longer, but it's a kinder, more compassionate approach. Withdrawal symptoms are less severe or avoided, so you're more likely to remain a productive, nicer human and succeed. Try reducing your daily intake by about 10–30 milligrams every few days—in practical terms, that's a quarter of a cup of coffee, a quarter of a can of energy drink, half a cup of tea or half a can of cola. You could try substituting one of your daily caffeine moments with a non-caffeine option—it's worth having a good alternative to slip into that habitual behaviour.

Whether you go cold turkey or reduce gradually to break your caffeine habit, put some thought into what you want your new habits to be. Critical moments throughout your day have been punctuated by caffeine—think about what you want to have or do in those times to satisfy the need behind the behaviour. Consider a fancy herbal tea or a decent-quality decaf. If your caffeine hit was about fortification, energy or enlivenment, can you pop out for a quick walk? Would an ice-cold sparkling beverage do the trick? Or a zesty orange juice? If it was about comfort, maybe a chai would work. If you're weaning off caffeine, consider a hot chocolate or mocha as a comforting alternative.

Alcohol: go easy (and go early)

At some point, the other 'friend' had to come up—alcohol. Your sleep diary may have already highlighted some patterns between your drinking and sleep. Patterns that you may have responded to, turned a blind eye to, or even made some elaborate rationalisations about to negate any need to do things differently. If you think drinking may be unhelpful for your sleep, try not to get annoyed or defensive—learn how alcohol actually affects sleep, instead.

The World Sleep Society includes a sleep commandment about alcohol—their recommendation is to avoid excessive drinking in the four hours before bed. They're not screaming stop, they're just saying ease up. Let's look at what's behind this.

In *Cognitive Behavioral Treatment of Insomnia*, the authors describe alcohol as 'the world's best and worst sleeping pill'.[9] On the one hand, having a drink in the evening feels helpful for many people. That glass (or two) of wine might seem to help you wind down, or take the edge off if you tend to feel irritated, upset or grumpy by the time the evening rolls around. With a drink in hand, it can feel like you relax and let go of your stress and worries for the day. It lifts your spirits and life seems good. What's more, it helps many people fall asleep more easily. (Hence the notion of having a nightcap before bed.) So far, so good.

Alcohol is the world's best and
worst sleeping pill.
—COGNITIVE BEHAVIORAL TREATMENT OF
INSOMNIA, MICHAEL PERLIS ET AL.

The problem is that, later in the night, alcohol can cause you to wake frequently and have difficulty falling back to sleep. It's associated with disturbances like sleeping lightly, nightmares, night sweats and dehydration headaches.[10] This rebound wakefulness occurs as the body metabolises the alcohol. Alcohol-induced troubled and fragmented sleep is especially likely if you've been drinking a lot or if you've been drinking later in the evening (even if it's only a glass or two).[11]

A shortcut is the longest distance
between two points.
—CHARLES ISSAWI

If you've been using alcohol as a sedative to induce sleep, be very aware that, while it helps many people get to sleep, it's very likely to be contributing to sleep dramas later in the night.

If you want to figure out if alcohol is messing with your sleep, you can experiment. From your sleep diary, you may have already collected data about what your sleep is like on the nights that you drink versus the liquor-free nights. See if you notice any patterns. This week, if you are curious, you can consciously explore what happens to your sleep with less or no alcohol. If you're up for it, try cutting back on alcohol and ensure that your drinking cut-off time is at least four hours before bed. Follow this approach for a week or two to get a sense of how drinking is impacting your sleep.

If you're accustomed to having several drinks each night (especially later in the evening) and find it challenging to break the habit, be gentle with yourself and take it slow. Get creative about modifying your habits. Once you start questioning automatic behaviour, it gives you some power and self-determination about habits that may not be serving you. Try pouring weaker or smaller drinks, substituting one of your drinks for a non-alcoholic option, checking out low-alcohol drinks or keeping less alcohol in the house.

If you'd like additional support to reduce your alcohol consumption, refer to Appendix III for some specific resources. Both New Zealand and Australia have local websites with excellent online tools to objectively review your current drinking patterns, and they can point you in the direction of information that will be helpful for your needs.

Smoking: create a cut-off time

Research shows that people who smoke tend to take longer to fall asleep, have shorter total sleep time and experience more frequent daytime sleepiness compared to non-smokers.[12] Of course, if you smoke, reducing or quitting is a massive endeavour in its own right. This is something to seriously explore down the track, for your overall health and quality of life; but one thing at a time. For now, focus on making some adjustments to your current smoking habits to support your sleep-improvement journey.

For someone who smokes, cigarettes can seem like they support sleep. But they, like alcohol, are not what they seem when it comes to getting a good night's kip. Some of you may smoke a cigarette before bed or when you wake in the night. Having that quiet, ritualised five or six minutes of inhaling and exhaling deeply feels relaxing and seems to set you up for sleep. But nicotine in cigarettes is a stimulant, and it messes with the sleep–wake cycle neurons. This affects sleep in several ways—difficulty falling asleep, sleeping more lightly, and waking in the night or very early in the morning. So what seems to make you calm and more likely to sleep actually disrupts sleep.

While, ultimately, it would be better to not smoke at all for your sleep, the process of stopping smoking is very likely to create sleep disturbances—one of the withdrawal symptoms is disrupted sleep.[13] If you stop smoking, you can expect sleep quality to deteriorate, night awakenings to increase and subsequent bad moods to ensue. These nicotine-withdrawal effects can last from a few days to twenty days, depending on how much and for how long you've smoked.

Instead of adding this challenge and complication to your sleep-improvement journey, consider avoiding cigarettes in the four hours before bed and abstaining overnight. As with other habit changes, it's easier to substitute one habit for another than go without and feel deprived. The critical moments are before bed and when you wake in the moonlight. Bear in mind the core of those habitual moments—you want to feel calm, relaxed and make it easier to fall asleep. Fortunately, your smoking behaviour has created the bones of an excellent habit for helping you feel calm and relaxed: sit quietly, and take a ritualised five or six minutes of inhaling and exhaling slowly and deeply. That behaviour sounds staggeringly like a meditation.

Alternatively, find something else that will help you relax in those moments—listening to music or reading. It's important to be kind to yourself and find something enjoyable to distract you from your usual habit, take your mind off any temporary cravings, and satisfy the underlying emotional need.

Later, if you do choose to quit smoking, know that your sleep is likely to be temporarily disrupted (for up to three weeks) before you start to reap the sleep benefits that non-smokers enjoy, like longer sleep durations. There are resources available in Appendix III to support you, if or when you choose to stop smoking.

Physical activity: a daytime and night-time advantage

You will already know that integrating physical activity or exercise into your weekly routine has numerous health and well-being benefits. What you might not know is that it helps you sleep better. Studies have shown that, for people with chronic insomnia, regular exercise can shorten the time it takes to get to sleep and reduce the amount of time awake during the night.[14] Exercise also helps alleviate symptoms of tiredness and fatigue during the day and reduces some of the symptoms of anxiety and depression. Given that it decreases pre-sleep anxiety and improves sleep, it's worth considering giving physical activity a go, if you aren't already.

In both New Zealand and Australia, it's recommended that you tally up 150 minutes of moderate-intensity activity each week for your general health. That's also what's recommended if you want to use exercise to help you sleep. This works out at half an hour a day for five days a week, or a bit over twenty minutes a day.

You've been doing fifteen-minute wake-up walks most mornings, so you've established a good base already. If you want to check out how physical activity can further support your sleep, you may need to pick up the pace a little to shift from light exercise to moderate intensity. To gauge whether an activity counts as moderate intensity, look out for the following cues:[15]

- your breathing quickens, but you don't feel out of breath
- you have a light sweat after ten minutes of the activity
- you can carry on a conversation, but it would be difficult to sing.

Moderate-intensity activities include things like brisk walking, hiking, swimming, biking, dancing and active yoga, as well as household chores like mowing lawns, vacuuming and mopping.

Build towards a regular habit of moderate-intensity physical activity: 30 minutes a day, five days a week.

There are different views about the best time to do physical activity. While sleep researchers are trying to come to a consensus, let's not get hung up on scheduling and let's just get moving. The priority is to create an exercise habit and make it sustainably happen in your life. Remember—done, not perfect. The only proviso: if you're going to exercise in the evening, don't do vigorous activity right before bed. It elevates your body temperature, which makes it hard to fall asleep.

Some of you will have collectively moaned at the prospect of exercise. (I did when I was really sleep deficient.) When you're feeling dog-tired, it can be a challenge to get your body moving. It makes sense to want to slow down, try to rest and conserve energy for the essentials. The prospect of exercise can feel daunting, even impossible.

When you're feeling this way, remind yourself that, despite how it seems, a bit of activity will help your mood, lift energy levels and support your sleep. Expect mild resistance and have an option that feels doable (and hard to argue with). Break it down to a 20-minute chunk, so it can be over and done fast, and make sure to choose the most enjoyable option (or the one that inspires the least resistance).

Daniel Ford, a behavioural sleep psychologist from The Better Sleep Clinic, suggests trying a little experiment if you're unconvinced about the value of exercise in your current condition. To challenge the thought *I need a good night's sleep to not feel fatigued*, consider that the fatigue may be related to not being sufficiently active. Maybe sleep is not the only way to generate energy. Test the possibility that exercise may boost your energy level—rate your energy before moderate-intensity exercise and predict how you'll feel afterwards. Then, once you've done the exercise, rate your energy level again and compare it to your prediction.

If you decide to explore improving your sleep with physical activity, start building a regular habit. Return to the notes on habit building in Chapter 3 to give yourself a good chance of making it an ongoing thing. It helps to have a plan of what you intend to do and when. Make sure you choose activities that you genuinely like to do and feel enthusiastic about—being physically active is not meant to be a chore. If you're walking or biking, plan some routes that you really enjoy, or pair the walking up with something else that you value—listen to podcasts, music, make phone calls or, if you're on a stationary bike, try binge-watching Netflix! It could also be helpful to arrange your activity sessions with someone else—for company, as a catch-up or to fortify your commitment.

Of course, life will be life—there will be days when the planets don't align and your activity session gets missed. Have a backup plan for this scenario. For example, if you miss a workout during the week, you can always catch it up on the weekend.

Our lifestyles have so many habits in play—dietary habits, water consumption, caffeine hits, drugs of choice (alcohol, nicotine, cannabis), physical activity. Once these habits have worked their way into your life and become automatic, they don't get much consideration. They're just what you do. This week is a chance to look at these choices in light of the impact they have on sleep. You'll know which of your lifestyle choices are working in harmony with your sleep and which ones are likely to be putting your sleep at risk.

This week, focus on reviewing your lifestyle habits. Congratulate yourself on what you're already doing well in nutrition and exercise to support your sleep, and scope out areas that may need review. Use the worksheet at the end of the chapter to note down the lifestyle areas where you're doing well, and any areas that could be holding your sleep improvement back. Once you've highlighted the area that's of most interest to you, create a plan based on what you've learned in this chapter to make adjustments. Start implementing these changes this week and observe how it affects your sleep. (Remember that some of these changes might make things worse before they get better and it might take a few weeks to start reaping sleep benefits.)

Plan Week Five

By now, you know the drill on what to do with your sleep–wake schedule for the week ahead. If your sleep-efficiency scores were 85 per cent or higher on four or more nights this week, do some rejoicing and allow yourself a bit more time in bed with an earlier bedtime. This is to allow your body the opportunity to increase its total time asleep overnight. Bring your earliest bedtime back by 30 minutes this week. Follow this plan for the whole week, and, even if your sleep is wobbly at first, stick with it and give yourself a chance to adjust to the new schedule.

If your sleep-efficiency scores were under 85 per cent on most nights of the week, accept that it is what it is, and stay with the same sleep–wake schedule as last week. Sometimes it takes a bit longer for sleep to consolidate. Lifestyle factors may be at play, and the adjustments you explore this week could hold the key to progress for you.

As you did last week, continue with stimulus control. Meaning, if you haven't fallen asleep or fallen back to sleep within fifteen minutes, get up, go to your cosy night-time haven, relax until you experience the symptoms of being sleepy, then return to bed for sleep. Keep reinforcing the association between your bed and falling asleep quickly and with ease. Hopefully you're having to get out of bed in the night less frequently now. (I remember feeling like such a yo-yo during this part of the process, but it was worth persisting.)

Let's plan your Week Five sleep–wake schedule overleaf and then get prepared for exploring lifestyle options.

It's understandable to experience some resistance to reviewing your lifestyle choices. Often the things we get most belligerent and defiant about are the things we most need to re-evaluate. I was adamant that coffee wasn't a problem for me for the longest time. Eventually I stopped being defensive and conceded to at least experiment with less coffee. That reduced-coffee fortnight was enlightening. The first week was pretty rough, to be honest—I was grumpy and the initial withdrawal headache was intense. But, after that, I really started reaping the benefits. My sleep improved noticeably, and I no longer felt edgy throughout the day. Win–win. Through this trial-and-error process, I found the point where I could enjoy my coffee without compromising my sleep.

This is your week to start experimenting with your lifestyle choices (and vices) to establish what truly works for you. Once you know what these things do to *your* sleep, you genuinely have freedom of choice.

Schedule your wake-up time

Keep this the same as every week.

My morning wake-up time I'm still committed to is _____ a.m.

Schedule your earliest bedtime

If your sleep-efficiency scores were 85 per cent or above on four or more nights last week, make your earliest bedtime 30 minutes earlier than last week. Otherwise, keep it the same as last week. Remember, this is the earliest time that you can go to bed.

My new earliest bedtime is _____ p.m./a.m.

Schedule time to prepare for bed

Continue to allow fifteen minutes to prepare for bedtime.

Schedule time to wind down

Continue to allow 60 to 90 minutes to wind down each night.
    Summarise your schedule below.

My sleep–wake schedule for Week Five
Wind down (60–90 minutes): _____ p.m.
Prepare for bed (15 minutes): _____ p.m.
Earliest bedtime: _____ p.m./a.m.
Morning wake-up time: _____ a.m.

Week Five recap: what you can do

1. Summarise your Week Five plan on the next page. Write it out again to reinforce your commitment.

2. Review lifestyle factors that may be impacting your sleep, including food, hydration, caffeine, alcohol, nicotine and physical activity.

3. Use the lifestyle-choices worksheet to decide which lifestyle adjustments to explore. Don't be too ambitious—focus on changing one factor at a time. This way, it's easier to see what makes a difference for you.

4. Implement the change as best you can. Remember, improving sleep is a journey. It takes the time that it takes. Don't put unnecessary pressure on yourself.

5. Update Week Five of your sleep diary. Jot down your daily sleep info and, at the end of the week, work out your sleep-efficiency scores. Note any lifestyle changes and track the impact they have on your sleep after a week.

6. Keep reading, keep learning and stay curious about your sleep.

My sleep–wake schedule for Week Five

Wind down (60–90 minutes): _____ p.m.

Prepare for bed (15 minutes): _____ p.m.

Earliest bedtime: _____ p.m./a.m.

Morning wake-up time: _____ a.m.

- Continue building on your **sleep–wake schedule** habits from previous weeks.
  - Maintain a consistent sleep schedule.
  - Enjoy your wind-down time (include your mindfulness meditation).
  - Go to bed when you're sleepy (at or after your earliest bedtime).
  - No clocks, phones or screens in the bedroom.
  - Get up ASAP after wake-time.
  - Get fifteen minutes of daylight and exercise in the morning.
  - Only nap if you genuinely have to (brief and completed by 4 p.m.).
- Continue with **stimulus control** (the 'out of bed' protocol) if needed.
  - Get up if you're not asleep within fifteen minutes.
  - Relax in your night haven.
  - Return to bed when you're sleepy.
  - Repeat the process until you fall asleep easily—within fifteen minutes.
- Keep up the great work with your **cognitive training**.
  - Keep reinforcing your helpful sleep thoughts.
  - Work through any unhelpful sleep thoughts that have surfaced.
  - Identify, accept, challenge and replace the unhelpful sleep thoughts with helpful sleep thoughts.
- Make some adjustments to your **lifestyle choices**.
  - Consider which lifestyle factors could be impacting your sleep.
  - Decide which aspect to explore this week.
  - Choose the changes you'd like to try and plan them.
  - Implement these for at least a week and track what happens.

LIFESTYLE-CHOICES WORKSHEET

This worksheet provides a summary of the lifestyle choices that support sleep. Tick those areas you're interested in exploring in your journey towards sleeping with ease.

Nutrition

- ☐ Consume a healthy diet, high in vegetables, fruit, fibre, legumes and fish, and low in red meat, saturated fat, sugar, carbs and processed food.
- ☐ If you're eating foods that are rich, heavy, spicy or high in sugar, consume them at least four hours before bedtime.
- ☐ If needed, have a *small* bedtime snack that's supportive of sleep, e.g., a few grainy crackers and cheese, unsweetened muesli with yoghurt, wholegrain toast with nut butter, two kiwifruit, a banana or a glass of milk.

Hydration

- ☐ Stay well hydrated throughout the day.
- ☐ Drink a volume of water appropriate for your bodyweight, increasing it in the heat or if physically active.
- ☐ Pace your water-drinking throughout the day.

Caffeine

- ☐ Keep caffeine levels below 400 milligrams per day (find the threshold that's okay for your sleep).
- ☐ Have a caffeine cut-off time appropriate to your caffeine sensitivity.

Alcohol

- ☐ Curb drinking to at least moderate levels.
- ☐ Keep the four hours before bedtime alcohol-free (no nightcaps).

Nicotine

- ☐ Keep the four hours before bedtime nicotine-free.
- ☐ Remain nicotine-free throughout the night.

Physical activity

- ☐ Create a regular habit of moderate-intensity physical activity, e.g., brisk walking, hiking, biking, dancing, swimming, lawn-mowing.
- ☐ Work towards 30 minutes, five days a week.

Decide which lifestyle area you will focus on this week. Create a plan of what you'll do differently and how you'd like to go about implementing these changes.

This week I'm going to make some adjustments to (choose one):

- ☐ Nutrition
- ☐ Hydration
- ☐ Caffeine
- ☐ Alcohol
- ☐ Nicotine
- ☐ Physical activity

What might not be working for me:

Write down habits in this lifestyle area that you suspect are hampering your sleep.

_____

_____

_____

_____

_____

Changes I want to explore:

Write down the changes you're interested in checking out.

_____

_____

_____

_____

_____

_____

_____

**How I plan to create and stick to these
new lifestyle habits this week:**

_____

_____

_____

_____

_____

_____

_____

_____

_____

_____

_____

_____

_____

SLEEP DIARY

Fill out your sleep diary every morning. Guess the approximate times, there's no need for clock-watching. On the next page, note any factors that helped with sleep or may have been unhelpful for your sleep. You're looking for clues and patterns . . .

Week Five	Night 1	Night 2	Night 3	Night 4	Night 5	Night 6	Night 7
Start Date _____ Day of Week							
What time did you go to bed?							
What time did you first try to go to sleep?							
What time did you fall asleep?							
How many times did you wake in the night?							
How long did these awakenings last in total?							
What time did you wake for the final time this morning?							
What time did you get out of bed for the day?							
How would you rate the quality of your sleep? (1 Terrible, 2 Bad, 3 OK, 4 Good, 5 Great)							
Total Sleep Time In total, how many hours' sleep did you get?							
Total Time in Bed In total, how long were you in bed?							
Sleep Efficiency % (Total Sleep Time ÷ Total Time in Bed X 100 = %)	%	%	%	%	%	%	%

SLEEP DIARY

Week Five	Night 1	Night 2	Night 3	Night 4	Night 5	Night 6	Night 7
Start Date _____ Day of Week							
Any factors that may have been unhelpful for your sleep last night?							
Any factors that may have helped with sleep last night?							

Observations & Insights:

Mindfulness, stress management and relaxation

When you come out of the storm you won't be the same person who walked in. That's what this storm's all about.

—HARUKI MURAKAMI

Y ou made it! Even with the best of intentions, it's easy to fizzle out on a self-help programme. Yet here you are, one of the irrepressible crew, who's up for *finishing strong*. I applaud you. You're reading this chapter, and that tells me you care deeply about your well-being and the days and nights beyond this book.

Mindfulness, stress reduction and relaxation are easy to brush aside. But they are crucial tools for consolidating your sleep-improvement progress and for protecting and preserving it into the future. All too often these things get the classic Kiwi 'yeah, yeah, nah'. We understand the value of this stuff in theory and know we should do it, but in our super-busy, time-poor lives everything else takes priority and acts of self-awareness and self-care get the flick.

Some of you may have already adopted a few of the principles of mindfulness and self-compassion when they were introduced earlier in the book, and even practised them a little throughout the programme. But others of you have likely let it ride. You might be tempted to skip over this stuff because at first glance it seems pretty lightweight—a nice to have, not a need to have—compared with some of the heavy-duty CBTi work you've done over the last month. But, trust me, it matters.

Emerging scientific research on the value of restoring the balance between the sympathetic nervous system (the stress response) and the parasympathetic nervous system (the relaxation response) is profound. You've seen how being stressed and wired ruins your sleep—it also interferes with other critical aspects of your biology. While some stress is common in life and is healthy, unrelenting stress is destined to damage your health down the track—it's linked with anxiety, depression, heart disease, high blood pressure, diabetes and cancer. Sure, you can try to push on as though you are invincible, but Mother Nature seems to have a way of keeping score.

This week you'll explore a variety of options to help you work more intentionally with your body's nervous system, learning how to avoid setting off your stress response and how to nurture and develop your relaxation response. Understanding your options and developing new habits or practices gives you the choice to relax your body and calm your mind. Some of the approaches will be familiar. Now, you will establish which one(s) you want to experiment with and figure out how to integrate them into your life.

First, let's recap your experiences last week.

Week Five review

You have made it through five weeks of the programme and you're back for more, so you've likely experienced some significant progress in your sleep and will be enjoying the flow-on effects to your days. Sleep consolidation will be getting easier as your sleep-efficiency improves, and your bedtime will be getting closer to the time that you genuinely want to go to bed. You won't be needing to get up in the night as often for stimulus control, as your bed is becoming a stronger and more reliable cue for sleep. With another week of conscious repetition of helpful sleep thoughts under your belt, these new messages will be getting etched into your brain as happy little goat tracks. Meanwhile, unhelpful neural pathways will be fading with time and intentional neglect.

The amendments you made to one of your lifestyle choices last week—nutrition, hydration, caffeine, alcohol, nicotine or exercise— may have revealed useful insights. Already there may be enough evidence for you to adjust your rules of engagement with this choice going forward, or the jury may still be out on how it helps or harms your sleep. If you're not convinced of the role the choice plays in your sleep, keep experimenting next week to test the boundaries, so you know for sure and can make a call.

Alternatively, you may want to check out the downstream effects of another lifestyle choice. Remember, it's easier to explore lifestyle changes one at a time, so you can get clarity on how they impact your sleep.

In this final week of the programme, you will bring together the CBTi, mindfulness and self-compassion techniques you've learned. You have done the heavy lifting on your sleep-improvement journey— the hard stuff is behind you. This week, open your mind and your heart to practices that will not only support your sleep but also alleviate the pressure on your hamstrung days.

The body's stress and relaxation responses

Let's do a quick refresher on the nervous system. Your body is wired to automatically react to anything it perceives as a threat in order to protect you. Your sympathetic nervous system kicks into top gear, and your stress response gets switched on. When the threat has passed, the body switches back to the parasympathetic nervous system. This cues the relaxation response, reassuring you that all is well and you don't need to worry. Both systems are vital for your welfare and survival, but it's essential that they operate in harmony.

Stress response	Relaxation response
Sympathetic nervous system	Parasympathetic nervous system
Revs you up so you can fight, freeze or flee	Calms you down so you can rest, digest and restore
Heart beats faster Breathing is fast and shallow Blood rushes to muscles for action Gut is less active—digestion difficult Stress hormones (adrenaline and cortisol) increase Expends or depletes your energy	Heart beats slow and rhythmically Breathing is deep and slow Blood flows to the gut and lungs Gut is more active—digests, absorbs nutrients Levels of adrenaline and cortisol lower Conserves your energy

The stress-response system is designed to be self-limiting. When the threat is over, the body should calm down again. The stress response was never intended to be left switched on most of the time. The trouble is, there doesn't have to be a significant threat to trigger it. The body doesn't muck around—if it senses danger, it mobilises to protect you. With hectic lives and busy minds, our bodies can feel like they're under threat a lot of the time. Threats can range from life-or-death stuff to minor hassles like running late for work, getting a parking ticket or arguing with a workmate. The risks don't even need to be real—the body responds in the same way to perceived and imagined threats! If the body thinks there's danger, even fleetingly, the stress response is up in arms instantaneously. While it's great to know it has your back, this hypervigilance can be overkill.

The stress response has a hair trigger. It takes so little to set it off. A whiff of danger, real or imagined, is enough for it to mobilise the troops.

In modern society, it's easy to feel like you are under siege most of the time. While the threats may not be biggies, there's often a barrage of them, and it can seem like there's no let-up. It's common to be very familiar with experiences like:

- frequently running late
- feeling frustrated, irritated or edgy
- being overextended with responsibilities
- having an eternal to-do list
- doubting your ability to do or complete a task
- feeling put upon with additional requests
- feeling a sense of burden or overwhelm
- believing there are not enough hours in the day.

Being in a relentless state of stress is draining and intense, and, as you know all too well, it takes a toll on your sleep. If the stress response accidentally becomes a default setting in your life, it's not psychologically or biologically sustainable. Something will give out. You have experienced that with your sleep difficulties. Dr Bruce Arroll explains, 'We all have warning lights on our dashboards, and insomnia is one of them.' (I love this analogy, maybe because I'm the daughter of a mechanic.) Poor sleep is a warning—your body is asking you to be aware of it, and to review the way you are choosing to think, behave and live.

You have taken heed of the warning provided by insomnia with everything you've done to support yourself with sleep. From here on, reducing stress is an essential part of preserving your sleep and looking after your well-being. It's not just about toning down or switching off your stress response—you must also do what you can to proactively encourage your body's relaxation response. To do those things, first and foremost, you need to start being aware of what's going on.

It's easy to ride roughshod through the day, tangled in the relentless noise of your busy mind, oblivious to the sensations and signals of your body. Yet you always have the option to tune in to what's really going on, here and now. Once you truly know what's happening in the moment, it's as though time slows down and you give yourself more choice.

Mindfulness matters

The core principles of mindfulness have been woven throughout the pages of this book. Mindfulness is a learned skill, developed through meditation and regular practice. This book only scratches the surface, to help you see the potential value it has for sleep and in other areas of your life. Think of this as a sampler. It takes learning from an experienced teacher and your own dedicated practice for mindfulness to come naturally and deliver its full benefits, but you've made a start.

While mindfulness has been on the periphery of your learning journey so far, now it's time to put it front and centre. Mindfulness is instrumental in enabling you to become aware of what's happening in your body and mind at any given moment. This insight will let you know, authentically, the answer to the question: 'How am I, really?' This is the starting point for relaxing your body and calming your mind.

In my hobby as an actor, I was introduced to the expression 'let the stone hit the bottom'. It means that you must put down your guard and become fully aware of how things genuinely are—how they land with you. It's not enough to generally know what's happening around you; it's about becoming aware, very specifically, of what you are experiencing and how these experiences reverberate in your body and mind. Mindfulness encourages you to be still inside, become aware, and check in with how you are in the moment. Mindfulness is bare-naked awareness—there's nowhere to run, nowhere to hide. It's just you, fully exposed in all your vulnerability and possibility in that one moment.

Mindfulness is bare-naked awareness.

Knowing mindfulness theoretically and truly living it are very different experiences. I still grapple with mindfulness—and at times even white-knuckle resist it. Which of course tells me that it's an area that I truly need to embrace. When I practise mindfulness, something softens inside me, possibilities open up, I'm much kinder to myself and life is easier. Don't delay and dodge integrating mindfulness into your daily life like I did—it really is powerful, liberating stuff that will (at a minimum) support you in managing stress and bringing a state of calm to your world.

The seven core attitudes of being mindful

- **Beginner's mind.** Develop a mindset that's willing to see everything as though for the first time. Rather than forecasting, anticipating or expecting, be open and have a growth mindset.
- **Trust.** Develop trust in yourself, your sensations and feelings, your intuition. Trust the practice of mindfulness and the value of turning towards your inner wisdom.
- **Non-judgement.** Be an impartial witness to your experiences. Step back and observe with an open mind. Avoid judgement or criticism, liking or disliking.
- **Patience.** Accept that things unfold in their own time.
- **Non-striving.** Pay attention to the here and now, and let go of having a particular goal or outcome.
- **Acceptance.** Accept things as they actually are.
- **Letting go.** Allow things to be as they are, rather than grasping at some experiences to elevate them or pushing others away to diminish them.

Chapter 10 covered the seven core attitudes necessary for being mindful, according to mindfulness pioneer Jon Kabat-Zinn: beginner's mind, trust, non-judgement, patience, non-striving, acceptance and letting go.[1] Being mindful allows you to be non-judgementally aware of how you really are. You can be more accepting of your experiences, even when they are difficult—know that they are part of life and that the thoughts, feelings and sensations you have about them will pass. It gives you a moment of grace to discern what, if anything, you need to support yourself in the face of what you're experiencing. It gives you the opportunity to respond rather than react.

Being mindful doesn't make you relaxed or less stressed; it enables you to be aware. It is this awareness that gives you choice.

Mindfulness meditation

Throughout your sleep-improvement journey, you have quietly been exploring meditation. While mindfulness meditation has value in the treatment of insomnia,[2] its benefits extend beyond your sleep and into your waking life.

If you're keen to explore meditation further, there are many programmes available, from entry level to advanced. Some of the go-to places for guided meditations are apps, like Headspace, Calm, Buddhify or Smiling Mind. Remember that these options tend to provide a starting place. If you're committed to cultivating your own mindfulness meditation practice, it's worth finding a reputable programme with a qualified instructor who offers weekly instruction and daily practice. Several resources are listed in Appendix III.

If mindfulness is not for you at this juncture, know that it exists and you can turn towards it at any time. At a minimum, consider continuing with the starter-kit mindfulness meditation practices encouraged throughout the course. Even spending ten minutes a day quietly tuning in to yourself has value—at least give yourself that.

Yoga

Yoga is another option for cultivating mindfulness. With its use of gentle, physical movement and calming breath, yoga has been used for centuries to relax the body, calm the mind, create awareness and restore the spirit. Studies show that regular practice of yoga has value in supporting sleep quality and many other aspects of well-being.[3]

Gentler practices like hatha yoga, restorative yoga and yoga nidra are particularly valuable for supporting sleep. There are myriad in-person classes available these days and many online programmes (a lot of them free), which has made yoga very accessible.

If you're new to yoga, start with a foundation course to learn the principles of safe movement and conscious breath. They will support you as you develop your practice. Start easy. (And, if you haven't already, check out the YouTube channel Yoga with Adriene.)

I encourage you to explore mindfulness in some capacity to cultivate your inner awareness, and allow yourself to make better choices about how stress and relaxation fit into your life.

Stress-management options

So many of us need to find ways to dial down the stressors in our lives. We want a reprieve from the pressure while we establish a better balance between stress and relaxation. It would be fabulous if we could cut pressure out altogether, but there will always be some stress in life. Some degree of stress is useful—it motivates you, helps you achieve goals and enables you to deal with a crisis. It definitely has its place. You just don't want it to rule your life.

Some stressors are beyond your control, but others you have a choice about. You might be able to influence the number of stressors upon you, how intense the pressure is, how long it goes on for, or how much you let it affect you. The most stressful situations are the ones we have, or believe we have, no control over. It's worth putting some thought into the options you have for reducing stress and managing stressful situations.

Learn to say no

Most of us simply have too much on our plates. 'I'm so busy' or 'I don't have time' have become mantras to live by. There are things you can do to manage what you've already committed to, and ways to alter how you relate to and feel about these responsibilities, but at some point it's worth considering how much you actually take on.

I'm big on learning to say no. As is typical for women of my generation, I was instilled with a strong need to please from an early age. I spent decades doing what I was told—being 'good' and being 'nice'. The trouble with being so accommodating and compliant is that you end up taking on an awful lot.

Saying 'no' doesn't always come naturally. Not conforming with what's asked of you may make you feel bad, judged or guilty, which adds to your stress—you can feel like you're damned if you do and damned if you don't. But saying no is a learnable skill, and it will serve you well in your stress-reduction quest and your desire to continue sleeping with ease.

The power of no

Wielded wisely, No is an instrument of integrity and a shield against exploitation. It often takes courage to say. It is hard to receive. But setting limits sets us free.
—JUDITH SILLS

The trick is how you frame 'no' in your own mind and how you deliver the 'no' to others.[4] Saying no to someone tends to feel like you're failing to look after their needs or cooperate with their wishes. Heaven forbid you put yourself first. But saying no is about taking responsibility for yourself and having clear boundaries (it's yang self-compassion in action). Think about it as being clear on who you are and what you value. You're standing up for what you truly need or can realistically manage. It is as vital as putting on your own oxygen mask first. Saying no to someone else is saying yes to yourself. Your needs matter, too.

It can feel hard to do because it's unfamiliar. Answering 'Yes, sure thing' might simply be a habit that needs to be questioned and disrupted for your own sanity and welfare.

When people are accustomed to hearing you oblige their requests, your 'no' is likely to encounter some resistance. They're not going to like it. The negativity bias in the human mind means that negative experiences, which includes being told 'no', are felt more acutely and for longer than positive experiences. There might be resistance to your non-compliance, and at times this can create conflict. Know this, and be sensitive in how you communicate 'no' so that you are looking after your needs while reducing the impact on your relationships.

Here are a few pointers for mastering saying no.

- **Buy yourself some time.** Rather than answering yes automatically, let the person know you need time to think and tell them you'll get back to them. This prepares them for a possible no and allows you space to be clear on how you will say it.
- **Let them down easy.** Soften your language, so 'no' lands more gently, e.g., 'Thanks for the opportunity, I appreciate being asked, but I'll say no this time. Have you considered asking Alex?'
- **Remain calm.** Maintain a swan-like air of grace on the surface to show that you're crystal clear in your decision (even if you're paddling like hell underneath).
- **Mention conflicting commitments.** Strategically refer to existing obligations—it makes it tricky for the requester to contest, e.g., 'I'd love to help out, but I'm already booked to support my friend in hospital that day.'
- **Rehearse.** Plan what to say in advance and run through it in your mind before you have to deliver it.

I lived in Canada for some time, where I picked up a few quirks of the local lingo. Now, when I'm supposed to say yes to an unwanted request, favour or demand, I have one of their cunning little phrases at my disposal: 'You know what . . .' It's so harmless, and it buys me a few nanoseconds to draw strength before I let someone down. Then I simply say, 'You know what . . . I'm going to have to say no this time.'

Schedule a worry time

The number of responsibilities ahead is not the only thing that can create stress—the sense that you are not in control of a situation can also bring grief.[5] If you know things are not okay, feel that you aren't coping and can't do anything about it, you'll be highly stressed. Rather than panicking, freaking out, running in circles, working around the clock or lying awake at night, consider pushing pause. By scheduling time to step back, take a breath and look at everything objectively in the light of day, it's easier to make a plan.

Schedule a block of uninterrupted time, say 30 minutes, during the day or early evening (keep worry time away from your wind-down time and bedtime). Go someplace quiet where you can focus and do some planning. Take a moment to quiet yourself and take a few deep, slow breaths to centre and calm yourself. Acknowledge that you are stressed and struggling. Remind yourself that this is a common experience and that you're not alone in feeling overwhelmed. Be kind with yourself about how you're feeling and reassure yourself that it's going to be okay. Know that you are going to look after yourself. (It's reassuring to know that you've got your own back.)

Write down all the things that are bothering and stressing you. Include the stuff on the to-do list that's winding you up, as well as anything else that boils to the surface as you contemplate your woes and worries. Nothing is too big or small. If it's an issue for you, get it out of your head and on to the page.

There are many ways to get this stuff written down—a meticulously ordered list, recorded in an app, scrawled on a napkin in a cafe. The aesthetic doesn't matter—just do it. I opt for an A3 page and a messy spider diagram. I start with a bubble in the middle that says 'shit that's bothering me' and then pour everything out on the page in rough clusters of worries. It becomes a scribbly tangle, but it feels good to have it documented and out of my head.

Once you've done the brain dump, sit back and reflect. Gently figure out how you are going to work through these challenges. Be practical and realistic. Once you have a map, you will feel more in control. There are ways to lighten the load or make it more doable.

- **Prioritise.** Work through and give things a priority: A, B or C. Focus on the most urgent or important ones—the As. The others can wait their turn.
- **Delegate.** Can someone else do the task instead of you?
- **Get help.** If you're out of your depth, or if it'll be more efficient to use an expert, reach out and get the support you need.
- **Delay.** Does every task really need to be done now? Or can some be filed under 'do later' or 'do sometime'? Non-urgent stuff can wait, especially if the deadlines are self-imposed. Cut yourself some slack.
- **Ditch.** Forget about stuff that doesn't actually matter. To get perspective, ask yourself: 'Will this matter in a year? Five years? Will the sky fall if I don't do this?'
- **Organise.** Work out what you are going to do, when—make sure things genuinely feel manageable. (Do your shoulders drop? Does your breath lengthen when you think about how you're going to work through your tasks? Listen to your body.)
- **Plan.** Work out how you will tackle each thing with practical steps. Write down what you need to do first and schedule it in your diary.

By outing all your worries, it's easier to see what's really going on for you. If you give yourself the time, space and moral support to find your way through, you will feel a real sense of relief. Look after yourself, just as you would a friend who was feeling stressed out. It can be both reassuring and empowering to go through this process. Quieten down your stress response and regain a sense of being back on track.

Put the day to rest

If you don't get the chance to process the day before climbing into bed at night, the mind can set to work on this inevitable task the moment it finally has stillness and quiet. It churns through work dramas or relationship glitches, or tries to figure out problems, or makes plans for the day ahead—including trying to keep track of all those little details that must be remembered. This processing is necessary, but it makes the mind more alert and the brain aroused, which is the opposite of what you need when you place your head on the pillow.

Keep this busy-brain activity away from bedtime. Consider building a habit to do it at the end of your workday or, if you must, at the start of wind-down time. Dedicate time to reflecting and processing the day. Some people do this mentally, others like to keep a journal or diary, or make use of an app. Just go with what works best for you. In the process of putting the day to rest, cover off the following:

- **Triumphs and victories.** Think about what went well and what you did well. Make sure you high-five yourself for your wins to boost your happiness hormones. Remember, triumphs and victories come in all shapes and sizes. I even congratulate myself when I do the dusting (my least-likely-to-get-done job).
- **Struggles and troubles.** Work through the tricky bits. Make sure you focus on what can be done or how you plan to cope rather than remaining stuck in a disempowering cycle of rumination or worry.
- **Disappointments and defeats.** If there are disappointments, losses or hard times, be kind and compassionate with yourself. Acknowledge the hurt and suffering you're experiencing, and consider how you can console or nurture yourself through this.
- **Gratitude and appreciation.** Take a moment to reflect on what's good in your life. Acknowledge the people, experiences, qualities, things, opportunities or moments that you cherish. Even on a rough day, there will be tiny things that bring joy to your day.
- **Tomorrow's to-do list.** Be practical and plan ahead—map out what needs to be done and remembered for tomorrow. There's nothing like a good to-do list to help you feel organised and on your game.

Going through the process of putting the day to rest is like defragging your mind. Sift through everything, tidy it all up, and get things nicely aligned once more. While it's essential to sort through the woes and deal with the worries, make sure you also give plenty of attention to the positives in your life. Remember the brain has a bias towards the negative, so you need to intentionally outfox the system by dialling up your focus on the good in your life.

Time management

Be realistic in your expectations of yourself when writing your to-do list. Align your tasks with how much time actually exists in a day. Also, create some wiggle room—it gives you breathing space and allows for the inevitable wildcard.

For a while, I found that my to-do lists were working against me—winding me up and making me feel like a failure. When I did a reality check on my week's to-do list, I discovered that it would have required an eleven-day week to complete. How was I ever supposed to achieve a sense of calm accomplishment when I was asking the impossible of myself? My to-do lists are now lined up with real-time hours, not some mystical, nonsense clock!

Relaxation is a priority

Relaxation is more than an annual holiday and a couple of weekends away. It must be integrated into your days and evenings as part of the very fabric of life—view relaxation as being as essential as breathing rather than an optional extra.

There are loads of things you can do to support yourself in feeling relaxed. Exercising, spending time in nature, socialising, unstructured time (how novel!) and laughter can all help. Make plenty of space in your life for these necessities, where and when you can.

It can be challenging to prioritise relaxation—there are so many other responsibilities and commitments. Some people are low in self-compassion and may feel undeserving of a regular serenity break. There are so many practical and psychological barriers to embracing relaxation wholeheartedly.

But resistance to relaxation is a curious thing. Though you know that it feels good and will serve you, you might dodge, refuse or decline it, even dig your heels in. The paradox is that being able to relax ultimately strengthens and fortifies you. Learning to relax requires a leap of faith.

Key relaxation hacks

Once you have convinced yourself to trust that relaxation may actually safeguard you rather than leave you vulnerable, you can prioritise it. Fortunately, relaxation is a skill that can be learned. There are four relaxation hacks recommended by sleep experts, especially for use at night.[6]

- belly breathing (diaphragmatic)
- progressive muscle relaxation
- 'warm, heavy, relaxed' training (autogenic)
- visualisation imagery.

These brief, DIY techniques will get the relaxation response working in your favour. None of them will put you to sleep—remember, you can't 'make' sleep happen—but relaxation techniques do induce biological conditions that are more conducive to sleep. The goal of relaxation is always *relaxation*. Calm the body, ease the mind.

Once learned, these quick DIY relaxation techniques will give you the skills to relax on demand.

You don't have to love or use all of these techniques. Give them a go and suss out which ones *you* find easy to do and actually work to relax *your* mind and body. Each one takes a bit of practice to get the hang of, but, once you get it, you've got it for good. You can carry it with you at all times—the skill to relax on demand.

When you're starting out with these relaxation techniques, sample and practise them during the day or in the evening during your wind-down time (not in bed or your bedroom). Allow me to repeat it: the goal of relaxation techniques is relaxation. By experimenting with them away from sleep time, you are more likely to accept that you simply want to use them to relax (with no ulterior motives for falling asleep). This way, you'll have more chance of unwinding and letting go.

Once you've found a technique that works well, and you've practised it by day and can confidently create a relaxed state, then you can responsibly use it at bedtime or in the night to create conditions conducive to sleep. (Not to *make* you sleep.)

> **Keep going, because you didn't come**
> **this far to only come this far.**
> —UNKNOWN

Belly breathing

When the body is tense, breathing tends to be shallow and rapid. You breathe into the upper part of your chest rather than optimising your full lung capacity. The ribcage creates space for the lungs to inhale—you haul your shoulders up, and your little intercostal muscles move your ribs apart so the lungs can inflate. This gets the job of breathing done, but it makes the body work harder and you get less reward for your efforts. This way of breathing can pervade the day (and night) without you really noticing. It's not until your shoulders are perched up by your ears and your neck is screaming with tension that you register you might be a bit stressed.

Noticing what is happening with your breath and the basic mechanics of how your body is getting air is a useful check-in. Breathing in this shallow, rapid way means the body is operating in its stress-response mode for some reason (remember, it doesn't take much to trigger it).

Pay attention to your breath and take time out to consciously start breathing with your diaphragm to shift your body into a more relaxed state in just a few minutes.[7] To get the hang of diaphragmatic breathing, try the following.

- Find a quiet place, where you can be undisturbed for a while.
- Set a timer for five to ten minutes. (Then you can forget about the time.)
- Sit on a chair with good, upright posture and both feet planted on the floor. (Alternatively lie flat on the floor and feel the floor supporting your body.)
- Place one hand flat on your abdomen, below the navel, and the other on your upper chest.
- Close your eyes and, without judgement, check in on your breathing.
  - Notice its pace and depth.
  - Be aware of how your body is creating space for your lungs to expand. (Where's the action—ribcage, shoulders or abdomen?)
  - If your breathing is all coming from your ribcage and shoulders, it's time to give them a rest and encourage your diaphragm to lead the way. (This will feel like your abdomen or belly is moving with the breath.)
- Inhale slowly, deeply and quietly through your nose, allowing your abdomen to expand as your diaphragm extends downwards.
- Gently pause and hold for a few seconds.
- Allow your breath to slowly and completely release through your mouth. (You'll feel your abdomen deflate.)
- Repeat your inhalation, pause, then exhale, enjoying the sense of calm it restores.
- Continue relaxing into this belly breathing till the timer sounds.

While you're doing this exercise, your mind will inevitably go wandering. That's normal and to be expected. When you catch it thinking about booking your next haircut, or that workmate who was sarcastic this morning, gently escort your attention back to your breath. Give your mind an easy little task to focus on to keep yourself non-judgementally in the here and now. Try counting the seconds of your inhalations, pauses and exhalations, or count your full breaths. You could also get your mind to notice the temperature of your cool inhalations and your warm exhalations. These 'jobs' are simply to help your mind stay present with your breathing.

There are different approaches to counting diaphragmatic breathing that will help keep you centred on the task. You are consciously extending your breath, but you want your breathing to feel relaxed, comfortable and slow, and to follow a repeating pattern. Conscious awareness of breathing is known as *pranayama* in yoga. The term is derived from Sanskrit, with *prana* meaning 'life force' and *ayama* meaning 'extension'.

Dr Giselle Withers, creator of A Mindful Way, works with a lot of people with sleep difficulties and suggests box breathing as a good option. In yoga, it goes by the name of *sama vritti pranayama*, and involves inhaling for four seconds, pausing for four seconds, exhaling for four seconds and pausing for four seconds. It's easy to remember—count off the 4-4-4-4 pattern.

Another option is the 4-7-8 method, recommended by Dr Andrew Weil, director of the Andrew Weil Center of Integrative Medicine at the University of Arizona. This approach also has its origins in yogic pranayama breathing. Inhale for four seconds, pause for seven seconds, exhale for eight seconds, then repeat the cycle.

- **Box breathing:** inhale for four seconds, pause for four seconds, release for four seconds, pause for four seconds, repeat.
- **4-7-8 method:** inhale for four seconds, pause for seven seconds, release for eight seconds, repeat.

If these approaches don't work for you, Dr Weil suggests the Zen practice of breath counting to help keep your mind focused. With this approach, you count each exhale. After you have counted five exhales, start over at one. It sounds deceptively simple, yet sometimes your mind goes AWOL, and you find you've counted beyond ten. If this happens, just go back to counting exhalations from one to five.

Go with the approach that is easy for you. Be sure to slow your respiration rate down in a way that feels okay—you are learning to extend your inhalations, pauses and exhalations, but only to the point that feels right. Speed up your counting a little if needed so that you aren't straining or pushing. Start from where you are, and gradually extend what's comfortable.

While your body knows perfectly well how to breathe in the relaxed-response mode, when you have been living in a state of prolonged stress this slower, deeper diaphragmatic breathing can feel unfamiliar, even contrived. With continued practice, it becomes second nature and preferable.

Awareness of your breathing provides a quick check-in for how you are doing. Once diaphragmatic breathing becomes easy again, you can use your breath as a shortcut to relaxation, wherever and whenever. Get into the habit of checking in with your breathing multiple times a day, so you can quietly calm yourself down if needed rather than allowing tension to escalate throughout the day.

Progressive muscle relaxation

Tension builds up in the muscles throughout the day (and night) when you are agitated, frustrated or stressed. When the situation is dire, you will be very aware of it. However, your body can carry tension without you being conscious of it, too. Especially if you've been under prolonged stress and you have become accustomed to it—the discomfort feels familiar.

Progressive muscle relaxation helps you to become more aware of your muscle tension, and gives you a simple tool to release it.[8] To explore progressive muscle relaxation, try the following.

- Find a quiet place and allow yourself ten to fifteen uninterrupted minutes.
- Loosen any tight clothing, so your body is comfortable.
- Lie flat on the floor, feeling supported by the surface beneath you.
- Take a few minutes to centre yourself by focusing on your breathing—slow, deep, abdominal breathing.
- **Tense** all the muscles in your hands. Scrunch them up tightly.

- **Hold** for a few seconds, noticing the sensation.
- **Release** the muscles slowly on the exhalation. Silently say the word 'relax' as you let go.
- **Observe** and enjoy the sensation of the muscles letting go and tension draining away.
- Return your attention to your breathing—slow and deep.
- Repeat this process for another area of your body. Gradually progress through your entire body: arms, shoulders and neck, face and jaw, back, buttocks, belly, legs, feet, right down to your toes.
- When all your muscles have had a turn, take time to feel the relaxation flowing throughout your entire body. Tension has ebbed away.
- Be still and breathe. Take time to absorb the sensation so that it becomes familiar.

This exercise helps to release muscle tension that you are consciously or unconsciously holding. It allows you to become familiar with the physical sensation of tension versus release. Becoming accustomed to the feeling of physically holding on versus letting go allows you more choice—if you know when you're holding on, you can choose to let go.

'Warm, heavy, relaxed' training

This DIY autogenic (meaning 'coming from within') training technique reduces tension within the body and increases blood flow to the extremities. Once you've got the hang of it, your body ends up feeling warm, heavy and relaxed—a state of relaxation that feels lovely by day and can be conducive to sleep by night.

Have a go with autogenic training, following this approach.

- Find a quiet place and allow yourself ten to fifteen uninterrupted minutes.
- Lie flat on the floor, feeling supported by the surface beneath you.
- Loosen any tight clothing, so your body is comfortable.

- Focus on slow, deep, abdominal breathing to centre yourself.
- Bring your attention to one leg.
- Imagine your leg is feeling **warm, heavy and relaxed**.
- Say the words 'warm, heavy, relaxed' in your mind.
- Once you feel these sensations in the leg, focus on another limb and do the same.
- When all limbs feel warm, heavy and relaxed, repeat the process for your front torso, back torso, butt, neck and head.
- Be still and breathe—take time to absorb the sensation so that it becomes familiar.

Visualisation imagery training

For those of you who are more visual by nature, this is a handy technique to have in the toolbox. Create and capture an image in your mind of a place, scene or situation where you feel blissfully safe and peaceful, to use as a visual shortcut that inspires the relaxation response. Rehearse and fine-tune this visualisation in advance so that it's imagined vividly and can be brought to mind in a heartbeat when needed.

To create your own visual image for relaxation, try the following.

- Find a quiet place and allow yourself about ten to fifteen minutes of peace.
- Sit in a chair with both feet placed on the floor, or lie flat on the floor, feeling supported by the surface beneath you.
- Take a couple of minutes to centre yourself by closing your eyes and focusing on slow, deep, abdominal breathing.
- Clear your mind, then picture a place or scenario (real or imagined) where you feel very relaxed and at ease—e.g., a beach, a meadow, a forest.
- Visualise this scene in vivid detail—use all your senses to experience the place, including:
  - aromas in the air
  - colours and images you see
  - temperature and atmosphere

- ○ sounds you hear
- ○ tastes.
- Bring the scene to life, observing the movements and changes in this idyllic place.
- Imagine yourself in this scene and notice how your body relaxes and feels at ease.

Once you have created a visual image of your place of deep relaxation, revisit it often and practise bringing it to mind in full sensory detail. You want this image to be available to you on call. If you can conjure it at will, you will have a powerful tool for activating your relaxation response—wherever and whenever you need it.

These four relaxation techniques are recognised and doable options to explore. The very process of giving them a go and practising them will help you become more aware of muscle tension and the physical sensation of stress. They will wake you up to what stress feels like *within your body*, compared to a state of physiological relaxation.

Remember that relaxation is a skill that needs to be learned. Allow yourself to be truly terrible at these techniques for a while—this is normal. Relieve yourself of any performance pressure or expectation, quit judging yourself, let yourself be a beginner and give it a go. You'll need to be patient, as it takes time and practice to get the hang of relaxation. You don't need to master these techniques, and you don't have to be able to do them all. As you practise, you will find something that resonates with you. Use what works.

Once you are confident that you have a relaxation technique that works for you by day, use it at night if you need to relax your body and calm your mind when you are in bed. You can use it to relax before sleep or to calm yourself if you wake in the night. But always remember that you are using these tools merely for relaxation—they are to comfort and soothe you because you are awake. (If sleep happens to occur that's okay, but the intention is simply to rest in a relaxed way.)

The final week of the programme gives you a chance to experiment with dialling down your stress response and honouring your relaxation response. Use the week to see how these changes support your well-being and your ability to create the physical and mental conditions for sleep. Knowing how you really are and what you need is central to this.

Continue building mindful awareness into your life so you can non-judgementally bring your attention to how you are doing in the present moment. With this wisdom comes choice, and you have a lot of options open to you. Consider the stress-reduction and relaxation techniques covered in this chapter a big, beautiful buffet of possibilities to pick and choose from as you please. Some you will be drawn to more than others. This is a time to explore different techniques, find those that resonate and then practise them, so they get easier and more effective. These methods are the building blocks to continue and, importantly, to maintain your sleep improvement.

Plan Week Six

If your sleep efficiency is now around 85 per cent most of the time, your total sleep time is fairly consistently between 7 and 9 hours, and you wake feeling refreshed and well slept, this may be the amount of sleep that your body thrives on. Hallelujah! Time to celebrate. There's no need to keep extending your time in bed if you have found a sleep schedule that works well for you. Lock in this schedule and roll with it. (You can make your bedtime a bit earlier, but if your sleep starts to fragment or if it's difficult to fall asleep, go back to the bedtime that you know works.)

If your sleep-efficiency scores were 85 per cent or higher most nights last week, but you still feel that you need more sleep, increase the total time that you are in bed overnight to increase your opportunity for sleep. Bring your bedtime back by another 30 minutes this week. Be patient if your sleep goes a little wobbly initially—stick with this schedule for the week to allow time for your sleep to adjust and settle down.

If your sleep-efficiency scores were under 85 per cent on most nights of the week, stay with the same sleep schedule as last week until it improves. This week, as you continue with adjustments to lifestyle factors and explore stress reduction and relaxation, you're bound to see some progress.

If you need to, continue with stimulus control (the out-of-bed protocol) this week. If you are awake in bed for longer than fifteen minutes, get up and relax elsewhere until your body shows signs of being sleepy.

Keep reinforcing your helpful sleep thoughts and neglecting any counterproductive thoughts.

Let's plan your Week Six sleep–wake schedule on the pages ahead.

The notion that we are inadequate, insufficient or flawed in some way is a fear that resides in too many of us. Individually and collectively, we must find a way to accept ourselves as we are—gloriously imperfect. Giving yourself permission to simply be as you are (no more, no less) is an act of kindness and courage. It doesn't mean that you renege on your responsibilities or let go of your dreams. Instead, you pursue what matters in a physically and psychologically sustainable way. Learn to trust that you can be exactly who you are, work in harmony with your biology, and still thrive. This asks you to shift your mindset. Instead of believing you are not enough, open your heart to the possibility you are plenty.

Your job this week is to **finish strong**. You've come so far, this is not the time to renege on your commitment. If you need to rally the troops, double back to your true north in Chapter 7 and reacquaint yourself with the intentions you had for your sleep at the outset. Stay focused and stay true to what matters to you.

If you are a little bit resistant to exploring mindfulness, stress reduction and relaxation, know that you are not alone. Part of you might always kick and scream about slowing down and relaxing, but consider that, the more you're fighting it, the more you might need it. Resisting relaxation can be delaying the inevitable. The wisdom of mindfulness, stress reduction and relaxation is not just for your sleep but for your well-being now and in the future.

Schedule your wake-up time

Keep this the same as the other weeks.

My morning wake-up time I'm still committed to is _____ a.m.

Schedule your earliest bedtime

If your sleep-efficiency scores were 85 per cent or above on most nights last week, make your bedtime 30 minutes earlier than last week if you need to increase your opportunity for sleep. Otherwise, keep it the same as last week. Remember, this is the earliest time that you can go to bed.

My new earliest bedtime is _____ p.m.

Schedule time to prepare for bed

Continue to allow fifteen minutes to prepare for bedtime.

Schedule time to wind down

Continue to allow 60 to 90 minutes to wind down each night.
Summarise your schedule below.

My sleep–wake schedule for Week Six

Wind down (60–90 minutes): _____ p.m.

Prepare for bed (15 minutes): _____ p.m.

Earliest bedtime: _____ p.m

Morning wake-up time: _____ a.m.

Week Six recap: what you can do

1. Summarise your Week Six plan on the next page. Write it out again to reinforce it.

2. Consider how an activated stress response may be inhibiting your sleep. Review your ability to switch off stress and initiate your relaxation response.

3. Use the worksheet to map out the stress reduction and relaxation tools you will explore. Be realistic about what you plan to do.

4. Explore mindfulness further. Encourage yourself to practise a little each day.

5. Update Week Six of your sleep diary. Jot down your daily sleep info and, at the end of the week, work out your sleep-efficiency scores. Note any mindfulness, stress management or relaxation initiatives that you use.

6. Keep reading, keep learning and stay curious about your sleep.

WEEK SIX GUIDE

My sleep–wake schedule for Week Six

Wind down (60–90 minutes): _____ p.m.

Prepare for bed (15 minutes): _____ p.m.

Earliest bedtime: _____ p.m.

Morning wake-up time: _____ a.m.

- Keep maintaining a consistent **sleep–wake schedule**.
  - Continue the healthy sleep habits you've been building.
  - Consider adding 'letting go of the day' to your evening wind-down.
- Continue with **stimulus control** (the 'out of bed' protocol) if it's needed.
  - If you're not asleep within fifteen minutes, get up and relax.
  - Once you're sleepy, return to bed.
  - Repeat the process until you fall asleep easily in your bed.
- Keep up your **cognitive training**.
  - Etch those helpful sleep thoughts in your mind.
  - Identify, accept, challenge and replace any unhelpful sleep thoughts.
- Carry on making adjustments to your **lifestyle choices**.
  - If you're ready, experiment with another food, caffeine, alcohol or exercise adjustment to establish how it affects your sleep.
  - Make a plan: what do you want to do differently and how will you make it easy for yourself?
  - See what difference this makes to your sleep across the week.
- Practise **mindfulness**.
  - Check in regularly throughout your days and evenings (a pause for breath is a great practice for this).
  - Explore practising mindfulness meditation throughout the week— try basic mindfulness meditation, yoga, etc.
- Explore **stress-management and relaxation techniques** that resonate with you.
  - Select and try out some stress-management techniques.

- Practise some of the relaxation techniques during the day or at wind-down time.
- When you're confident with a relaxation technique, use it in bed at night to **relax**.

MINDFULNESS, STRESS-REDUCTION AND RELAXATION WORKSHEET

This worksheet is an opportunity to reflect on what you could do differently to be more aware of your experience, and to explore ways to reduce stress, relax your body and calm your mind.

Mindfulness

How mindful am I?
Reflect, without judgement, on how present you tend to be. Do you find it easy to be fully in the moment? Or do you tend to be lost in thoughts—distracted, planning ahead, worrying about the future, mulling over the past, struggling with a perpetually busy mind?

_____

_____

_____

_____

Practising mindfulness meditation
Write down how you might add a mindfulness meditation to your days.

_____

_____

_____

_____

Stress reduction

How stressed am I?
Consider your current stress levels and how this affects your body and mind. Does it affect how you feel?

_____

_____

_____

_____

Stress-reduction techniques to try
Write down techniques you could try this week: saying no, scheduling worry time, putting the day to rest, or time management.

_____

_____

_____

_____

Relaxation

What difference would it make if I was more relaxed?
How might this help you mentally, physically and emotionally?

_____

_____

_____

_____

Relaxation techniques to try
Write down techniques you'd like to try this week: belly breathing, progressive muscle relaxation, 'warm, heavy, relaxed' training or visualisation imagery.

_____

_____

_____

_____

SLEEP DIARY

Fill out your sleep diary every morning. Guess the approximate times, there's no need for clock-watching. On the next page, note any factors that helped with sleep or may have been unhelpful for your sleep. You're looking for clues and patterns . . .

Week Six	Night 1	Night 2	Night 3	Night 4	Night 5	Night 6	Night 7
Start Date _____ Day of Week							
What time did you go to bed?							
What time did you first try to go to sleep?							
What time did you fall asleep?							
How many times did you wake in the night?							
How long did these awakenings last in total?							
What time did you wake for the final time this morning?							
What time did you get out of bed for the day?							
How would you rate the quality of your sleep? (1 Terrible, 2 Bad, 3 OK, 4 Good, 5 Great)							
Total Sleep Time In total, how many hours' sleep did you get?							
Total Time in Bed In total, how long were you in bed?							
Sleep Efficiency % (Total Sleep Time ÷ Total Time in Bed X 100 = %)	%	%	%	%	%	%	%

SLEEP DIARY

Week Six	Night 1	Night 2	Night 3	Night 4	Night 5	Night 6	Night 7
Start Date _____ Day of Week							
Any factors that may have been unhelpful for your sleep last night?							
Any factors that may have helped with sleep last night?							

Observations & Insights:

PART 3

Maintenance and Follow-up

CHAPTER 11

Review, refine and keep moving forward

*Knowledge is only a rumour
until it lives in the bones.*

—ASARO TRIBE PROVERB

ongratulations! You have come a very long way on your sleep-improvement journey. Knowledge of how to sleep now lives within you—it's yours for keeps. It has been a privilege and an honour to be at your side as you've challenged your behaviours and your thinking to build a sustainable lifelong approach to better sleep. You will have battled your sheets and your beliefs to find your way to more peaceful and predictable sleep patterns. Kudos to you. Making transformational changes to your health, whether in the realm of exercise, nutrition or sleep, is an epic journey. What you have done is champion.

Review Week Six

Take stock of how far you have come. Go back to your original sleep review and your baseline sleep diaries to look at the state that you and your sleep were in six weeks ago. Reflect on the soft sleep goals you set for yourself in Chapter 9, and consider the improvements you've made in sleep efficiency, the time it takes you to fall asleep, awakenings in the night, total sleep duration and your sleep quality. There will have been some real shifts in how you sleep at night. Also notice how you feel these days—physically, mentally and emotionally.

You may feel you're now in better physical health than when you started. With more nutritious eating habits, improved hydration and more exercise in your weekly routine, along with easier sleep, you may feel that you now have more energy and are significantly healthier than when you started. Sleep improvement may have made a real difference to your workdays with improved motivation, productivity, concentration, memory or creativity. You may have noticed that anxiety has eased, you are calmer or your spirits have lifted. It is my hope that you are also being kinder and more compassionate with yourself, too.

These changes may be having fantastic flow-on effects in important areas of your life. Close relationships may be more relaxed, enjoyable and fulfilling. Your world may be opening up beyond the bare essentials once more—with time and capacity for socialising, leisure pursuits and fun. You may now have the mettle to make decisions that previously seemed too hard or too fraught to navigate. You may be looking ahead with ideas and plans for your future. You may have a greater sense of confidence, not just in your sleep but also in yourself.

The empowering experience of transforming my sleep—something that, for so long, seemed impossible—led to growth in almost all of these areas of my life. For me, learning to sleep was a game changer. I was no longer someone whose life and sense of self were strangled by sleep difficulties and feelings of powerlessness. Once again I was wholeheartedly and unapologetically me. The experience of teaching myself to sleep gave me a stronger sense of self and a real sense of agency. Ever since, I've been ready, able and up for actively propelling my life forward in directions that matter to me.

Creating the conditions that allow sleep to come to you is only the beginning. Sleep requires you to get core aspects of your life into a viable equilibrium—your sleep thoughts and habits, crucial lifestyle choices like nutrition and exercise, stress management and relaxation, as well as your practice of mindfulness and self-compassion. This has demanded a great deal of you, especially when you started the journey feeling compromised by sleep deficiency. You have achieved what you set out to do. From here, your possibilities are endless.

Refine

Even if you still have a little way to go with your sleep-improvement journey, feel confident that you now have the knowledge and essential tools to continue your progress. It may be that you'd like to practise or explore further some of the things you have learned. Use the worksheet at the end of this chapter to write down any aspects of the programme you want to continue exploring in your sleep-improvement pilgrimage. And remember: sleeping well is an ongoing journey, not a destination. Optimising sleep is about acquiring skills to have on hand along the way, applying them as you need, and honing them to suit your specific and ever-changing needs. All along the way, it's been about progress, not perfection. Continue to go at your own pace, with an ongoing sense of curiosity, and use trial and error to determine what supports you to more predictably experience the sleep of your dreams.

Consistent sleep–wake schedule

- Use your knowledge of your sleep needs to set a workable sleep–wake schedule to live by. When you reach a pattern of sleep that you thrive on, lock in your optimal bedtime and wake-time. These will be your centre of gravity for sleeping well. Remember: your wake-up time is an anchor for your body clock. Honour this as best you can. Your bedtime is a general guideline for going to bed, but listen to your body and watch out for signs of sleepiness. Go to bed when you are *sleepy*.

- From here, you don't have to be regimented about your sleep–wake schedule—you can probably sway half an hour either side with little impact on your sleep. From time to time, you can stray far from these thresholds if life asks this of you. Having a night off from your sleep–wake routine is no big deal. Just remember to return to your schedule on subsequent nights—you know it serves you well. Going off-piste for several days is where you may find yourself running into sleep difficulties. If this happens, don't panic or beat yourself up. Simply return to what you know works, and be aware that it may take a few nights for your sleep to settle back into your preferred pattern.
- Maintain the sleep-supporting habit of allowing yourself wind-down time each evening. Continue the habit of getting up at wake-time (or close to it). Support your body clock by getting outside into the daylight for fifteen minutes each morning. If you can, combine it with your walk.

Sleep consolidation

- If your sleep-efficiency scores aren't yet at 85 per cent or higher on most nights of the week, you may want to continue with your current sleep–wake schedule until this shores up. Once it has, change your earliest bedtime to 30 minutes earlier at night.
- There are more sleep diaries in Appendix IV if you would like to continue using them to keep an eye on your progress.
- Continue the sleep-consolidation process until your sleep efficiency is high pretty regularly (85 per cent or over on four or more nights of the week), and your sleep duration has consistently reached a level that feels great for you. Make sure your total sleep time is suitable for your age, and you wake feeling rested, restored and ready for the day. Remember, it's okay to thrive on less than 8 hours per night, but it's highly unlikely to be under 6 hours.

Stimulus control

- Once your bed and bedroom have become a strong cue for sleep, you will fall asleep or fall back to sleep easily (use fifteen minutes as your guide).
- If your bed or bedroom is not yet working as a trustworthy sleep cue, continue to use stimulus control to really strengthen that association between your bed and falling asleep with ease.

Cognitive training

- Continue reinforcing your helpful sleep thoughts. Repeat them to yourself at the times when they're needed until they become automatic responses.
- If any new unhelpful sleep thoughts materialise, be aware that the stress they create makes sleep elusive. Be sure to spot them, gently challenge them, and replace them with more accurate and helpful thoughts about sleep.

Nutrition and exercise

- Keep moving towards healthy eating habits—for most of us, this is an ongoing journey. Knowing that eating well supports your sleep is another sound reason to continue your endeavours. Keep building healthy food habits little by little— more fruit and veggies, fibre (e.g., whole grains), legumes, nuts and seeds, and fish, and reduce the saturated fats, simple carbs, sugar, red meat and processed food. Keep yourself well hydrated throughout the day.
- There may be other lifestyle choices (or vices) that you know you need to take care of for the sake of your sleep, or for your well-being generally. If you need to, keep exploring ways to curb your caffeine, alcohol, nicotine or cannabis habits.
- Maintain or build the amount of moderate-intensity activity you do each week. Make this an ongoing commitment to yourself for sleep and general health and well-being. Use 30 minutes a day, five days a week as your reference.

Mindfulness, stress reduction and relaxation

- Cultivate your own mindfulness practice—intentionally pay attention to the present moment without judgement. Use the starter kit provided: the one-minute meditation, a pause for breath, or the basic mindfulness meditation. You could also explore mindfulness through movement with some yoga. Yoga with Adriene on YouTube is a really accessible place to start.

- If you're ready to go deeper with your mindfulness, explore formally led meditation or yoga programmes. They will support you in cultivating a daily practice and integrating mindfulness into your life.

- Alongside mindful awareness, continue to practise self-compassion. Honour your needs and take care of yourself as you would a dear friend. Remember there are two strands of self-compassion: the gentle nurturing style (yin) and the confident, action-oriented style (yang).

- Use self-compassion to find your way through difficult times and experiences. Be aware of and accept when you're suffering, know that you're not alone with your struggles, and be supremely kind to yourself—either with gentle self-care or by using inner strength to stand up for what you truly need.

- Take steps to reduce the stressors in your life—learn the art of saying no, schedule a worry time if things are piling up on you, put your day to rest each night, be realistic about what to expect of yourself and manage your time accordingly.

- Make use of the relaxation techniques that you've learned—belly breathing, progressive muscle relaxation, 'warm, heavy, relaxed' training and visualisation imagery. Once you've mastered these by day, they can be used in bed to help your body and mind relax in preparation for sleep to come.

Sleep education and sleep hygiene

- Remind yourself how sleep works—understand your circadian rhythm and sleep pressure. Work with your biology, rather than against it.

- Maintain realistic expectations of what healthy sleep looks like. Sleep cycles mean there will be periods throughout the night where sleep is lighter, or you briefly wake. Know that there is monophasic sleep as well as biphasic. Interludes of wakefulness can be okay.
- Understand how insomnia evolves from an acute temporary situation to become more persistent. Be aware that many well-intentioned thoughts and behaviours unintentionally perpetuate insomnia. Remind yourself to intervene early— don't let chronic insomnia get its claws in.
- Continue to live by the World Sleep Society's ten commandments of sleep hygiene to support and maintain your sleep improvements. Remember, it's like the brushing and flossing of dental hygiene—boring but necessary to prevent cavities.
- Keep phones and devices out of your bedroom.

Embrace your days

- Sleep makes up about a third of our lives—around 25 years, in fact. So you have had good reason to commit to discovering how to sleep with ease. Your sleep has been difficult for so long that it's natural to put the focus on it that you have. By understanding your sleep, and being more at one with how to create the conditions for sleep, you can now broaden your focus to the other two-thirds of your life: your glorious waking hours. Fill them with what matters to you. Enjoy them. Live well to sleep well. And vice versa.

You have done so well, and I respect you for showing up and engaging with this programme in its entirety. The training wheels are off, and you can now ride solo. I'm confident that you have what you need to continue your sleep-improvement journey single-handed.

When you feel secure that your sleep efficiency is regularly above 85 per cent and your sleep duration is working well for you, it's time to throw away the sleep diary. You can stop monitoring and calculating.

Be relaxed and trusting of this beautiful biological phenomenon called sleep. You've put in the time to learn, and you now know what it takes to sleep with ease! Be sure to remind yourself often: 'I sleep well.' Start identifying yourself as someone who sleeps easily, or sleeps well, because you are.

Celebrate

Make sure you take time to acknowledge your motivation, commitment and progress in sleeping with ease. Brené Brown encourages us to practise gratitude and celebrate our milestones and our victories (even if our tendency historically has been to throw away opportunities for joy and recognition). In early chapters, you worked out why you embarked on this endeavour—your true north for sleep improvement—and you set some soft goals for your sleep. By now, you will be reaping these rewards. It's time to celebrate. When you achieve something that genuinely matters to you, it's worth celebrating.

Acknowledging and honouring how your relationship with sleep has changed shifts something inside of you—you feel empowered, have a sense of agency, and there's momentum in your life. It's incredibly fortifying and liberating. And it's a far cry from where you started—feeling frustrated, despairing, stuck, powerless, shackled by persistent and unpredictable sleep problems. That is behind you. Now you can trust that your body knows how to sleep, and you understand how to create the conditions for sleep. You've shown yourself that you can.

Celebrate your success in a way that's meaningful for you. (Just don't let it be a stiff whisky right before bed—you know the drill on nightcaps!) If you're not currently in the habit of rejoicing and basking in your accomplishments, consider some of the possibilities listed here. Use this as a springboard to come up with ideas that will infuse the experience in positivity for you.

Honour your sleep

One of the World Sleep Society's commandments for sleep is to make your sleep environment comfortable and inviting. Previously, your nights were in terrible shape so your bedroom probably had a bad vibe and you might have harboured some negativity towards your bed. Those days are gone now, thanks to the work you've done. Your bedroom is now a place of serenity, and your bed a cue for sleep.

A very tangible way to honour your sleep improvement is to give your sleep environment an upgrade. Now that you know the glories of sleeping well, you'll be more inclined to invest a bit of money, energy and flair into making this space a sanctuary of peace. Below are some areas worth considering.

Mattress

Consider your mattress an essential piece of sleeping equipment. A decent mattress lasts about seven to ten years, but often our beds get taken for granted and our mattresses are slept on well beyond their expiry date—often for decades. Mattresses physically wear out and become no longer comfortable, hygienic or supportive. On top of that, physical needs change over time. Bodies morph in shape and weight, fitness levels change, and issues with necks or backs may occur.

Mattress needs may also change with partners and pregnancy.

It's usually only when the situation gets dire that people are forced to investigate a replacement—a noticeable hollow, a maverick spring, or relentless back pain and broken sleep. Too many of us change our mattresses as a last resort. Quality mattresses are expensive, they are a hassle to research, choose and replace, and there are real consequences for sleep if you get it wrong. It's little wonder that people delay the purchase. But the mattress is the physical foundation for your sleep. It provides both comfort and support for your entire body every night— it's worth taking the time and spending the money. It's an investment in your health and well-being.

Pillows

The intended lifespan of a pillow is about eighteen months. Higher quality, natural-fibre ones last a bit longer, and memory-foam pillows last up to three years. This seems like a short product lifespan, but keep in mind that we lay our heads on them about 3000 hours a year! It's common not to give much thought to our pillows until they become a problem—discomfort, sore necks, stains, smells, even mildew. Consider your pillow another essential piece of sleeping equipment that's worth investing in regularly. It needs to be comfortable for your head to rest on and provide sufficient support for your shoulders, neck and head.

Bed linen and sleepwear

With your newfound respect and reverence for sleep, consider rewarding yourself with lovely new bed linen or sleepwear. I adore good bed linen and sleepwear, so could rave on about this forever. But when I distil it all down, there are really only two recommendations to make: choose what you truly love; and consider natural fibres as they are breathable and more eco-friendly.

Bedroom aesthetic

Surround yourself with what you love in your sleep environment. It is your sanctuary. You will spend about a third of your time in this room. It's your most private, intimate space, where you retreat from the world and can be your most authentic, vulnerable self. Make it beautiful to your eyes.

Beyond this, keep your bedroom clean, tidy and uncluttered. A National Sleep Foundation study shows that keeping your bedroom clean and tidy is associated with better sleep.[1] So Marie Kondo the space, or at least adopt the habits of making your bed daily and washing your linen, vacuuming and airing the room regularly.

Create meaningful bedtime rituals

Sleeping well is what you value and want for yourself from now on, so it's worth creating rituals that will help to settle you for the night. Use them to provide calming, quietening cues that gently remind you all is well and it's time for sleep. Most of us understand the value of bedtime rituals when we are settling young children for the night—a warm bath, cute PJs, a snuggly blanket or soft toy, warm milk, story time, a song and a kiss goodnight. A bedtime ritual can be just as beneficial for adults, but it has to be DIY.

Consider having a few bedtime rituals that are special to you. Choose a couple of little self-care things that will ease you into a peaceful state conducive to falling asleep. You know these things will not 'make' you fall asleep—they will simply help you relax before sleep.

Be guided by your senses to find things that inspire feelings of serenity and inner calm. Go with what is lovely for you. Consider these suggestions:

- ambient lighting from a muted lamp or candle
- the soft, comforting textures of a blanket or a wrap
- the relaxing aroma of a scented candle, diffuser or lotion, e.g., lavender, rose, geranium, jasmine, vanilla, sandalwood
- a warm, comforting drink, such as milk or herbal tea, e.g., chamomile, lavender, lemon balm, valerian
- a photo of people, places or moments that bring joy to your heart

- relaxing music
- a book you love
- a gratitude journal.

When creating a bedtime ritual, remember to keep everything as a nice-to-have, not a need-to-have. Enjoy things simply because you like them, and they support you in feeling relaxed, not because you have to have them or you won't sleep. These little rituals aren't to become presleep rules that cannot be broken. Avoid getting fretful, overattentive or attached. Keep them optional. The ability to sleep well lies within you—you don't *need* these external factors. They are little acts of self-care, self-nurture and self-love.

I value my sleep so much that, in the evenings, I really enjoy preparing my bedroom in advance. I draw the curtains early, adjust the thermostat on the heater or open the window a little so the temperature will be just right, turn on my bedside lamp and turn back the covers of my bed. When it's time to turn in, my bedroom and bed are welcoming. I nestle happily under the covers and many nights I light the rose-and-geranium serenity candle that my sister gave me. Sometimes I use a wrap to get cosy, or I massage my hands with a beautiful lotion (a gift from my other sister). Some nights I discover the 'Pillow Book' slipped into my bed. (This is a precious journal that my daughter and I have shared since she was six years old, a place where we write kind, heartfelt messages to one another.) I take a moment to appreciate my day and my life, then I pick up a marvellous novel from the tower beside me and get lost in it for half an hour. In doing these things, I feel cared for and loved, regardless of how my day has been. None of this makes me sleep, though. Nor can it. It's all optional. I do it because I enjoy it—I'm taking care of myself and supporting the possibility of a lovely night's sleep.

If you ever feel that your sleep rituals have accidentally morphed into sleep rules,[2] it's worth gently resolving it. Note any rituals you have become too attached to, or rules that have developed. Anything that belongs in the 'if I don't do this, I can't sleep' department. Then, without making a fuss or getting uptight about it, give yourself permission to let go of one rule. Try being non-compliant about it for a few days, and, if your sleep remains okay, gently let go of another until your sleep is no longer restrained by your self-imposed rules.

The hard work of CBTi is done. It's now time to do the fun stuff—review your progress, celebrate your accomplishments, and find ways to respect, honour and truly enjoy your sleep from now on. Acknowledging and rewarding yourself embeds these new thoughts, behaviours and healthy approaches to sleep. It imbues sleep with an optimistic sentiment that will endure long after you finish this book. My vision was to share what I've learned about sleep and to make the challenging journey doable for sleep-deficient people. I'm excited for you that you have built a better relationship with sleep and restored trust in this vital part of your life.

Chapter recap: what you can do

1. **Review your progress.** Go back to your initial sleep review, your baseline sleep diaries, your true north and your sleep goals. Look at how far you've come and the benefits you're experiencing.

2. **Celebrate your progress.** Do something to acknowledge the journey you have been on and rejoice in what you've accomplished.

3. **Honour your sleep.** As a mark of respect, upgrade your sleep environment. Invest in your mattress if needed, or at least replace your pillow. Unclutter and beautify your bedroom, so it becomes your sanctuary.

4. **Create bedtime rituals.** Imbue bedtime with some self-care options that bring you peace and a sense that you are loved.

5. **Keep reading, keep learning and stay curious about your sleep.**

HOW FAR I'VE COME

Progress I have made with my sleep and my relationship with sleep:

_____
_____
_____
_____
_____

Benefits I notice in myself and my life:

_____
_____
_____
_____

To celebrate my progress with sleep, I will:

_____
_____
_____
_____

I will honour my sleep by:

_____
_____
_____
_____

Optional bedtime rituals I'd like to create for myself:

_____
_____
_____
_____

ONGOING SLEEP-IMPROVEMENT PLAN

Use this worksheet to record any areas of the programme that you'd like to spend a little more time exploring as you continue your sleep-improvement journey.

- ☐ Consistent sleep schedule
- ☐ Sleep consolidation
- ☐ Stimulus control (the 'out of bed' protocol)
- ☐ Cognitive training
- ☐ Nutrition and exercise
- ☐ Stress reduction and relaxation
- ☐ Sleep education and sleep hygiene
- ☐ Mindfulness and self-compassion

Write down what you want to explore and how you will do this:

_____

_____

_____

_____

_____

_____

_____

_____

_____

_____

There are additional sleep diary pages included in Appendix IV, if you need them.

_____

My sleep–wake schedule moving forward

Wind down (60–90 minutes): _____ p.m.

Prepare for bed (15 minutes): _____ p.m.

Earliest bedtime: _____ p.m.

Morning wake-up time: _____ a.m.

CHAPTER 12

What to do when things go wobbly

Just take this step ... The horizon will look after itself.
—CHARLIE MACKESY

ou've worked diligently to restore your precious sleep, and you're committed to doing what you can to maintain and protect it. Your sleep confidence is back, and there's a sense of calm about your nights. Even so, you need to anticipate curveballs. Things will happen that derail your sleep, and that's life being life. Even the best sleepers have times in their lives when their sleep goes haywire. You will be okay.

Chapter 6 covered the precipitating factors of insomnia—things that can trigger sleep difficulties. These can include medical illness or injury, acute stress, the onset of or changes to a mental-health issue, a new job involving shift work, a new partner with different sleep patterns, pregnancy, care for an infant, or menopause. So many factors can set off a bout of acute insomnia. Some of these things you'll have some control over, but some things are entirely out of your hands. The Covid-19 pandemic, for example, hit the world hard and fast. It intensified stress levels, created global uncertainty and changed our ways of life. It caused a profound increase in rates of disturbed sleep, especially insomnia and nightmares.[1]

As someone who has already experienced chronic insomnia, you might be more susceptible to further triggers and episodes of sleep difficulties in the future. It's not written in your destiny, but having been there before means you may have somewhat higher chances of sleep problems occurring again. So you're not out of the woods. This is fine as long as you are a good scout and remain prepared for what may lie ahead.

As you know, there are things you can do to maintain your sleep health and minimise the risk of self-imposed insomnia. This makes sense, and you will have already built these habits into your daily routines. Keep them up—they will serve you well. But throughout your life, there will be events and situations that are entirely beyond your control that can seriously disturb your sleep. Instead of living in fear, you're going to look ahead, have a plan and know what to do to manage.

I'm restless. Things are calling me away.
My hair is being pulled by the stars again.
—ANAÏS NIN

If and when your sleep unravels in the future, the critical thing is to remain calm. Know that this is probably going to happen at some stage. It may be a voluntary choice ('Hell, yes, pour me another wine even though it's midnight') or accidentally self-inflicted ('I'm almost certain I asked the barista for decaf this afternoon!'). Or it may genuinely be through no fault of your own. However sleep difficulties emerge, simply accept them for what they are—common, temporary and transient.

Your job is to intercept them early. You want to nip issues in the bud to prevent chronic insomnia from taking hold like it did last time. You will not participate in any insomnia-perpetuating factors now that you know what they are—no going to bed super early to catch up on sleep, no sleeping in on the weekend, no long afternoon naps, no nightcaps. You know better. From what you've learned in this programme, you have the knowledge and the tools to help yourself and prevent insomnia persisting. Your plan is to keep short-term insomnia short term.

When sleep difficulties happen, get this book out again, dust it off and go back to the basics—going into a tailspin will only feed the monster. Make sure that you're following the fundamentals of sleep hygiene. Refresh your memory about how sleep works and insomnia takes hold. Use the CBTi principles you've learned to support yourself. Check that you have a consistent sleep schedule. Consider compressing your sleep, like you did in Week One. Preserve a strong association between your bed and sleep. Make sure your sleep thoughts are helpful. Fine-tune your nutrition and exercise to your advantage. Manage your stress levels and make good use of your relaxation strategies. Strengthen, return to or start mindfulness and self-compassion practice.

You may want to reach out for some herbal support, even if the science is deemed not strong yet. While it may not be essential, herbal remedies can be helpful, even psychologically. For me, they can provide natural support while I get on with the things that I know need recalibrating.

If your symptoms feel different from the insomnia that you've been dealing with here, double back to Chapter 2 to reread about other sleep disorders and take the appropriate action based on a self-diagnosis. If your sleep troubles have been triggered by a new life stage or a lifestyle change, check the additional resources in Appendix I for more information on specific sleep challenges such as sharing a bed, snoring, pregnancy, shift work, menopause and ageing.

If you feel like it's a sleep emergency that you can't manage yourself, and you're freaking out despite everything you've learned, contact your doctor to discuss your situation and the possibility of a prescription for sleeping medication. You may need to use sleeping medication to get through the worst of it, alongside mindful self-compassion and the implementation of healthy sleep thoughts and behaviours. Make sure you get the lowest dose and shortest course required for the scenario and, in consultation with your doctor, make a plan of how and when to come off them. Use them while you deal with the stressor in your life, and until you get your healthy sleep habits back on track.

While some triggers can't be anticipated, other potential sleep-busters occur each year—daylight saving and summer heat. Rather than let these sneak up on you and upset your nights, take action to get through these times with your sleep unscathed.

Daylight saving

Daylight saving is observed in New Zealand and across parts of Australia (it is not observed in Queensland, the Northern Territory and Western Australia). Every spring, the clocks spring forward one hour to create 'summer time', and every autumn the clocks fall back an hour. This seasonal time shuffle was pioneered in New Zealand to provide more daylight in the evening. Even though it's been around for over 40 years in its current form, it's still one of those things that can trip up sleep at changeover time.

Given the gains that you've made with your sleep, you don't want to let daylight saving throw you off your game. So here's the lowdown on what to anticipate sleep-wise and how best to prepare yourself for this annual occurrence.

Spring: clocks spring forward

This is the time change to pay attention to—it's the one most likely to muck up your sleep as it's a bit harder for the body to adjust to than the autumn transition. The most common issues that you'll run into include: not feeling tired at your normal bedtime, staying up late, getting out of bed feeling rugged in the morning, or getting anxious because you anticipate that you're going to have sleep problems. With the change and your response to it, there's a risk that you can lose some sleep.

You know that the body operates on an internal body clock (circadian rhythm) and that's pretty well in sync with the 24-hour cycle of light and dark. So, when the government artificially shifts time for six months, you can expect your body to scramble a bit initially as it adjusts to the change. While there definitely can be sleep problems, there doesn't have to be. You just need to do a bit of preparation, so your body doesn't have to make the adjustment in one night.

If you're naturally a night owl, the start of daylight saving can be particularly challenging, so make sure you take steps to help your body to synchronise more easily.

What you can do

The guts of it is, you need to fall asleep an hour earlier and wake up an hour earlier than what your body is accustomed to. To support your sleep, try the following:

- Bring bedtime and wake-up time forward by fifteen to twenty minutes per day for a few days before daylight saving and on the Saturday night of the official clock change.
- Go to bed at the earlier bedtime and get up at the earlier wake-up time.
- Get plenty of exposure to sunlight first thing in the morning— hurl those curtains back and go for a fifteen-minute walk without sunglasses.
- Avoid caffeine in the afternoon and the evening, and avoid nicotine in the evening.
- Don't use alcohol (or cannabis) to help you fall asleep.

Easing into daylight saving across a few days makes for a smoother transition that's less likely to upset your sleep. Even so, you can anticipate it taking about a week for your body to completely acclimatise to the change.

Autumn: clocks fall back

The end of daylight saving in April is less disruptive to sleep. It's a much smoother transition for the body, and generally takes only a day or two to adjust. After the clocks change, it's darker earlier and more conducive to putting yourself to bed. Plus, it's lighter in the morning, so you may be more inclined to get up and get moving. Some people find that the end of daylight saving actually helps improve their sleep.

New Zealand daylight saving time	Australia daylight saving time
STARTS IN SPRING	**STARTS IN SPRING**
Clocks spring forward one hour from 2 a.m. to 3 a.m. on the last Sunday in September.	Clocks spring forward one hour from 2 a.m. to 3 a.m. on the first Sunday in October.
ENDS IN AUTUMN	**ENDS IN AUTUMN**
Clocks fall back one hour from 3 a.m. to 2 a.m. on the first Sunday in April.	Clocks fall back one hour from 3 a.m. to 2 a.m. on the first Sunday in April.

Summer heat

In Australia and some parts of New Zealand, summer heat can add a challenge to sleeping conditions. As you know, temperature affects the ability to fall asleep and stay asleep. When it's just too hot, it takes longer to fall asleep and sleep can be fragmented.

If it's scorching hot, you need to adjust your expectations of sleep and do what you can to make the night easier for yourself. While some people have temperature-controlled homes, the rest of us have to improvise to make sleeping in the heat tolerable. Sleep Health Foundation,[2] National Sleep Foundation,[3] and SleepHub[4] have some practical tips on their websites. Their suggestions include the following.

What you can do

- Keep well hydrated throughout the day and don't get sunburnt.
- Prevent heat building up in your bedroom.
  - In the daytime, close curtains or blinds and windows if it's hotter outside than in.
  - At night, open the windows if it's cooler outside (and it's safe).
- Don't go to bed too early. Wait till you're sleepy or the temperature has come down a bit.
- A cool shower or bath before bed may help (or in the night if it's crazy hot).
- Sleep naked or wear as little as possible—light cotton sleepwear, not sweaty synthetics.
- Use 100 per cent cotton bed linen, rather than blends that include synthetics.
- Try to get air circulating over your skin—use a fan or open window to create a breeze.
- Keep your hands and feet cool by keeping them out from under the sheets.
- Have chilled water in a drink bottle at your bedside.
- Have a cold pack on standby to cool your face, hands and neck, e.g., a hot-water bottle with icy cold water, a cold facecloth or ice packs.
- Have another layer of bedding on standby, as you may feel cold when your body temperature drops between 3 a.m. and 5 a.m.
- Attitude matters. Accept that it's hot and that everyone's sleep will be a bit sketchy for now. Use your newly developed

skills to keep your body relaxed and your mind calm and understanding. Trust that it's okay to just doze and rest.

- If you get agitated and frustrated, it's better to get up than wrestle in your bed. (You want to keep your bed associated with sleep, not wakefulness.) Find a way to cool your body and calm down before returning to bed when you feel sleepy.

Jet lag

Travelling across time zones can play havoc with your sleep. Jet lag means there's a mismatch between the local time and the time your body thinks it is. With your body clock out of whack, sleep goes to hell and daytime fatigue makes life in the new city or country feel somewhat surreal. Knowing what to expect and what you can do about it can help.

The nature, severity and duration of jet lag depend on the number of time zones crossed as well as the direction of travel (eastward or westward). Some folk are more susceptible to jet lag than others, but, as a general rule of thumb, the human body can adjust to two time zones of travel in the westward direction per 24 hours and one time zone of travel in the eastward direction per 24 hours.[5] For casual short-distance travellers, jet lag can be all part of the fun and adventure, but for people flying frequently or doing long-haul flights, jet lag is definitely not fun. And, for those of us with a history of insomnia, we want to avoid jet lag triggering what we know can become an ongoing problem.

If you're concerned about the impact a flight may have on your sleeping patterns, it's worth talking to a doctor in advance to make a plan for how best to manage the upcoming flight and the potential fallout. Treatment can involve strategically using melatonin and exposure to light and dark to outfox the time-zone changes and speed up your body's adaptation to the local schedule. Stimulants (caffeine) or sleeping pills can also be used strategically to help manage the symptoms of jet lag while your body is aligning with the clock.

If you're travelling westward across time zones, your body clock is going to be ahead of the locals. You'll want to crash out before everyone else, and you'll be bright-eyed and bushy-tailed while others are still fast asleep in the morning. (You're like a morning lark in this new habitat.) If you are travelling east, the opposite happens. You'll be wide awake well into the night and will struggle to drag yourself out of bed in the morning on local time. (You become like a night owl at your destination.) The table below, based on the reference book *Sleep Medicine*,[6] provides some general guidelines for supporting your sleep when you're jet-setting.

	Flying west	Flying east
Symptoms to expect when you get to your destination	Crashing out before the locals and waking too early in the morning	Staying awake longer than the locals and difficulty getting out of bed in the morning
Prepare before departure	Go to bed and wake up an hour later eaoh day	Go to bed and wake up an hour earlier eaoh day
Daylight hacks when you get there	Exposure to bright light in the evening and avoid sunlight in the morning	Avoid light in the late evening and get exposure to bright light in the morning
Melatonin?	Consider melatonin in the morning	Consider melatonin in the evening

There will always be events and times that throw off your sleep schedule, but do what you can to look after it. You will know how much sleep disruption you can tolerate before your sleep is really at risk.

A couple of years ago, I was invited to be interviewed for a TVNZ documentary, *The Curious Mind*. It explored the miracle of the human mind and the fascinating neuroscience that is emerging. Naturally, there was an episode on how crucial sleep is for the brain. Nigel Latta, a celebrity psychologist, was to speak with me about my experiences living with insomnia and the profound benefits I'd gained by restoring my sleep. In the setup for the show, the production team went through my home with me discussing the locations required for the shoot. When it came to my bedroom, I went cold. This was my private sanctuary, the altar of my glorious, hard-won sleep. I didn't feel comfortable with cameras, lights and crew in there. However, I needed to put my big-girl undies on, as the story was important and for the greater good. But when they suggested that I lie in bed *pretending not to sleep*, I drew the line. As a bit-part actor, I'm familiar with living in imaginary circumstances, and this scene was well within my skillset. But faking insomnia was too raw and too real. This was my bed, my haven, the place where I had diligently created helpful sleep associations. It felt like they were asking an alcoholic to have just one little sip of whisky. I have lived with chronic insomnia, I know that the price is extraordinarily high. It's a price I paid for far too long. I will never, ever go back there.

Times of unsettled sleep are part of life's rich tapestry. Our job is to take them in stride and proactively manage them when they occur. Having navigated your way through chronic insomnia, you are well equipped with the mindset and tools to confidently attend to a temporary bout of unsettled sleep. Recognise it early, accept that it happens to everyone, be gentle with yourself, and take the necessary steps to calmly and patiently steer your way back to your body's preferred sleeping pattern. Keep in mind that, like us, sleep is organic and ever-changing. As we grow and age, our bodies change, and our sleep needs and patterns will alter with them. This is an opportunity for us to stay curious about the mysterious and miraculous natural process that is sleep.

Get the jump on sleep health

To get fresh insights in sleep health and timely reminders to prepare for seasonal changes that interfere with sleep, drop your details at my website Sleep Haven. Let's stay in touch beyond the book, I'd love to help you to continue to sleep easy.
www.sleephaven.co.nz

CHAPTER 13

Better nights and better days

Live in the sunshine, swim in the sea, drink the wild air.

—RALPH WALDO EMERSON

L ike breathing, sleeping is one of the most essential rhythms of life. It's a changing tide, restoring and refreshing. As a biological necessity, it deserves reverence and respect. You are wise to have recognised the value of being able to sleep easy, and it was courageous to have embarked on this journey to rebuild your relationship with sleep, at a time when everything felt like a struggle.

Along the way, you've had to unlearn what you thought you knew about fixing the problem and making yourself sleep. You've had to let go of a need to control and make change through effort, at the same time as implementing new ways of thinking and behaving. You've had to learn to be flexible and allow things to unfold in their own way and time. As much as this journey has been about CBTi, the principles of mindfulness and self-compassion are perhaps the most meaningful.

The path to sleeping easy isn't always easy. There are some inner battles to be resolved—I definitely had my share. Experiencing sleep difficulties seems to insist on us better understanding ourselves to allow sleep to come.

When I was a child, I spent a lot of time at a family friend's farm on the outskirts of my hometown, Ōamaru. Their cat had a litter of kittens deep in the crawl space under the shed. Born a cat-lover, I wanted those kittens with all my heart. I longed to touch them, hold them. I needed those kittens. Yet the more I tried to lure them, coax them, encourage them out from their hiding place, the more they resisted. They knew I was there and knew that I wanted them. My urgency and wanting made them stay away.

One day, beside myself with frustration and failure, I gave up. I surrendered my efforts and no longer cared whether I got those kittens or not. Defeated, I sat with my back against the wall of the run-down shed and cried with self-pity. When I was done, I closed my eyes and rested quietly, enjoying the sunshine on my face and the smell of the warm, dry grass beside me.

Then, I sensed a presence. I didn't dare look. There was warmth near my hand and a tender brush of what could only be tiny whiskers. Tentatively, I opened my eyes to see not one but two wee tabby kittens staring up at me with curiosity.

With sleep, our yearning and our battle to have it often make it elusive. Learning to trust that nature has your back and that sleep will come if you stop trying so damned hard is quite the lesson. It took me the longest time to learn it, but I got there in the end. It's inspiring to experience what's possible, once we know to get out of our own way.

Sometimes I feel sad about the years I lost in the fog of insomnia, the moments I missed with my husband and my daughter because I was just too tired, the opportunities that passed me by while I was trying to get through my insomnia-addled days. But there's little value in looking back. My attention is better placed on what is right here with me now, in the present. A present that I'm able to experience wholeheartedly and with gratitude, thanks to the life-changing difference it makes to be at one with my sleep.

Since finding my way home to myself and my sleep, life has really opened up for me. I don't know whether this is from the rejuvenation provided by sleep itself or from the empowerment and confidence that came with resolving a major difficulty in my life. Maybe it's both.

By day, I'm now experiencing things that several years ago were beyond the realm of possibility. This, my first book, is one of them. Another first is funding for a short-film script that I wrote. Last year I went skateboarding with my daughter (I'm very sensible now that I'm in my fifties).

A few months ago, between lockdowns, my family took a brief holiday at a remote farm in Northland—a magical place with horses. Lily is a great rider, and my husband, John, is much further ahead than me in his horse confidence. I do what I can to hang on and not be too afraid. We went on a stunning bareback trek through native bush and along secluded streams. When we came to a clearing, we halted our horses at the foot of a steep hill.

The decision was made to canter to the top. Having never cantered before, my heart was in my mouth. But our wise guide, Ellen, was confident. I took a pause for breath, acknowledged my fear and chose to relax, trust and go with it. Holding on to my horse's long mane, we took off in a heartbeat. Pounding hooves and the power of 500 kilograms of muscle beneath me, my husband on a bay beside me, and our daughter ahead on a grey, cantering bareback, I was filled with exhilaration, joy and absolute triumph.

We paused at the hillcrest in silence, taking in the majesty of the view. Seeing the farmhouse in the distance, I thought, *Look how far we've come.* There I was, with plenty of energy, in this extraordinary place, living in the present moment with the people I love, experiencing life in full glory.

It's been a privilege to share my experience in overcoming insomnia with you, and what I've learned since. Not just about sleep, but also about our need to be mindful and compassionate with ourselves so we can sleep and live well. The more I read and explore, the more I am blown away by sleep and the discoveries that sleep professionals continue to make in this fascinating field of human health. In the scheme of things, sleep is a relatively new branch of medicine. While mindfulness and compassion are, by comparison, an even younger branch of Western medicine, their origins are ancient. It's clear that we have so much to learn.

Fortunately, we are blessed with an international community of dedicated, passionate and accomplished experts in these fields, so there is much knowledge already. My intention with this book and our time together has been to share their wisdom, passing knowledge, principles and practical how-to insights into your hands and your heart, so you too can find your way to sleep easy.

ACKNOWLEDGEMENTS

Every book finds its own way. I have deep gratitude for the early believers, who gave me the courage to propel the idea of a local DIY sleep manual from dream to reality. The briefest conversations helped allay reservations, instil confidence and build momentum. Rachel, from the local bookshop Dear Reader for her genuine exuberance when I first gave voice to wanting to write an insider's guide to sleep. The esteemed Dr Lee Mathias for letting me know that this work mattered. Michael Saccente, whose heart-warming anecdote put my imposter syndrome to bed. The entrepreneurial and ever-practical Hannah McQueen for telling me to just get a proposal on the page. Megan Nicol Reed for describing a sample paragraph as beautiful, and surreptitiously making a connection that ultimately led the project to the perfect publisher.

The team at Allen & Unwin have been an incredible, streamlined force to work with. From the very outset, I knew, this story and I were in exceptionally safe and capable hands. I give a heartfelt thanks to Michelle Hurley, publisher, for seeing the value in this book, for believing in me, and for encouraging me to stretch the geographical boundaries of this opportunity. My appreciation goes to Jenny Hellen, publishing director, for seeing the vision, knowing the timing was right and taking a punt on a rookie (who still can't touch-type). I give thanks to the competence and kindness of project editor Leonie Freeman, to publicity manager Abba Renshaw and to the whole team.

A special thanks goes out to our remote editor from the beautiful south, Claire Davis, for her insight, discretion and eternal good humour. The art of slashing and burning, while leaving an author's dignity and integrity intact, is nothing shy of remarkable. Thanks to Megan van Staden, for bringing this non-fiction book to life through inspired design. My gratitude is also with those invisible yet instrumental forces that are our proofreaders Mike Wagg and Matt Turner and to Carol Dawber for the indexing to ensure our sleep-deficient readers can easily find their way.

This book would not be of the calibre that it is without the incredible encouragement and expert advice I have received from the sleep community through its inception and development. My deep appreciation and respect go firstly to two outstanding professionals in the field. I thank Dr Tony Fernando, who so generously shared his learned wisdom, practical insights, and valuable networks with grace and equanimity throughout this entire journey – from our first meeting as a patient, to his encouragement to aim higher in my requests for *Sleep Easy*'s endorsements. For Dr Moira Junge, there are barely words to capture the gratitude I have for her chapter-by-chapter involvement in this book's creation. Taking on the project, when we had only met via Zoom amidst the first Covid lockdown, was an extraordinary act of faith that I remain humbled by. Her wealth of knowledge on sleep and extensive experience treating people suffering insomnia lifted the bar on the content and brought important subtleties and nuances to the language we used.

Other highly regarded practitioners I would like to thank for their involvement and support are: Dr Giselle Withers for the valued expertise she brought to the chapters and resources on mindfulness; Dr Anna Friis for her insight into the role of self-compassion in the sleep improvement journey and for so vividly bringing to life yang compassion; Dr Bronwyn Sweeney for her overview of the New Zealand sleep improvement landscape and review of specific sleep challenges; Daniel Ford for the unique experience he brings with his credentials in performance psychology and sleep; Dr Bruce Arroll for his research and insight on the interface between sleep improvement and general practice. My thanks also go to Dr

Alex Bartle and Dr Karen Falloon for the insightful interviews and conversations we shared on the state of sleep issues and solutions currently available to the public.

Writing my first book, through these unprecedented times, has been both inspiring and challenging. I am blessed to be surrounded by colleagues, and friends who have championed the cause and fortified my resolve. Thanks for the verve and camaraderie of my petri-dish friends, Kim Tay, Sally Wyatt, Shannon Brown and Carol Ferguson, who nurture new ideas and endeavours. Special thanks to Kim for her energy and optimism, and teaching me that resilience is as much about bouncing forward as it is about bouncing back. Thanks to Selina Joe, Kathryn Thomas, Bridget Lowry, Elizabeth Brown, Bridget O'Toole, Jane Healy, Julie Clark, Lauren Gunn, Jac Wilson, and Cheri Inoue, who have all inspired and encouraged me in unique ways at pivotal moments on this journey.

For my family, I thank each of them for being who they are to me. My southern family, Mum, Dad, and my glorious and inspirational sisters Bronwyn and Megan, I thank them for believing in me and trusting this shift in my purpose. To my extended whānau in the north, south and the UK in all their iterations, including in-laws and out-laws; I appreciate their interest and encouragement in this endeavour.

I have tremendous gratitude for my husband, John, for leaning in on the home front and surrendering his share of the office for most of the year, creating space both literally and figuratively for me to pursue something beyond my day job, a goal that truly matters. Our daughter, Lily, has been the eternal believer in me and my book. Her thoughtful and well-timed words of kindness have spoken volumes along the way. I thank them both for their patience and understanding as I dedicated so much of myself to the research and writing of this book. I trust that it aligns with the values we hold as a family:

*Be brave and true, and just do
what needs to be done.*

It has been a privilege to have this time to write and do something of value for others. I thank you, the reader, for recognising the value of your sleep and giving this book your time and your attention. I hope with all my heart that you are sleeping easier these days and that you feel inspired, like I did, to encourage others to do what they can to discover how to sleep easy.

—Bernice Tuffery, 2021

Appendices

APPENDIX I

Specific sleep challenges

Different life stages and lifestyles can interfere with sleep. The following specific sleep challenges could be exacerbating your sleep difficulties—it's worth understanding why and what you can do to help.

- Sleeping with a bed-partner
- Snoring
- Sleep during pregnancy
- Sleep and menopause
- Sleep and shift work
- Sleep and ageing

Sleeping with a bed-partner

Sharing a bed with your partner has pros and cons for sleep. The presence of another person can be warm, comforting and reassuring, which supports the body's relaxation response and makes it easier for sleep to occur. But this all changes if there's tension in the relationship, it's a hot night, someone's a blanket hog, sleep schedules clash, or if one or both bedfellows experience sleep difficulties. Whether there's insomnia, snoring, restless legs or general fidgeting, fussing, mumbling or coughing, the behaviour of one partner can affect the sleep of the other.

Just as importantly, a sound sleeper can make matters worse for a person with insomnia. When you're awake in the night for extended periods, hearing your partner sleeping peacefully beside you can exacerbate feelings of frustration and loneliness. And elevated anxiety makes it more difficult to sleep.

When you're experiencing sleep problems, your wakefulness and restlessness can be annoying for your partner, but their insight into your sleep can help you figure out the problem. Ask if they've noticed things like long pauses in your breathing, gasps for breath or heavy snoring. If they have, get the possibility of sleep apnoea checked out as soon as possible. Partners can also make observations about other sleep-disorder symptoms, like tooth-grinding, restless legs, sleep-talking and walking.

If you have chronic insomnia and decide to use a CBTi programme, keep your partner in the loop. They will probably support you taking action to improve your sleep, but let them know it's a journey—things may get worse before they get better. They may find some CBTi techniques more disruptive than your usual night-time antics. Reassure them that it's temporary and ultimately for the greater good—of your well-being and the relationship.

If the sleep-improvement programme might create stress in your relationship, consider sleeping in separate rooms over the coming weeks while you get your sleep back on track. Sleeping apart doesn't mean your relationship is falling apart. It can be a conscious act of sleep-care for both of you.

Snoring

Snoring is really common—according to the Sleep Health Foundation, 30–40 per cent of adults snore from time to time.'The adults most likely to snore are middle-aged. Men are somewhat more likely to snore than women, but, even so, about one in three women snore some nights. Women have a higher chance of snoring when they're pregnant and during menopause. Habitual snoring—snoring most nights—affects about 15 per cent of people. It's a problem shared by many.

If you're not sure if you snore, there are snoring apps available (such as SnoreLab) that will give you an indication of what's going on. You can record yourself sleeping for a few nights to provide an indication of your snoring behaviour, capturing overnight data on when, for how long, and how loudly you snored. (SnoreLab even highlights if any snoring in the vicinity reaches 'epic' levels!)

Snoring can be a symptom of obstructive sleep apnoea. This condition can be serious and needs attention. About 10 per cent of regular snorers have sleep apnoea, so it's worth checking with your doctor to get a clinical diagnosis or to rule it out. Once you're confident that you're dealing with garden-variety snoring, there are things you can do to help yourself.

Snoring occurs when there's a narrowing in your upper airway at the back of your throat. This happens when muscles in this area including your tongue relax, restricting the pathway for breathing. With less room for air to get through, the air vibrates the soft tissues as you breathe, creating the snoring sound—the narrower the airway, the more 'epic' the snore.

Many things can contribute to your chances of snoring. Physical factors include the bone structure of your face, the soft tissue in the throat (including tonsils and adenoids), and carrying extra weight (although thin people do snore, too). How deep you sleep or how relaxed your muscles in this area are when you sleep can affect snoring. Alcohol and some medications can lead to more or louder snoring. Body position comes into it—sleeping on your back restricts the air passage more than sleeping on your side. Having a blocked nose, allergies or hay fever can exacerbate snoring. And smoking can make things worse, too.

There are myriad gadgets for sale promising salvation from snoring. (Lots of them are probably purchased by the partners of snorers, desperate for a reprieve!) Reviews of anti-snoring devices are pretty mixed in terms of their effectiveness and what they are like to use.

If snoring is bothering you or your partner, there are some

practical things you can try. Think through the possible contributing factors and deal with them. Dr David Cunnington at SleepHub has the following suggestions: lose a few kilos if you're carrying extra weight, or try changing your sleeping position to side-sleeping if your snoring is worse when you lie on your back.[2] If drinking is the culprit, consider making some changes to see how that affects your snoring—try reducing your intake and avoiding alcohol for four hours before sleeping. If a blocked nose is hampering your airflow, talk to your chemist or doctor for support for your cold, allergies or hay fever.

Sleep during pregnancy

Sleep is essential for the health of a mother and her baby's development. Throughout pregnancy, sleep is essential, yet it's a time when physical and hormonal changes make sleep more challenging.

Pregnant women often feel tired, and this is especially prevalent in the first and last trimesters. As pregnancy progresses, sleep is less deep and waking in the night occurs more frequently. Physical changes and discomfort contribute to these disruptions—peeing often, heartburn, back pain, whumping around to change position, as well as foetal movements in the second and third trimesters. Hormonal changes, including those that set off nausea and vomiting, also add sleep challenges.

It's common for women to snore during pregnancy. It's okay if it's occasional, but if your snoring is loud or disrupting sleep, it's worth checking with your doctor or midwife. Snoring can be indicative of night-time breathing problems or an increase in blood pressure. Some pregnant women (or their partners) may notice pauses in their breathing during sleep—the occasional brief pause is okay, but, if the pauses are frequent or extended or end with a gasp, snore or snort, it's time to get it checked out. These patterns can cause excessive sleepiness during the day and can be a clue that there's a serious breathing disorder such as obstructive sleep apnoea. Prioritise getting on to it and getting a diagnosis and treatment plan if required.

Another possible sleep change during pregnancy is an increase in leg movements during the night. It may be the odd twitch, kick or jerk, or quite dramatic limb movements that go on throughout the night. If periodic limb movements or restless legs interfere with sleep during your pregnancy, talk with your doctor, or get more of an insight on these symptoms from the Sleep Health Foundation or SleepHub websites.

Getting sufficient sleep throughout your pregnancy is critical for the healthy development of your baby and for your own physical and mental well-being. Expectant mothers who are struggling with untreated sleep disorders may have increased health risks, such as high blood pressure, diabetes, even pre-eclampsia. Lack of sleep during pregnancy can increase the chances of anxiety or depression, which can persist after the baby is born. From your sleep review, if you suspect your sleep struggles are more than chronic insomnia, be sure to seek professional help. Becoming a new parent is a precious but challenging time, and taking care of your sleep is a priority.

If you are pregnant and have chronic insomnia, a mindfulness-based approach to CBTi is a preferable option for sleep improvement in my view. While the sleep education in this book will be informative, the programme itself may be too demanding. Some CBTi techniques that reduce your sleep temporarily, including sleep consolidation and stimulus control, may be too tough while you're carrying a baby. Instead you may prefer to explore a psychologist-developed mindfulness and CBTi programme for sleep. A Mindful Way's online programme is currently being tailored for pregnant women, with a clinical trial planned. Their website will have updates on when this version is available.

While it's generally advised to avoid napping when you are trying to improve your sleep, if you are pregnant or a new parent, naps become your new best friend—allow yourself to have short naps during the day to help with your tiredness. You may find you can't actually fall asleep during the day, but it is still worth taking opportunities to rest.

If you're looking for more information on how you can support your sleep during pregnancy and as a new parent, the Sleep Health

Foundation offers some practical tips in the fact sheets on their website. Dr David Cunnington also covers this topic on his site, SleepHub. You could also check out *Sleeping Better in Pregnancy* by Clare Ladyman with Leigh Signal, from the Sleep/Wake Research Centre at Massey University.[3] This book provides an understanding of sleep during pregnancy based on the latest research and offers a trimester-by-trimester guide to getting better sleep.

Pregnancy was what triggered my sleep difficulties, and becoming a new mum perpetuated the cycle of insomnia. I wish I had known more about sleep at the time and had sought help earlier. It's brilliant that you are already taking your sleep seriously and are actively looking for ways to improve it. You don't want your sleep difficulties to unravel the way mine did—your little one needs you. Continue reading and learning, do what you can to improve your sleep with the information offered here, but make sure you get professional help if you get any whiff that you need it.

Sleep and menopause

When I started drafting this book, I was in the early stages of menopause and symptoms weren't a biggie for me. I have been pretty lucky so far, which I thank in part to the lifestyle clean-up I undertook over the last five years (one of the upsides of my experience with cancer). Even so, over the last year, overheating in the night has been waking me up, and it has threatened to unravel my ability to sleep well. Menopause definitely adds a layer of complexity to the process of sleep improvement, but progress can absolutely be made. Sleep changes occur throughout life, and we need to continually adjust our expectations of what a good night's sleep looks and feels like.

Body temperature plays a big part in the sleep problems experienced throughout menopause. It influences our ability to fall asleep and stay asleep, so when you're experiencing menopausal thermostat issues, and your temperature cranks up, it's little wonder that your sleep goes to hell.

Yet menopause is a natural biological process. (I've seen it referred to as a 'medical condition' and a 'disorder' while researching, which I try to remain calm about instead of becoming a ranting wild woman!) Throughout these transitional years, the body goes through a multitude of hormonal changes, and the related night sweats, hot flashes and mood changes can generate or exacerbate sleep problems. About 38 per cent of women in perimenopause experience sleep disturbance, so it's pretty damn common.[4] The types of sleep issues experienced throughout menopause can be complicated and can include hot flashes, night sweats, insomnia, restless-leg syndrome, snoring and obstructive sleep apnoea. On top of that, mood changes and depression can make sleep more difficult.

If your sleep disruptions are dire, it can be complicated for even a sleep specialist to diagnose what's going on, so it's imperative you get medical advice. For severe menopausal symptoms, hormone-replacement therapy (HRT) can be an option. But weigh up the pros and cons in consultation with your GP. The research on HRT's effect on sleep disturbance shows mixed results, although, generally, it can provide help with hot flashes and night sweats.[5]

There are a lot of self-care options to support your sleep throughout menopause. The CBTi-based sleep-improvement programme in this book is entirely workable throughout perimenopause and menopause, and it can help minimise the effects of your symptoms on your sleep. However, because of what your body is going through, there are certain areas where you will need to pay special attention. No scrimping and cutting corners—you really must put your own needs first.

Bedroom environment
- Keep your bedroom temperature at around 18 degrees Celsius.
- Ventilate your room if possible—a latched open window or a fan.
- Use bed linen and sleepwear made from natural, breathable fabrics.
- Be prepared for overheating—have a change of bedding, fresh sleepwear, chilled water on standby.

Tropical moments

- When you wake in the night with overheating, don't fight it. It's a natural biological process, and it will pass.
- Accept these phases of wakefulness in the night. Your job is to look after yourself *while* they pass.
- There is no point 'trying' to sleep. Remain calm and relaxed as you nurture yourself because you are awake.
- If needed, change the bedding and sleepwear to freshen up.
- To bring your temperature down, have a cool shower, use an ice pack or drink chilled water.
- Leave the bedroom and relax in another room until your temperature cools down (ensure that your bed remains a cue for sleep, rather than wakefulness).
- Return to bed when your temperature feels okay, and you physically show signs of being sleepy—yawning, rubbing your eyes, heavy eyelids, etc.

When you wake in the night with menopause-related 'hot spells', it's worth keeping in mind that biphasic and polyphasic sleep provides a different yet acceptable sleep option. Based on how your sleep has been in the past, it's easy to think of menopausal nights as 'broken sleep'. If you use monophasic sleep (sleeping in one long stretch) as your reference point, it's easy to become distressed about your changed sleeping pattern. This anxiety and stress exacerbate sleep difficulties. Instead, you could consider that you're transitioning into a different style of sleeping now—biphasic (sleep is in two chunks with a relaxing wakeful time in between) or polyphasic (sleep is in multiple parts, interspersed by quiet periods of wakefulness). Sleeping in phases is popular in some cultures and stages of life. Where biphasic or polyphasic sleep works well, pauses of wakefulness can be used as peaceful, restorative periods of quiet time for the individual. If you've been struggling with interrupted sleep, consider accepting a new normal rather than trying to hold on to monophasic sleep.

Throughout the six-week programme, make sure you prioritise your sleep and practise plenty of self-compassion. Think about the support and kindness you would offer a dear friend going through menopause and suffering these sleep problems. Make sure you nurture yourself with the equivalent.

Starting this evening, allow yourself a decent amount of wind-down time before bed. As busy women in midlife, we're often responsible for teenagers and ageing parents, as well as all the other relentless 'adulting' tasks. Amid all this, it's easy to let your own needs slide down the list. If you want to improve your sleep, aim to prioritise yourself. Start allowing yourself a minimum of an hour of non-negotiable quiet time before you turn in each night.

While sleep can frequently turn to custard leading up to and throughout menopause, it's important to keep it in perspective. A six-year study exploring the sleep of women transitioning from premenopause through menopause showed that the women had shorter sleep times, more awakenings and more time awake overnight compared to their premenopause sleep.[6] This sounds worse than it is. Yes, they did sleep less, but, on average, it was only 23 minutes less per night, and their awake time during the night was only 27 minutes. What's more, there were indications that the women had an increased amount of deep sleep, which may be the body compensating for the new sleep–wake patterns. So, yes, your sleep isn't going to be the same as it used to be, but if you take care of what you can and seek help if you need to, sleep throughout the transition is doable.

Rather than resisting the changes to your sleep, understand and accept these inevitable changes with grace. (In the same way we make peace with our ever-deepening character lines!) Obviously, depending on which way your mood is swinging, you'll have times when you're more gracious about these changes than others.

If you want more information on sleep throughout menopause, there are helpful resources available on the Sleep Health Foundation and SleepHub websites.

Sleep and shift work

Shift work has the potential to create so many challenges to a person's sleep.[7] In fact, sleep disorders as a result of shift work get their own classification in the ICSD-3: shift work disorder (SWD). SWD is also recognised by the *Diagnostic and Statistical Manual of Mental Health Disorders* (DSM-5). It's not to be taken lightly.

SWD is a type of circadian-rhythm disorder, where insomnia or excessive daytime sleepiness occurs as a result of a person's shift work schedule not lining up with the standard night-time sleep. The work roster conflicts with a person's natural biological clock and the 24-hour light–dark cycle. Short and disturbed sleep can result in a lack of energy, difficulty concentrating, headaches and irritability during wake-time. It can also impact a person's wake-time functioning, affecting work performance and safety, and can be detrimental to their home life. When these disrupted sleep patterns and daytime symptoms are experienced for more than a month, the problem is recognised as shift work disorder (assuming other causes are ruled out).

SWD is hard to live with and, longer term, there are elevated health risks to consider—anxiety, depression, obesity, diabetes, high blood pressure and cancer.

Long shifts (e.g., twelve to fourteen hours) and rotating rosters are the most challenging for a body to deal with and adjust to, meaning they pose a higher risk to sleep than others. Some people are more susceptible to the impact of shift work than others. Tolerance to shift work tends to be lower among older people and those with physical or mental-health conditions.

SWD is relatively common, and it's estimated to affect about one in ten shift workers. If you suspect that you have reached the threshold of a shift work or two disorder, contact your GP or a sleep specialist with the information that you've gathered in your sleep review. (It's also worth completing a week or two of your sleep diary to take to the appointment.)

If you're a shift worker and want to look after your sleep, the following websites provide practical information and resources: Sleep Health Foundation, SleepHub and Sleepio.

Sleep and ageing

It's a commonly held belief that sleep becomes terrible with age. I hear things, like, 'You hardly sleep at all,' 'You need much less sleep,' 'You only sleep lightly,' 'You wake up often in the night,' 'You need long naps during the day' or 'You definitely need sleeping pills.' Sleep patterns and needs indeed change with age, but it helps to have an understanding of what normal sleep looks like in *healthy* older people. Understand what's within the realm of okay and have realistic sleep-improvement aspirations for your age.

The clinical reference book *Sleep Medicine* provides a helpful overview of normal age-related sleep changes in healthy individuals.[8] Obviously physical and mental-health conditions, chronic pain and medication all have the potential to alter and impact sleep. Many older adults deal with health issues alongside sleep challenges. If other variables are in the mix, especially if they are complex, it's best to discuss how they may be affecting your sleep with your GP or specialist. They may be able to provide direction for sleep improvement in your particular scenario.

For those who aren't dealing with other health conditions, the following sleep changes tend to occur naturally as we age.

Sleep duration

While there is a reduction in total time asleep at night as a person ages, the decrease is small and gradual across a lifespan. Healthy adults lose about ten minutes for each passing decade up to midlife, then just shy of half an hour each decade from mid-forties to eighties. So, for me, I was a pretty consistent eight-and-a-bit-hour sleeper in my twenties (not that I counted or cared as sleeping was such a non-issue), but, now that I'm in my early fifties, 7.5 hours a night feels fine.

Waking after falling asleep

There may be a bit more waking in the night or early in the morning as you get older, but it's nothing radical. These awakenings tend to reduce overall sleep duration. So, while you might go to sleep and wake at similar times, you may be awake a bit more in the night as you get older. These night-time awakenings are all part of a natural sleep cycle. Young adults experience brief awakenings throughout the night as they transition from one stage of sleep to another, but they barely notice them. As an older adult, you may wake a bit more often or stay awake a bit longer throughout the night. It's not a lot of time in total, but it will feel different because you're more aware of when you surface throughout the night.

Less deep sleep

The amount of deep or slow-wave sleep that occurs overnight gradually reduces with age. It comes down by about 3 per cent per decade as you age from twenty to 60 years, then it continues to decline. Slow-wave sleep tends to be replaced by lighter stages of sleep. Deep sleep plays a role in keeping you asleep, hence the gradual increase in overnight awakenings as you age.

Falling asleep

The time it takes to fall asleep gets a little longer throughout life. But the changes are tiny—only a ten-minute increase is expected from twenty years to 80 years!

Reduced sleep efficiency

Sleep efficiency refers to the percentage of time in bed that you're asleep. With increased awakenings and decreased sleep duration, sleep-efficiency scores do come down over a person's lifetime. Again, in healthy adults, these decreases are very gradual—about 3 per cent per decade.

Body-clock changes

From around middle age, the body's circadian rhythm starts to change—body-clock time shifts to an earlier clock time. As with other changes, Mother Nature is kind and the changes happen gradually. As you get older, your body will start signalling for you to go to sleep a bit earlier and you're likely to feel like getting up earlier than when you were a young adult.

Napping

With decreased sleep duration and somewhat more fragmented sleep, it seems logical to think that there'd be more daytime sleepiness and more intentional or unintentional daytime napping among older people. There definitely is a lot of napping action among older adults. But, among healthy older adults, napping is not inevitable—it can be a lifestyle choice.

Knowing how sleep naturally changes with age can help align your thoughts and behaviours more closely with your biological sleeping needs. Relying on common but somewhat misguided beliefs about sleep in older people can make you think and behave in ways that perpetuate or aggravate insomnia. For instance, staying in bed longer than your body needs you to, napping more frequently or for longer than is required, or taking sleeping pills long term to try to achieve the sleep of youth rather than what your body needs now.

If you're a healthy older adult, it's worth using this information to align your sleep aspirations with human biology. You may discover that you are sleeping just fine for someone your age. Or you may find that, even based on these age-adjusted norms, you have sleep difficulties. In which case, it's worth considering whether there is a sleep disorder.

There are many medical conditions common in older people that interfere with sleep. These include arthritis, osteoporosis, Parkinson's disease, heart disease, lung disease (like asthma or chronic obstructive pulmonary disease), indigestion and incontinence. The pharmaceuticals used to help manage or treat these medical issues can further interfere with sleep. Pain makes sleep worse, and insufficient sleep can make the experience of pain worse. Anxiety, depression, dementia and Alzheimer's may all make sleep worse. Indeed, there are many age-related physical and mental-health conditions associated with old age that can have an impact on sleep.

Some sleep disorders are more prevalent among older people, too. According to the Sleep Health Foundation, at least one in four older adults has obstructive sleep apnoea or periodic limb-movement disorder (such as restless-leg syndrome). Around 40 per cent of older people have insomnia, with about 10 per cent of older people having chronic insomnia (where it persists for more than three months).

The CBTi-based programme in this book can be helpful for older adults with chronic insomnia who are otherwise healthy. But, if other medical conditions—mental or physical—and medications are involved, it's recommended that you discuss your sleep challenges with your healthcare professional to determine the most effective and safest approach to improving your sleep.

Sleep Health Foundation and SleepHub provide some helpful information about sleep and ageing on their websites.

Sleep resources

Online sleep resources

Sleep Health Foundation
www.sleephealthfoundation.org.au
Useful resource for general information on sleep and sleep disorders.

SleepHub
www.sleephub.com.au
Useful resource for general information on sleep and sleep disorders.

Sleepio
www.sleepio.com
Useful resource for sleep information and an online CBTi-based sleep-improvement course.

This Way Up
www.thiswayup.org.au
Offers an online CBTi-based sleep-improvement course.

A Mindful Way
www.amindfulway.com.au
An online MBTI-based sleep-improvement course.

Specialist sleep clinics and professionals

This is not a full directory but it provides a place to start. Some clinics accept patients by referral only (from a GP or healthcare professional), but other clinics and psychologists with sleep expertise welcome self-referrals.

New Zealand

Sleep clinics
New Zealand Respiratory & Sleep Institute (Auckland)
www.nzrsi.co.nz
Appointment by referral only.

Practice 92 (Auckland)
www.practice92.co.nz
Appointment by referral only.

Sleep Well Clinic (nationwide)
www.sleepwellclinic.co.nz

Health professionals with a special interest in insomnia
Dr Tony Fernando (Auckland)
Psychiatrist, Sleep and Insomnia Specialist
Practice 92
www.practice92.co.nz

Dr Kimberly Falconer (Auckland)
Psychologist
New Zealand Respiratory & Sleep Institute
www.nzrsi.co.nz

Dr Bruce Arroll (Manurewa)
General practitioner
Greenstone Family Clinic
www.greenstoneclinic.co.nz

Daniel Ford (Auckland)
Psychologist
The Better Sleep Clinic
www.thebettersleepclinic.com

Dr Bronwyn Sweeney (Wellington)
Psychologist
Tend Psychology
www.tendpsychology.com

Australia

Australasian Sleep Association (ASA)
www.sleep.org.au
The ASA provides a directory of sleep services and professionals:
www.sleep.org.au/Public/Public/Resource-Centre/Sleep-services

Clinics

Victoria
Melbourne Sleep Disorders Centre
www.msdc.com.au

Yarraville Health Group
www.yarravillehealth.com.au

Alfred Hospital
www.alfredhealth.org.au

Respiratory Sleep Disorder Centre
www.rsdc.com.au

New South Wales
Illawarra Sleep Psychology
www.illawarrasleeppsychology.com.au

Sydney Sleep Centre
www.sleepcentres.com.au

Woolcock Institute of Medical Research
www.woolcock.org.au

Sydney Adventist Hospital
www.sah.org.au

University of Sydney, Charles Perkins Centre
www.sydney.edu.au/charles-perkins-centre

South Australia
Adelaide Insomnia Clinic
www.insomniaclinic.com.au

Adelaide Institute for Sleep Health
Flinders University
www.flinders.edu.au/adelaide-institute-sleep-health

Western Australia
Sleep Matters Perth
www.sleepmattersperth.com.au

Queensland
Sleep Disorders Centre
Princess Alexandra Hospital
www. metrosouth.health.qld.gov.au/sleep-disorders-centre

Books

Mindfulness for Insomnia: A four-week guided program to relax your body, calm your mind, and get the sleep you need, Catherine Polan Orzech and William H. Moorcroft

Quiet Your Mind and Get to Sleep: Solutions to insomnia for those with depression, anxiety, or chronic pain, Colleen E. Carney and Rachel Manber

Sleeping Better in Pregnancy: A guide to sleep health for New Zealand women, Clare Ladyman with Leigh Signal

The Sleep Revolution: Transforming your life, one night at a time, Arianna Huffington

Why We Sleep: Unlocking the power of sleep and dreams, Matthew Walker

APPENDIX III

Other resources

New Zealand

Anxiety and depression support
Anxiety NZ Trust
www.anxiety.org.nz
24-hour helpline: 0800 269 4389

www.depression.org.nz
24-hour helpline: 0800 111 757 or text 4202

Lifeline
www.lifeline.org.nz
24-hour helpline: 0800 543 354 or text 4357

The Lowdown
www.thelowdown.co.nz (for young people)
24-hour helpline: 0800 111 757 or text 5626

Mental health or addictions support
Need to Talk?
www.1737.org.nz
24-hour helpline: 1737 (text or call)

Alcohol and drug support

Alcohol Drug Helpline
www.alcoholdrughelp.org.nz
0800 787 797

Community Alcohol and Drug Services (CADS)
www.cads.org.nz
0800 787 797 or 09 845 1818

Nicotine support

Quitline
www.quit.org.nz
0800 778 778 or text 4006

Australia

Anxiety and depression support

Black Dog Institute
www.blackdoginstitute.org.au

This Way Up
www.thiswayup.org.au

Beyond Blue
www.beyondblue.org.au
24-hour helpline: 1300 22 46 36

Lifeline
www.lifeline.org.au
24-hour helpline: 13 11 14

Alcohol and drug support

Alcohol & Drug Information Service (ADIS)
1 800 250 015 (National alcohol and other drug hotline. You will be automatically directed to the ADIS in the state or territory you are calling from.)

Your Room
www.yourroom.health.nsw.gov.au

Nicotine support
Quitline
www.quitlinesa.org.au
13 78 48

Your Room
www.yourroom.health.nsw.gov.au

Mindfulness and self-compassion resources

Mindfulness training (MBSR: mindfulness-based stress reduction)
Mindfulness Training Institute
www.mtia.org.au
Find a qualified teacher in Australia or NZ.

Mindfulness Auckland
www.mindfulnessauckland.co.nz

Mindfulness Aotearoa
www.mindfulnessaotearoa.com

Openground Mindfulness Training
www.openground.com.au

Self-compassion
Center for Mindful Self-Compassion
www.centerformsc.org

Dr Kristin Neff
www.self-compassion.org

Tara Brach
www.tarabrach.com

Meditation apps
Headspace
www.headspace.com

Calm
www.calm.com

The Mindfulness App

www.themindfulnessapp.com

Smiling Mind

www.smilingmind.com.au

Online yoga

Yoga with Adriene

www.youtube.com/user/yogawithadriene

APPENDIX IV

Additional sleep diaries

SLEEP DIARY

Fill out your sleep diary every morning. Guess the approximate times, there's no need for clock-watching. On the next page, note any factors that helped with sleep or may have been unhelpful for your sleep. You're looking for clues and patterns . . .

Week _____	Night 1	Night 2	Night 3	Night 4	Night 5	Night 6	Night 7
Start Date _____ Day of Week							
What time did you go to bed?							
What time did you first try to go to sleep?							
What time did you fall asleep?							
How many times did you wake in the night?							
How long did these awakenings last in total?							
What time did you wake for the final time this morning?							
What time did you get out of bed for the day?							
How would you rate the quality of your sleep? (1 Terrible, 2 Bad, 3 OK, 4 Good, 5 Great)							
Total Sleep Time In total, how many hours' sleep did you get?							
Total Time in Bed In total, how long were you in bed?							
Sleep Efficiency % (Total Sleep Time ÷ Total Time in Bed X 100 = %)	%	%	%	%	%	%	%

SLEEP DIARY

Week _____

Start Date _____ Day of Week _____

	Night 1	Night 2	Night 3	Night 4	Night 5	Night 6	Night 7
Any factors that may have been unhelpful for your sleep last night?							
Any factors that may have helped with sleep last night?							

Observations & Insights:

SLEEP DIARY

Fill out your sleep diary every morning. Guess the approximate times, there's no need for clock-watching. On the next page, note any factors that helped with sleep or may have been unhelpful for your sleep. You're looking for clues and patterns . . .

Week _____	Night 1	Night 2	Night 3	Night 4	Night 5	Night 6	Night 7
Start Date _____ Day of Week							
What time did you go to bed?							
What time did you first try to go to sleep?							
What time did you fall asleep?							
How many times did you wake in the night?							
How long did these awakenings last in total?							
What time did you wake for the final time this morning?							
What time did you get out of bed for the day?							
How would you rate the quality of your sleep? *(1 Terrible, 2 Bad, 3 OK, 4 Good, 5 Great)*							
Total Sleep Time In total, how many hours' sleep did you get?							
Total Time in Bed In total, how long were you in bed?							
Sleep Efficiency % (Total Sleep Time ÷ Total Time in Bed X 100 = %)	%	%	%	%	%	%	%

SLEEP DIARY

Week _____

Start Date _____ Day of Week

	Night 1	Night 2	Night 3	Night 4	Night 5	Night 6	Night 7
Any factors that may have been unhelpful for your sleep last night?							
Any factors that may have helped with sleep last night?							

Observations & Insights:

NOTES

Introduction

1   M. Ree, M. Junge & D. Cunnington, 'Australasian Sleep Association position statement regarding the use of psychological/behavioral treatments in the management of insomnia in adults,' *Sleep Medicine*, 2017, vol. 36, S43–S47.

2   Sleep Health Foundation, *Chronic Insomnia Disorder in Australia—A report to the Sleep Health Foundation*, 2019, July, sleephealthfoundation.org.au/pdfs/Special_Reports/SHF_Insomnia_Report_2019_Final_SHFlogo.pdf

3   D. Riemann, C. Baglioni, C., Bassetti, et al., 'European guideline for the diagnosis and treatment of insomnia', *Journal of Sleep Research*, 2017, vol. 26, no. 6, December, pp. 675–700.

4   M.J. Sateia, D.J. Buysse, A.D. Krystal, et al., 'Clinical practice guideline for the pharmacologic treatment of chronic insomnia in adults: an American Academy of Sleep Medicine clinical practice guideline', *Journal of Clinical Sleep Medicine*, 2017, vol. 13, no. 2, February, pp. 307–49.

5   C.A. Espie, '"Stepped Care": A health technology solution for delivering cognitive behavioral therapy as a first line insomnia treatment', *Sleep*, 2009, vol. 32, pp. 1549–58.

6   M. Walker, *Why We Sleep*, London: Penguin Random House, 2018, p. 23.

7   If you have health insurance, check in with your provider to see if you have cover for sleep disorders.

8   J.C. Ong, S.L. Shapiro & R. Manber, 'Mindfulness meditation and cognitive behavioral therapy for insomnia: a naturalistic 12-month follow-up', *Explore*, 2009, vol. 5, pp. 30–6.

9   A. Qaseem, D. Kansagara & M.A. Forciea, 'Management of insomnia disorder in adults: A clinical practice guideline from the American College of Physicians', *Annals of Internal Medicine*, 2016, July.

10 Qaseem, Kansagara & Forciea, p. 676.

11 World Sleep Society, *Prevalent, Significant, Costly: The chronic inability to sleep*, World Sleep Society, 8 March 2018.

12 World Sleep Society, *Prevalent, Significant, Costly*.

13   M. Zucconi, & R. Ferri, 'Assessment of sleep disorders and diagnostic procedures', in *ESRS Sleep Medicine Textbook*, 2014, p. 96. ICSD-3 is one of a number of respected classification systems to diagnose sleep disorders—others include the *Diagnostic and Statistical Manual of Mental Disorders* (DSM-5), often used by psychologists and psychiatrists, and the *International Classification of Diseases* (ICD-11) from the World Health Organization.

Part 1

Chapter 1: Review your sleep—screen for 'insomnia'

1   B. Arroll, A.T. Fernando, K. Falloon, et al., 'Development, validation (diagnostic accuracy) and audit of the Auckland Sleep Questionnaire: A new tool for diagnosing causes of sleep disorders in primary care', *Journal of Primary Health Care*, 2011, vol. 3, no. 2, June, pp. 107–13.

2   C.M. Morin & J. Carrier, 'The acute effects of the COVID-19 pandemic on insomnia and psychological symptoms', *Sleep Medicine*, 2020, June.

3   C. Samaranayake & A.T. Fernando, 'Insomnia classification, features, diagnosis, and evaluation', in D. Mansfield (ed.), *Sleep Medicine*, Melbourne: IP Communications, 2017, p. 304.

4   Sleep Health Foundation, *Herbal Remedies and Sleep*, retrieved from sleephealthfoundation.org.au/pdfs/HerbalRemedies-D713.pdf

5   Online programmes are evolving … Internationally, Sleepio, designed by the esteemed sleep expert, Professor Colin Espie, is currently being rolled out as a free service for most areas of the UK (via NHS), and is offered free by some US employers. The best antipodeans can get at this stage is to get access by registering your interest as a research participant. Somryst (formerly Shuti) is now FDA approved in the US and available on prescription by healthcare professionals. This Way Up is an Australian offer sponsored by St Vincent's Hospital, offering self-directed and clinician-supported online CBTi options. A Mindful Way, developed by clinical psychologist Dr Giselle Withers in Melbourne, combines mindfulness with CBTi.

6   www.mentalhealth.org.nz/assets/Uploads/MHF-Quick-facts-and-stats-FINAL-2016.pdf

7   www.beyondblue.org.au/media/statistics

8   As defined by Te Hiringa Hauora/Health Promotion Agency New Zealand and based on Australian and Canadian guidelines for low-risk drinking.

9   Sleep Health Foundation, *Sleep tracker technology*, 2015, February, retrieved from sleephealthfoundation.org.au/pdfs/SleepTracker-0215.pdf

Chapter 2: Other sleep disorders to consider

1   M. Zucconi & R. Ferri, 'Assessment of sleep disorders and diagnostic procedures',
    in European Sleep Research Society, *European Sleep Medicine Textbook*,
    Regensburg: ESRS, 2014, pp. 95–109.

2   D. Cunnington, What is sleep apnea?, SleepHub, 2017, July, retrieved from www.
    sleephub.com/what-is-sleep-apnea

3   P.H. Gander, G. Scott, K. Mihaere, et al., 'Societal costs of obstructive sleep apnea
    syndrome', *New Zealand Medical Journal*, 2010, vol 123, no. 1321, August.

4   M. Zucconi & R. Ferri, 'Assessment of sleep disorders and diagnostic procedures', in
    European Sleep Research Society, *European Sleep Medicine Textbook*, p. 100.

Chapter 3: Create a sleep-diary habit

1   C.B. Samaranayake & A.T. Fernando, 'Insomnia classification, features, diagnosis,
    and evaluation', in Mansfield, p. 301.

2   B. Gardner, P. Lally, & J. Wardle, 'Making health habitual: The psychology of "habit-
    formation" and general practice', *British Journal of General Practice*, 2012, vol. 62,
    no. 605, December, pp. 664–6.

3   B. J. Fogg, *Tiny Habits: The small habits that change everything*, New York:
    Houghton Mifflin Harcourt, 2019.

4   J. Clear, *Atomic Habits: tiny changes, remarkable results*, New York: Avery, 2018.

5   G. Rubin, *Better Than Before*, London: Two Roads, 2015.

6   P. Lally, C.H.M. van Jaarsveld, H.W.W. Potts, et al., 'How are habits formed: Modelling
    habit formation in the real world', *European Journal of Social Psychology*, 2010, vol.
    40, no. 6, October, pp. 998–1009.

7   M. Bateson, D. Nettle & G. Roberts, 'Cues of being watched enhance cooperation in
    a real-world setting', *Biology Letters*, 2006, vol. 7, no. 3, September .

8   P. Lally & B. Gardner, 'Promoting habit formation', *Health Psychology Review*, 2013,
    vol. 7, pp. 137–58 .

9   J. Clear, 'Plan for failure: Being consistent is not the same as being perfect', www.
    jamesclear.com/plan-failure

10 B.J. Fogg, 'Rewire Your Brain', www.tinyhabits.com/rewire

Chapter 4: Learn the fundamentals of sleeping

1   Jade Wu, 'Sleep hygiene doesn't cure insomnia', scientificamerican.com/article/
    sleep-hygiene-doesnt-cure-insomnia-do-this-instead

2   World Sleep Society, *10 Commandments of Sleep Hygiene for Adults*, retrieved
    from worldsleepday.org/10-commandments-of-sleep-hygiene-for-adults

3   *The Global Pursuit of Better Sleep Health*, Philips Global Sleep Survey, 2019, March.

4   Sleep Health Foundation, *Caffeine, Food, Alcohol, Smoking and Sleep*, 2013, May.

5   My wonderful publisher, Allen & Unwin, obviously with vested interests, wondered if
    reading books was a permissible activity in the bedroom. While it's not on the World
    Sleep Society's list of ten commandments, Dr Gregg Jacobs' *Clinical Training Manual*

for CBTi says that reading can be used as a relaxation activity in bed. That's provided you don't overdo it—limit reading in bed to 20–30 minutes in the evening to wind down. Of course, this means an actual, real-life book, not something on a screen. Oh, and it needs to be relaxing, pleasurable reading—not work or anything overstimulating!

6   This is the World Sleep Society's recommendation for children up to twelve years, but for adults with chronic insomnia it's seriously worth doing this while you are restoring your sleep.

Chapter 5: You are not alone

1   Walker, p. 240.

2   Y. Furman, S.M. Wolf & D.S. Rosenfeld, 'Shakespeare and sleep disorders', *Neurology*, 1997, vol. 49, no. 4, October.

3   New Zealand Ministry of Health, *Health and Independence Report 2017*. The Director-General of Health's Annual Report on the State of Public Health, Wellington, 2018, pp. 36–7.

4   Sovereign, *A Third of Kiwis are Sleep Deprived*, www.sovereign.co.nz/about-us/media

5   Southern Cross Healthcare Group, *Shocking Sleep Stats*, 2015, https://www.southerncross.co.nz/group/media-releases

6   C.H. Lee & C.G. Sibley, 'Sleep duration and psychological well-being among New Zealanders', *Sleep Health*, 2019, vol. 5, no. 6, December, pp. 606–14.

7   Sleep Health Foundation, *Chronic Insomnia Disorder in Australia*.

8   National Sleep Foundation, *The National Sleep Foundation's 2020 Sleep in America® Poll Shows Alarming Sleepiness and Low Levels of Action*, 7 March 2020, press release.

9   C.M. Morin, M. LeBlanc, L. Belanger, et al., 'Prevalence of insomnia and its treatment in Canada', *Canadian Journal of Psychiatry*, 2011, vol. 56, no. 9, September, pp. 540–8.

10   K. Morgan, A. Luik, & R. Sharman, 'Clinical review: Insomnia', *GP Online*, 2017, July.

11   *The Global Pursuit of Better Sleep Health*, Philips Global Sleep Survey, 2019.

12   World Sleep Society, *World Sleep Day 2020*, Talking Points.

13   M. Maria Calem, J. Bisla & A. Begum, 'Increased prevalence of insomnia and hypnotics use in England over 15 years', *Sleep*, 2012, vol. 35, no. 3, March, pp. 377–84.

14   S. Pallesen, B. Sivertsen, I.H. Nordhus, et al., 'A 10-year trend of insomnia prevalence in the adult Norwegian population', *Sleep Medicine*, 2014, vol. 15, no. 2, pp. 173–9.

15   Morin & Carrier, 'The acute effects of the COVID-19 pandemic'.

16   *The Global Pursuit of Better Sleep Health*.

17   Sleep Health Foundation, *Chronic Insomnia Disorder in Australia*.

18   B. Arroll, & A.T. Fernando, 'Prevalence of causes of insomnia in primary care: A cross-sectional study', *British Journal of General Practice*, 2012, vol. 62, no. 595, February, pp. 99–103.

19   H. Meaklim, L. Jackson, D. Bartlett, et al., 'Sleep education for healthcare providers: Addressing deficient sleep in Australia and New Zealand', *Sleep Health*, 2020, May.

20   Y. Chong, C.D. Fryar & Q. Gu, 'Prescription sleep aid use among adults: United States, 2005–2010', *National Centre for Health Statistics*, 2013, vol. 127, August

21   Sleep Health Foundation, *Chronic Insomnia Disorder in Australia,* p. 20.

22 National Sleep Foundation, *Sleep in America® Poll 2020, Americans Feel Sleepy 3 Days a Week, With Impacts on Activities, Mood & Acuity*.

23 Walker, p. 137.

24 Walker, p. 145.

25 C. Morin & C. Espie, *Insomnia: A clinical guide to assessment and treatment*, New York: Springer Science+Business Media, 2004, pp. 95–6.

Chapter 6: Understanding sleep and insomnia

1 Walker, p. 53.

2 M.L. Perlis, C. Junquist, M.T. Smith, et al., *Cognitive Behavioral Treatment of Insomnia*, New York: Springer, 2008, p. 39.

3 Sleep Foundation, Stress and Insomnia, 2020, September.

4 Samaranayake & Fernando, 'Insomnia classification features, diagnosis, and evaluation', p. 300.

5 R.E. Schmidt, D.S. Courvoisier, S. Cullati, et al., 'Too imperfect to fall asleep: Perfectionism, pre-sleep counterfactual processing, and insomnia', *Frontiers in Psychology*, 2018, vol. 9, p. 1288.

6 Meaklim et al.

7 Morin & Espie, p. 98.

Chapter 7: Finding your true north—prioritising sleep improvement

1 The CBTi success rate is around 70 per cent, so you want to do what you can to support your probability of being among the majority for whom it works.

2 Walker, pp. 107–89.

3 E. Van Cauter, K. Spiegel, E. Tasali, et al., 'Metabolic consequences of sleep and sleep loss', *Sleep Medicine*, 2008, vol. 9, no. 01, September, pp. S23–S28.

4 F.A.J.L. Scheer, 'Hungry for sleep: A role for endocannabinoids?', *Sleep*, 2016, vol. 39, no. 3, March, pp. 495–6.

5 C.E. Kline, 'The bidirectional relationship between exercise and sleep: Implications for exercise adherence and sleep improvement', *American Journal of Lifestyle Medicine*, 2014, vol 8, no. 6, November–December, pp. 375–9.

6 Walker, p. 134.

7 New Zealand Ministry of Health, *Major Causes of Death 2010–2012*.

8 New Zealand Ministry of Transport, *Fatigue Report 2016*.

9 A.A. Prather, D. Janicki-Deverts, M.H. Hall, et al., 'Behaviorally assessed sleep and susceptibility to the common cold', *Sleep*, 2015, vol. 38, no. 9, September, pp. 1353–9.

10 R. Leproult & E. Van Cauter, 'Effect of 1 week of sleep restriction on testosterone levels in young healthy men', *JAMA*, 2015, May, vol. 305, no. 21, pp. 2173–4.

11 D. Cunnington, *Sleep and Depression. What's the link?*, SleepHub, 2015, March, sleephub.com.au/sleep-and-depression-whats-the-link

12 Diabetes NZ, *Type 2 Diabetes Outcomes Model 2018*, September, www.diabetes.org.nz/news-and-update/2018

13   Australian Institute of Health and Welfare, *Diabetes*, www.aihw.gov.au/reports/diabetes

14   M. Irwin, A. Masoovioh, J.C. Gillin, et al., 'Partial sleep deprivation reduces natural killer cell activity in humans', *Psychosomatic Medicine*, 1994, vol. 56, no. 6, November–December, pp. 493–8.

15   World Health Organization, *Dementia*, 2019, www.who.int/news-room/fact-sheets/detail/dementia

16   If wholehearted living strikes a chord, I recommend Brené Brown's books *Daring Greatly*; *The Gifts of Imperfection*; and *Braving the Wilderness*.

Chapter 8: Sleep medication—to take or not to take

1   Walker, p. 283.

2   D. Cunnington, *Medication for Insomnia*, SleepHub, 2019, February , sleephub.com.au/medication-for-insomnia/sleep-medication

3   D. Cunnington & M. Qian, 'Pharmacotherapy for insomnia', in Mansfield, pp. 311–17.

4   Walker, pp. 284–5.

5   Combining sleeping pills with alcohol can be dangerous, and is not advised.

6   C.M. Morin, A. Vallieres, B. Guay, et al., 'Cognitive-behavior therapy, singly and combined with medication, for persistent insomnia: Acute and maintenance therapeutic effects', 2011, *JAMA*, vol. 301, no. 19, May, pp. 2005–15.

7   D. Gardner & A. Murphy, *Stop Sleeping Pills Guide*, SleepWell, mysleepwell.ca/wp-content/uploads/2019/03/Stop-Sleeping-Pills-Guide-and-Planner.pdf

8   Harvard Health, 'The Savvy Sleeper—wean yourself off sleep aids', 2013, health.harvard.edu/staying-healthy/the-savvy-sleeper-wean-yourself-off-sleep-aids

9   D. Cunnington, *Is Melatonin Helpful for Sleep?*, SleepHub, 2015, July

10   E. Ferracioli-Oda, A. Qawasmi & M.H. Bloch, 'Meta-Analysis: Melatonin for the treatment of primary sleep disorders', *PLOS One*, 2013, vol. 8, no. 5, May

11   D. Cunnington & M. Qian, 'Pharmacotherapy for insomnia', p. 314.

12   D. Cunnington, *Is Melatonin Helpful for Sleep?* SleepHub, 27 July, 2015.

13   Australian Institute of Health and Welfare, *National Drug Strategy Household Survey 2019*, p. 33, aihw.gov.au/reports/illicit-use-of-drugs/national-drug-stradegy-household-survey-2019/content/table-of-contents

14   New Zealand Ministry of Health, *Cannabis Use 2012/13: New Zealand Health Survey* , health.govt.nz/publication/cannabis-use-2012-13-new-zealand-health-survey

15   D. Cunnington, *Cannabis and Sleep: What are the effects?*, SleepHub, 2017, March, sleephub.com.au/cannabis-and-sleep

16   K.A. Babson, J. Sottile & D. Morabito, 'Cannabis, cannabinoids, and sleep: A review of the literature', *Current Psychiatry Report*, 2017, vol. 19, no. 23, March, p. 2.

17   R.P. Ogeal & A.C. Young, 'Drugs of abuse and sleep', in Mansfield, p. 511.

18   Perlis et al., p. 39.

19   Babson et al., p. 2.

20   Babson et al., p. 3.

21   Sateia et al.

22   Sleep Health Foundation, *Herbal Remedies and Sleep*.

Chapter 10: Sleep—the inside job

1   J.C. Ong, S.L. Shapiro, R. Manber, et al., 'Mindfulness meditation and cognitive behaviour therapy for insomnia', *Explore*, 2009, vol. 5, no. 1, pp. 30–6.

2   J.C. Ong, *Mindfulness-Based Therapy for Insomnia*, Washington: APA, 2017.

3   C. Polan Orzech & W. Moorcroft, *Mindfulness for Insomnia*, Oakland: New Harbinger, 2019, p. 76.

4   A. MacBeth & A. Gumley, 'Exploring compassion: A meta-analysis of the association between self-compassion and psychopathology', *Clinical Psychology Review*, 2012, vol. 32, no. 6, August, pp. 545–52.

5   K. Neff, *Cultivating Kindness and Strength in the Face of Difficulty: Yin and yang of self-compassion*, Center for Mindful Self-Compassion, 2019, October.

Part 2

Week One: A consistent schedule and permission to wind down

1   G. Jacobs, *Say Goodnight to Insomnia*, Pennsylvania: Rodale, 2009, pp. 87–8.

Week Two: Sleep consolidation—less, but better

1   A.J. Spielman, P. Saskin & M.J. Thorpy, 'Treatment for chronic insomnia by restriction of time in bed', *Sleep*, 1987, vol. 10, no. 1, pp. 45–56.

2   Samaranayake & Fernando, p. 306.

Week Three: Your bed as a cue for sleep

1   P. Hauri & S. Linde, *No More Sleepless Nights*, US: John Wiley, 1996, p. 87.

2   C. Morin, R.R. Bootzin, D.J. Buysse, et al., 'Psychological and behavioral treatment of insomnia: update of the recent evidence (1998–2004)', *Sleep*, 2006, vol. 29, no. 11, November, pp. 1398–1414.

3   Perlis et al., pp. 12–14 .

4   Hauri & Linde.

Week Four: Operation mind shift—dispel your sleep myths

1   Morin & Espie, pp. 77–99.

2   National Institute for the Clinical Application of Behavioural Medicine, *How Does Neuroplasticity Work?* nicabm.com/brain-how-does-neuroplasticity-work/

3   Positive Psychology, *Cognitive Distortions: When your brain lies to you*, 2020, September, positivepsychology.com/cognitive-distortions/

4   Positive Psychology, *What is the Negativity Bias and How Can it be Overcome?*, 2020, September, positivepsychology.com/3-steps-negativity-bias

5   T. Brach, *Radical Compassion*, London: Ebury, 2020.

6   Morin & Espie, pp. 80–3.

7   C.M. Morin, A. Vallières & H. Ivers, 'Dysfunctional beliefs and attitudes about sleep (DBAS): Validation of a brief version (DBAS-16)', *Sleep*, 2007, vol. 30, no. 11, November, pp. 1547–54.

8   A. Huffington, *The Sleep Revolution*, London: Allen, 2017, p. 74.

9   G.D. Jacobs, *Say Goodnight to Insomnia*, London: Rodale, 2009, p. 75.

Week Five: Use nutrition and exercise to your advantage

1   This is my spin on the quote, sometimes attributed to Abraham Lincoln, 'Discipline is choosing between what you want now, and what you want most.' I prefer to loosen it up and look at it as freedom, rather than discipline.

2   M. St-Onge, A. Mikic, & C. Pietrolungo, 'Effects of diet on sleep quality', *Advances in Nutrition*, 2016, vol. 7, September, pp. 938–49.

3   Sleep Foundation, *The Best Foods to Help You Sleep*, 2020, August, sleepfoundation.org/articles/food-and-drink-promote-good-nights-sleep

4   American Sleep Association, *Top 10 Foods that Help You Sleep*, sleepassociation. org/about-sleep/top-10-foods-help-sleep

5   Sleep Foundation, *The Connection Between Hydration and Sleep*, 2020, July.

6   B. Warren, 'The importance of hydration', *BePure*, bepure.co.nz/blogs/news/importance-hydration

7   Sleep Health Foundation, *Caffeine and Sleep*, 2018, sleephealthfoundation.org.au/caffeine-and-sleep

8   Coffee and Health, *Coffee and Fatigue*, n.d., www.coffeeandhealth.org/topic-overview/coffee-and-fatigue/

9   Perlis et al., p. 77.

10   Sleep Health Foundation, *Caffeine, Food, Alcohol, Smoking and Sleep*, 2013, May, sleephealthfoundation.org.au/pdfs/CaffeineAlcohol-0713.pdf

11   Hauri & Linde, p. 61.

12   M. Costa & M. Esteves, 'Cigarette smoking and sleep disturbance', *Addictive Disorders & Their Treatment*, 2018, vol. 17, no. 1, March, pp. 40–8.

13   R.P. Ogea & A.C. Young, 'Drugs of abuse and sleep', in Mansfield, p. 512.

14   D. Cunnington, *Does Exercise Help Sleep?*, SleepHub, 2016, December, sleephub. com.au/does-exercise-help-sleep

15   Mayo Clinic, *Exercise Intensity: How to measure it*, 2019, August, www.mayoclinic. org/healthy-lifestyle/fitness/in-depth/exercise-intensity/art-20046887

Week Six: Mindfulness, stress management and relaxation

1   J. Kabat-Zinn, *Full Catastrophe Living*, revised edtition, London: 1: Piatkus, 2013, pp. 21–31.

2   J.C. Ong, R. Manber, Z. Segal, et al., 'A randomized controlled trial of mindfulness meditation for chronic insomnia', *Sleep*, 2014, vol. 37, no. 9, September, pp. 1553–63.

3   B.J. Stussman, L.I. Black, P.M. Barnes, T.C. Clarke & R.L. Nahin, 'Wellness-related use of common complementary health approaches amongst adults: United States,

2012', *National Health Statistics Report*, 2015, no. 85, November 4 .

4　J. Sills, 'The power of no' , *Psychology Today*, 2013, November 5, psychologytoday. com/us/articles/201311/the-power-no

5　Hauri & Linde, pp. 110–15.

6　Perlis et al., p. 19.

7　Mayo Clinic, *Decrease Stress by Using your Breath*, 2017, March.

8　Morin & Espie, pp 55–9.

Part 3

Chapter 11: Review, refine and keep moving forward

1　Sleep Foundation, *2011 Bedroom Poll*, 2011, sleepfoundation.org/professionals/ sleep-american-polls/2011-bedroom-poll

2　D. Cunnington, *What are Your Sleep Rules?* SleepHub, 2015, September, sleephub. com.au/sleep-rules

Chapter 12: What to do when things go wobbly

1　Morin & Carrier.

2　Sleep Health Foundation, *Hot Nights—How to Help Sleep*, 2016, December.

3　Sleep Foundation, *How to Sleep When It's Hot Outside*, 2020, July, sleepfoundation. org/articles/sleeping-when-is-blistering-hot

4　D. Ounnington, *Sleeping in the Heat*, SleepHub, 2019, December, sleephub.com.au/ sleeping-in-the-heat

5　D. Cunnington, *How Do I Manage Jet Lag*, SleepHub, 2015, June, /sleephub.com.au/ jet-lag

6　J.J. Gooley, 'Jet lag', in Mansfield, pp. 353–7.

Appendix I: Specific sleep challenges

1　Sleep Health Foundation, 'Snoring', 2011, October, sleephealthfoundation.org.au/ snoring.pdf

2　D. Cunnington, *Snoring Devices: What Works*, SleepHub, 2016, July, sleephub.com. au/snoringdevices

3　C. Ladyman, *Getting Better Sleep in Pregnancy*, Wellington: Massey University Press, 2020.

4　J. Goldin, C. Choy & M. Hickey, 'Sleep and the menopause', in Mansfield, p. 490.

5　Goldin et al., p. 492.

6　L. Lampio, P. Polo-Kantola, S-L Himanen, et al., 'Sleep during menopausal transition: A 6-year follow-up', *Sleep*, 2017, vol. 40, no. 7, July .

7　S. Ferguson & J. Paterson, 'Shift work sleep disorder', in Mansfield (ed), pp. 347–52.

8　A. Scovelle & C. Anderson, 'Normal sleep in the elderly', in Mansfield (ed), pp. 417– 22.

INDEX